Medical Informatics
An Executive Primer

Second Edition

Edited by
Ken Ong, MD, MPH

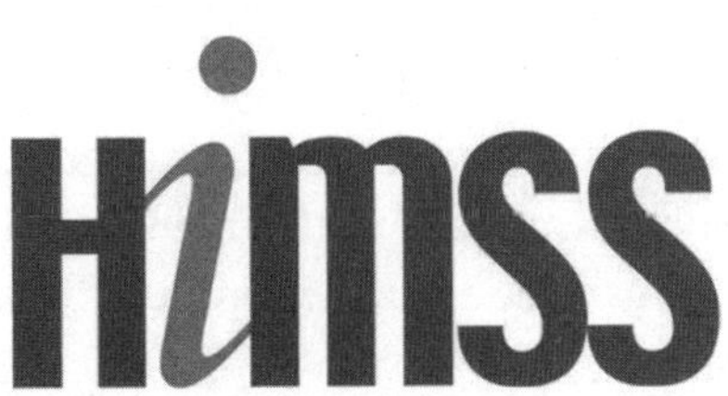

HIMSS Mission

To lead healthcare transformation through the effective use of health information technology.

Printed in the U.S.A. 5 4 3 2 1

Requests for permission to make copies of any part of this work should be sent to:
Permissions Editor
HIMSS
230 E. Ohio, Suite 500
Chicago, IL 60611-3270
nvitucci@himss.org

ISBN: 978-0-9844577-0-0

The inclusion of an organization name, product or service in this publication should not be considered as an endorsement of such organization, product or service, nor is the failure to include an organization name, product or service to be construed as disapproval.

For more information about HIMSS, please visit www.himss.org.

About the Editor

Ken Ong, MD, MPH, is the Chief Medical Informatics Officer of New York Hospital Queens, an urban teaching hospital serving the most diverse county in the nation and an affiliate of the New York-Presbyterian Health System. His current responsibilities include achieving Meaningful Use of the electronic health record (EHR) for both acute and ambulatory care. Dr. Ong serves as chair of the hospital's Clinical Informatics Committee and leads its core informatics workgroup. He has worked in many hospitals in the New York metropolitan area. His past projects include developing and implementing the acute care EHR with computerized practitioner order entry; clinical decision support for the acute care and ambulatory EHRs; a hospital pharmacy system; web-based results review, and mobile physician charge capture. Dr. Ong is a former deputy commissioner in the New York City Department of Health and Mental Hygiene.

Active in a number of professional groups, Dr. Ong is a member of the Healthcare Association of New York State's Health Information Strategy Group, a member of the Greater New York Hospital Association Health IT Steering Committee, a past president and former at-large board member of the New York State chapter of the Healthcare Information and Management Systems Society (HIMSS) and past president and current board member of Medical Informatics New York.

Dr. Ong serves as a reviewer for the *Informatics Review* and the *International Journal of Medical Informatics*. In addition, he served as editor of the first edition of *Medical Informatics: An Executive Primer*, which received the 2007 HIMSS Book of the Year Award. Dr. Ong is a previous recipient of the AMDIS Award In Applied Medical Informatics and the Centers for Disease Control and Prevention Charles C. Shepard Science Award.

Dr. Ong enjoys teaching and currently serves as an adjunct faculty member at Columbia University's Mailman School of Public Health and School of Medicine. His medical informatics seminar is a popular offering each fall semester.

Residency trained and board certified in family practice, internal medicine and infectious diseases, Dr. Ong is a fellow of the American College of Physicians, the Infectious Disease Society of America, HIMSS, and the New York Academy of Medicine. He received his MPH at Columbia University in New York, his MD at Wayne State University in Detroit, Mich., and his BS at the University of Michigan in Ann Arbor.

About the Authors

Abha Agrawal, MD, FACP, serves as the Interim Medical Director of Kings County Hospital Center in Brooklyn, New York. Dr. Agrawal is an Associate Professor of Medicine and Medical Informatics at the State University of New York Downstate Medical Center. Previously, she served as Chief Medical Information Officer of the Central Brooklyn Family Health Network (CBFHN) and the Associate Medical Director of Kings County Hospital. Prior to coming to Brooklyn, she was the Informatics Coordinator for the VISN1, an integrated network of hospitals and clinics in six New England states. Dr. Agrawal was appointed as a Clinical Faculty Member at Harvard Medical School and as a Research Scientist at the Brigham and Women's Hospital, both in Boston. She is a nationally recognized leader in health information technology and serves on important national and regional organizations, including as a Commissioner on the Certification Commission on Healthcare Information Technology (CCHIT) and a Board Member on New York Clinical Information Exchange (NYCLIX). Dr. Agrawal was also elected as the 2008 President of Medical Informatics New York, an association of physician leaders in informatics from hospitals, academia and corporations. She has received numerous awards in health IT, including the 2007 National Association of Public Hospitals Safety Net Award in the patient safety category for her work on electronic medication reconciliation and the 2006 *IndUS Business Journal* award for innovation in healthcare. She is a physician trained in Internal Medicine (SUNY Downstate) and Medical Informatics (Yale School of Medicine).

Rachel Block is Deputy Commissioner for Health Information Technology Transformation in the New York State Department of Health, where she oversees development and implementation of New York's statewide health information technology strategy. Before joining the Department in May 2009, she served as the founding executive director for the New York eHealth Collaborative (NYeC), a statewide multi-stakeholder organization committed to advancing health information technology adoption and use in New York. From August 2003 to March 2008, Ms. Block was the project director for the United Hospital Fund's Quality Strategies Initiative where she developed several initiatives to coordinate improvements in healthcare delivery and outcomes across the healthcare system in New York, including the planning process which led to creating NYeC. Prior to joining the United Hospital Fund, she worked in the public and private sectors leading strategic planning and policy development efforts to improve the effectiveness and efficiency of state health programs. She served as a vice president for health services at Maximus from 2002 to 2003. From 1994 to 2002, Ms. Block held several senior management positions at the Centers for Medicare & Medicaid Services (previously Health Care Financing Administration) where she directed policy development and operations of Medicaid, State Children's Health Insurance, and Federal Survey and Certification Programs, with particular emphasis on quality improvement, data and systems issues. Ms. Block is the immediate past president of the board for the eHealth Initiative.

Adam Cheriff, MD, is a graduate of Harvard College, one of two schools within Harvard University in Cambridge, Mass. After receiving his medical degree from Johns Hopkins School of Medicine in Baltimore, Maryland, he completed a residency in Internal Medicine at New York Presbyterian Hospital (Weill Cornell Campus). In 2001, Dr. Cheriff joined the faculty within the Department of Medicine at Weill Cornell; he currently is an Associate Professor. He has maintained an active internal medicine practice at Weill Cornell Internal Medicine Associates while overseeing clinical IT operations for the Weill Cornell Physician Organization. Dr. Cheriff led the implementation of Weill Cornell's shared ambulatory electronic health record (EHR). In 2009, Dr. Cheriff was appointed the Chief Medical Information Officer for the Weill Cornell Physician Organization. In addition to managing the ongoing support of the EHR, he is responsible for Weill Cornell's data warehouse, data dictionary, online physician directory and patient portal. Dr. Cheriff's interests include clinical system usability, provider productivity and process improvement. His recent research efforts have centered around measuring the effects of the EHR on provider productivity and medication prescribing accuracy and safety.

Curtis Cole, MD, is the Chief Information Officer for Weill Cornell Medical College in New York City where he is an Associate Professor of Clinical Medicine and Public Health. He practices Internal Medicine at Weill Cornell Internal Medicine Associates at New York Presbyterian Hospital. Dr. Cole is the acting co-Director of the Clinical & Translational Science Center Bioinformatics Core, a partnership with Memorial Sloan Kettering Cancer Center, the Hospital for Special Surgery and Hunter College, all located in New York City. After medical school at Cornell and residency at the then New York Hospital, Dr. Cole served as a Clinical Investigator in Medical Informatics at the hospital. He joined Cornell as the Director of Information Services and later became the Chief Medical Information Officer. He has led the implementation of several clinical information systems including outpatient and inpatient EMRs, diagnostic, procedural and revenue cycle systems. Dr. Cole has led the development of Weill Cornell's data dictionary called TruData, as well as the clinical data warehouse.

Joseph Conte, MPH, is the Executive Vice President for Corporate Services at Catholic Health Services of Long Island (CHSLI) in New York. Mr. Conte is responsible for Finance, Information Technology and Performance Improvement/Quality Management for the system. The direct reports to the position are the Chief Financial Officer, Chief Information Officer, Chief Medical Officer of CHS and VP of Mission & Ministry. Under Mr. Conte's leadership, CHSLI earned the Pinnacle Award for Quality and Patient Safety from the Hospital Association for New York State. Mr. Conte was with the North Shore-Long Island Jewish Health System for 15 years prior to assuming his new role in 2008 at CHSLI. He was most recently CHSLI's Senior Vice President of Systemwide Quality Management. Prior to that, he served as the Chief Quality Officer at Staten Island University Hospital for six years; during that time, the organization was a top performer in the nation in the CMS Pay for Performance Project, won the Codman Award for Quality from The Joint Commission and the Pinnacle Award for

Patient Safety from the Healthcare Association of New York State. Mr. Conte has an appointment in the department of Biologic Sciences at Wagner College in Staten Island, New York and teaches in the college's PA and MBA programs. He is also on the adjunct faculty at Columbia University's Mailman School of Public Health in New York City.

Leanne M. Currie, RN, DNSc, is Associate Professor in the School of Nursing at the University of British Columbia in Vancouver, Canada. Dr. Currie received her Master's of Science in Nursing Informatics degree from University of California, San Francisco, and her Doctorate in Nursing Science degree from Columbia University School of Nursing (Hons) in New York City. While at Columbia, she was a National Library of Medicine Trainee in Informatics via the Department of Biomedical Informatics. In 2008, she was named Columbia's Distinguished Young Researcher. Currently, Dr. Currie is a member the Nursing Informatics Special Interest Group Science Program Committee for NI2012, to be held by the International Medical Informatics Association. Previously, she has served as Chair of the Nursing Informatics Work Group for the Fall Nursing Informatics Symposium presented by the American Medical Informatics Association (AMIA) and Co-Chair of the Nursing Informatics track for AMIA's Spring Nursing Informatics Symposium.

Deborah Johnson-Ingram is a Senior Program Manager on the Performance Improvement Team with Primary Care Development Corporation (PCDC) in New York City. She provides consultative support to community health centers and private physician practices on achieving National Committee on Quality Assurance Physician Practice Connections®-Patient Centered Medical Home™ recognition and implementing electronic health records. Prior to joining PCDC, Ms. Johnson-Ingram worked for IPRO, the New York State Quality Improvement Organization, as a Senior Clinical Practice Advisor. Her work included performing individual site assessments on practice redesign with a focus on healthcare quality improvement, EHR optimization; she extracted and analyzed practice level data on clinical quality metrics. She has also consulted with EHR vendors on their systems reporting and registry capabilities. Ms. Johnson-Ingram has more than 15 years of experience in healthcare quality, including seven years of facilitating the implementation of EHRs in both small and large practice settings. She has served as a presenter at meetings of local health departments and health insurance institutions on Academic Detailing, a method of educating and partnering with healthcare providers by bringing education to their work sites. Ms. Johnson-Ingram served on two major immunization coalitions: the Nassau/Suffolk Adult Immunization Coalition and the New York City Department of Health and Mental Hygiene Adult Immunization Coalition. She has a BA in Sociology from New York University.

Joseph Kannry, MD, has dual appointments in IT and Medicine at Mount Sinai Medical Center in New York City. He is the Lead Technical Informaticist on the EMR Clinical Transformation Group at Mount Sinai. Dr. Kannry is an Associate Professor of Medicine and a practicing board certified internist at Mount Sinai's Internal Medicine Associates (IMA). He is a graduate of the Yale Center for Medical Informatics in New Haven, Connecticut, a National Library of Medicine training program in Informatics. Dr. Kannry is an active member of the American Medical Informatics Association (AMIA) and the Healthcare Information and Management Systems Society (HIMSS).

He has served as a member of AMIA's Task Force on Guidelines for the Clinical Use of Electronic Mail with Patients, Task Force on Applied Informatics and Education Committee and Public Policy Committee. He also has served as a member of the HIMSS Ambulatory EMR Knowledge Resource Task Force, the HL7 EHR Ambulatory Care Large Minimum Function Set: Ambulatory Care-Large, the Healthcare Information Technology Standards Panel, and the Greater New York Hospital Association IT Steering Committee. Dr. Kannry has served as the Chairman of the Clinical Advisory Group for the New York Clinical Information Exchange (NYCLIX), in addition to serving on NYCLIX's Steering Committee/Board. He was a member of the Program Committee for the 2007 Information Technology and Communications Conference at the University of Vancouver. In 2009, Dr. Kannry was elected Chair of the AMIA Clinical Information System Working Group, with the term beginning in 2011. He was also invited to join the NYS ACP Health Information Technology Committee.

Ross Koppel, PhD, has taught sociology, research methods, medical sociology and statistics in the Sociology Department at the University of Pennsylvania in Philadelphia for the past 18 years. At the university's School of Medicine, Dr. Koppel is the principal investigator at the Center for Clinical Epidemiology and Biostatistics study on hospital workplace culture. In addition, he is the co-principal investigator at the Rand Corporation, where he directs studies on the unintended consequences of health information technology. Dr. Koppel also served that role for a National Science Foundation study of the cyber connections among medical devices worn by patients and operated within hospitals. He has authored or co-authored more than 160 academic papers and articles, several monographs, and several books and book chapters. In the past four years, he has published 24 papers—many of them in leading medical journals, primarily on medication errors and the use of technology. Much of Dr. Koppel's work focuses on the use of health IT. His articles in *JAMA* (*The Journal of the American Medical Association*) on the role of computerized practitioner order entry systems in facilitating medication errors and on hold-harmless clauses in vendor contracts received wide notice. More recently, Dr. Koppel's work has focused on ways to improve understanding of and methods to correct health IT difficulties. His recent key work includes a model of how health IT interacts with socio-technical systems and the built environment and a study of nurses' and physicians' workarounds associated with the use of automated medication bar coding administration.

Gilad Kuperman, MD, PhD, is the Board Chair and Executive Director of NYCLIX, a health information exchange serving Manhattan and other parts of New York City. He is also the Director for Interoperability Informatics at New York Presbyterian Hospital. Dr. Kuperman is on the faculty of Biomedical Informatics at Columbia University Medical School in New York City. The author of 60 articles related to various aspects of informatics, Dr. Kuperman is a member of the Board of AMIA and is on the Editorial Board of *JAMIA*. He served as the Scientific Program Committee Chair for AMIA's 2010 Annual Symposium.

Andre Kushniruk, PhD, MSc, is a Professor at the School of Health Information Science at the University of Victoria in British Columbia, Canada. Dr. Kushniruk previously served as the Director of the School of Health Information Science. A fellow of the American College of Medical Informatics, Dr. Kushniruk is known internationally for his work. He has published more than 100 articles on health informatics and has served as an advisor on a variety of national and international committees and projects. Dr. Kushniruk recently co-edited a book entitled *Human, Social, and Organizational Aspects of Health Information Systems.* He has held academic positions at a number of Canadian universities and worked with a number of major hospitals in Canada, the United States and other countries. Dr. Kushniruk has taught a number of courses in health informatics in the areas of system design and evaluation. In addition, he has worked on developing innovative health informatics educational programs and curricula in Canada and internationally. Dr. Kushniruk holds undergraduate degrees in Psychology and Biology, as well as an MSc in Computer Science and a PhD in Cognitive Psychology from McGill University in Montreal, Quebec, Canada.

Jonathan Leviss, MD, is the Director of Clinical Solutions for Microsoft Health Solutions Group and an internist at the Thundermist Health Center in Woonsocket, Rhode Island. As a physician, Dr. Leviss has used advanced healthcare technologies for more than 15 years and served as the first CMIO at the New York City Health and Hospitals Corporation. He was the Vice President and Chief Medical Officer at Sentillion prior to its acquisition by Microsoft in 2010. Dr. Leviss also held leading positions at Cerner and Deloitte Consulting and faculty positions at New York University School of Medicine and Columbia University College of Physicians and Surgeons, both in New York City. He co-chairs the Rhode Island HIT Physician Advisory Committee, which advises the Rhode Island Quality Institute on key statewide health IT initiatives. Dr. Leviss regularly writes and presents on health IT and edited the recently published book *HIT or Miss: Lessons Learned from Health Information Technology Implementations.*

G. Daniel Martich, MD, FACP, has led the University of Pittsburgh Medical Center's (UPMC) efforts in deploying clinical information technology for one of the nation's largest integrated delivery networks. During his tenure as Chief Medical Information Officer, UPMC has gained a reputation as the nation's premier innovator in leveraging new products, processes and technology to solve various information technology needs for the betterment of patient care. Dr. Martich has a long history with UPMC, having joined the second largest non-governmental employer in Pennsylvania in 1992 as a critical care physician. He has served as an intensivist and co-director of the cardiothoracic intensive care unit, winning awards for his clinical acumen and teaching abilities. Dr. Martich started the critical care information system department shortly after joining UPMC and has served as its only medical director. That department provides for all the bedside integration of information systems for each of the more than 150 critical care patients at UPMC. In 1999, he began serving in a similar capacity for all clinical information systems at the 19 hospitals of UPMC; he is responsible for developing standards of information sharing and display among the multiple care sites. In 2003, Dr. Martich was appointed Vice President and Chief Physician of the UPMC eRecord, the health system's enterprise aggregation of all EHR applications.

Glenn Martin, MD, is Director of Medical Informatics for the Queens Health Network (QHN) in New York, a winner of the Nicholas E. Davies Award of Excellence. QHN is comprised of the two public hospitals in the borough of Queens. While providing clinical direction for implementation of the EHR, Dr. Martin has also been actively involved in deploying smart card technology in the form of patient ID cards with extracts of their medical record. He is currently medical director of the Interboro health information exchange, which covers Queens and parts of Brooklyn, NY. Dr. Martin is a practicing psychiatrist and President of the New York State Psychiatric Association. He also serves as Associate Dean for Research at the Mount Sinai School of Medicine in New York City and as the school's Associate Director for its Program for the Protection of Human Subjects.

Denni McColm, MBA, is Chief Information Officer for Citizens Memorial Healthcare in Bolivar, Miss. Ms. McColm has been at Citizens Memorial since 1988, serving as Director of Human Resources and Director of Finance before moving into the CIO role in June 2003. She served as a Commissioner for the Certification Commission for Health Information Technology from 2006 to 2008. She also served on the Nicholas E. Davies Award of Excellence Organizational Selection Committee from 2006 to 2008 and again in 2010. Ms. McColm is a member of the Board of Directors for the Medical Users Software Exchange (MUSE) and the Editorial Board for *Healthcare IT News,* published in partnership by MedTech Media and HIMSS. She holds a Master of Business Administration degree from the University of Missouri-Columbia.

Pravene Nath, MD, MSE, FACEP, is Chief Medical Information Officer at Stanford Hospital and Clinics and Clinical Assistant Professor of Emergency Medicine at Stanford University School of Medicine in Palo Alto, Calif. Dr. Nath oversees physician informatics, nursing informatics, and clinical transformation teams, with a particular focus on the enterprise EHR. He previously served as Chief Medical Information Officer, Senior Director of Clinical Information Systems, and Assistant Professor of Emergency Medicine at NYU Langone Medical Center in New York City, where he managed informatics and clinical system initiatives from 2003 through 2008. Dr. Nath is board certified in emergency medicine, with a background in biomedical engineering and over seven years of leadership experience in health information technology.

Yvette A. Ortiz, MD, has been practicing Internal Medicine in the South Bronx since 1994. Dr. Ortiz received her Bachelor Degree from Hunter College in New York City. She worked as a biller and accounts analyst at Mount Sinai Hospital in New York City while completing her major in Physics and pre-med requirements. Dr. Ortiz received her MD degree from Albert Einstein College of Medicine of Yeshiva University in Bronx, NY, and then completed her residency in Internal Medicine at New York City's Bellevue Hospital. During her training, she specialized in Primary Care and the management of patients with HIV/AIDS. Dr. Ortiz was born in the Washington Heights neighborhood of New York City; her parents were immigrants from Colombia and Ecuador. Growing up in a bilingual household in a largely Hispanic and medically underserved community, she developed a strong desire to serve her community and provide high quality and culturally competent care. Over the years, Dr. Ortiz has served as a mentor and role model to dozens of young Hispanic students interested in healthcare careers. She served as the model and spokesperson for the National Hispanic Scholarship fund and continues to mentor and inspire students at NEST+m Middle School and Stuyvesant High School in New York City. Her lifelong dream has been fulfilled by founding, developing and running a successful private practice in an underserved Hispanic immigrant community. Dr. Ortiz was one of the early adopters of the eClinical Works EHR and has collaborated closely with the New York City Department of Health and Mental Hygiene (NYDOHMH) in a variety of care management and quality improvement activities. Her practice was designated as a Level III Medical Home by the National Committee for Quality Assurance.

Amanda Parsons, MD, MBA, joined NYDOHMH in January 2008. She is currently the Assistant Commissioner, overseeing all of the activities of the Primary Care Information Project (PCIP). Previously, Dr. Parsons was the Director of Medical Quality where she was responsible for creating and leading the Quality Improvement, Billing Consulting and EHR Consulting teams deployed to PCIP's small physician practices. Prior to joining PCIP, Dr. Parsons spent four years at McKinsey & Company as an Engagement Manager, serving clients in the Pharmaceutical & Medical Products and Global Public Health sectors. She received her MD and MBA degrees from Columbia University and completed medical post-graduate training at Beth Israel Medical Center in Internal Medicine, both located in New York City. She completed her undergraduate studies at Boston College in Mass., where she was a Presidential Scholar. Dr. Parsons is a frequent presenter and panelist, focusing on quality improvement, EHR adoption, the patient-centered medical home and extension center activities. She serves on the Board of Directors of VIP Community Service and the New York eHealth Collaborative (NYeC).

Robin S. Raiford, BSN, RN-BC, CPHIMS, FHIMSS, has more than three decades of nursing experience and over 17 years in healthcare informatics. Currently, she is Executive Director of Federal Affairs at Allscripts, where she is responsible for review of government initiatives and their impact on the company's customers and product direction. Previously, she served in this role at Eclipsys. Ms. Raiford closely follows the Office of the National Coordinator for Health Information Technology, the HIT Policy Committee and the HIT Standards Committee regarding the meaningful use of EHRs.

She previously held informatics positions at the Smithsonian Institution, Kaiser Permanente and Microsoft, in addition to serving as a senior consultant for the Department of Defense Health Affairs on the worldwide Computerized Patient Record Project. She also volunteered in the Clinton Administration on healthcare reform. Ms. Raiford has served as chair of the HIMSS Patient Safety and Quality Outcomes Steering Committee and the Public Comments Work Group. She is a former member of the HITSP Education, Communication and Outreach Committee, a two-time recipient of the Spirit of HIMSS Award, and a 2008 recipient of the HIMSS Distinguished Fellow Service Award.

Bertram S. Reese is Senior Vice President and Chief Information Officer of Sentara Healthcare, an integrated not-for-profit health system in southeastern Virginia and northeastern North Carolina. Sentara is comprised of nine acute care hospitals, a health plan with 300,000 covered lives, seven nursing centers, three assisted living centers and a 400-member physician medical group. Sentara has continually ranked as one of the most integrated healthcare networks in the United States by *Modern Healthcare* magazine and is the only healthcare system in the nation to be named in the top 10 for seven consecutive years. Mr. Reese is responsible for the Information Technology, Process Improvement, Information and Supply Chain Management for the health system. Most recently, this group has implemented an EHR across the enterprise, resulting in significant financial savings and improved clinical outcomes. The group has received many national awards, including Most Wired from *Hospitals & Health Networks* magazine, Top 100 Innovations, Best Employer in Information Technology and achieved Stage 7 on the HIMSS Analytics Electronic Medical Record Adoption Model℠, its highest level.

Jason S. Shapiro, MD, is a board certified practicing emergency physician, and a fellowship-trained informatics expert who has specialized in health information exchange and evaluation of health information technology systems implementations. Dr. Shapiro serves as a Postdoctoral Research Scientist in Biomedical Informatics at Columbia University and an Assistant Professor in Emergency Medicine at Mount Sinai School of Medicine, both located in New York City. He is the Chair of the Clinical Advisory Committee and Co-chair of the Evaluation Committee for Mount Sinai's health information exchange, NYCLIX. Dr. Shapiro has mentored numerous residents, informatics graduate students, informatics fellows and students and others participating in short-term internships. He earned his MD degree from Columbia University College of Physicians and Surgeons in New York City. He completed an internal medicine internship at the University of California, San Francisco and an emergency medicine residency at Mount Sinai School of Medicine.

Alan L. Silver, MD, MPH, is currently a Medical Director at IPRO and an Associate Professor, Departments of Medicine, Epidemiology and Population Health, Albert Einstein College of Medicine of Yeshiva University in Bronx, New York. He has been at IPRO since 1994 and has been involved with the Health Care Quality Improvement Program since its inception. Dr. Silver received his undergraduate degree, master's degree and general preventive medicine residency training at the University of Michigan in Ann Arbor, and his medical degree and internal medicine residency training at Wayne State University in Detroit, Mich. He subsequently became a fellow in community medicine at New York City's Mount Sinai School of Medicine and is board certified in internal medicine and general preventive medicine/public health. In 1980, Dr. Silver helped found a general internal medicine group practice at Mount Sinai Medical Center in New York City and worked there for 17 years. He then spent over 10 years at the North Shore-Long Island Jewish Health System, where he served as Medical Director in Quality Management and an assistant attending in medicine at Long Island Jewish Medical Center. In 1984, he received a three-year WK Kellogg National Leadership Fellowship. He has also been awarded mini-fellowships in medical ethics at the Kennedy Institute of Ethics at Georgetown University in Washington, DC, and in medical informatics at the National Library of Medicine in Bethesda, Maryland. He is currently a fellow of the New York Academy of Medicine. Dr. Silver has studied quality-of-care practice patterns and their relationship to organizational structure and physician behavior for a variety of clinical conditions. He has authored or co-authored papers and reports in medical care organization, clinical practice evaluation, medical education, preventive services and medical ethics.

Mytri Pritam Singh, MPH, is the Executive Director of Implementation at the Primary Care Information Project (PCIP), a Bureau within the New York City Department of Health and Mental Hygiene (NYCDOHMH). She manages a team that helps implement electronic health records at private physician practices, health centers and hospital out-patient departments in New York City. Prior to joining PCIP, Ms. Singh worked in the Bureau of HIV Prevention and Control from 2001 to 2006 as the Project Director in the Office of Outcomes Evaluation. Her team provided capacity building technical assistance to help community-based organizations develop, sustain and evaluate their HIV prevention interventions. Later, as the Deputy Director of the HIV Testing Unit, she provided guidance and funding oversight to programs that integrated routine rapid HIV testing in emergency departments and community-based clinics. From 1998 to 2001, Ms. Singh managed multiple HIV research grants at The Baron Edmond de Rothschild Chemical Dependency Institute at Beth Israel Medical Center in New York City. The research focused on HIV prevention studies and behavioral interventions for injection drug users who were attending syringe exchange and methadone maintenance treatment programs in New York City. Ms. Singh has a master's degree in Public Health in Infectious Disease Epidemiology from Yale University's School of Public Health in New Haven, Conn.

Thomas W. Smith is the Chief Information Officer for NorthShore University HealthSystem (formerly Evanston Northwestern Healthcare) in Evanston, Ill. NorthShore is an integrated delivery network with four hospitals, more than 650 employed physicians, home care services and a research institute. Mr. Smith has more than 30 years of hospital administration and information systems management experience, including more than 20 years as a CIO at two different multi-hospital corporations. He has led the IT efforts at NorthShore since 1989. He is a member of ACHE, CHIME and HIMSS. The winner of HIMSS' Nicholas E. Davies Organizational Award of Excellence in 2004, NorthShore (then ENH) was recognized as the first organization to have both hospital and physician office data combined in a single EHR database. In 2009, NorthShore University HealthSystem was one of the first two health systems in the United States to achieve Stage 7 (the highest level) on the HIMSS Analytics Electronic Medical Record Adoption Model^{SM}, which represents best practices in the implementation of its electronic medical record systems. In addition, in 2010, for the seventh consecutive year, NorthShore was named one of the Most Wired Hospitals in the U.S. by *Hospitals & Health Networks* magazine. NorthShore also has been named one of the Top 100 Hospitals/Top 15 Major Teaching Hospitals in the nation for 14 of the last 16 years by Thomson Reuters, a leading provider of information and solutions to improve the cost and quality of healthcare.

Salvatore Volpe, MD, FAAP, FACP, CHCQM, has 20 years of primary care practice experience. He is one of the few physicians in the country to have successfully become board certified in Pediatrics, Internal Medicine, Geriatrics and Quality Assurance. Dr. Volpe is a national lecturer on such diverse topics as consumer health software, E-prescribing, electronic health records, patient centered medical home, physician-patient communication and smartphones. His blogs and podcasts are often referenced by the media and his peers. Dr. Volpe currently serves on the medical editorial board of *Medical Economics* magazine, as a member of the AMA Health Information Technology Advisory Panel, as Chairman of the NYS Medical Society HIT committee and as the 2009–2011 President of the New York State Chapter of HIMSS. In 2009, Dr. Volpe's practice became the first solo practice in the state of New York to achieve Level 3 NCQA Patient Centered Medical Home Certification. He currently serves as the Physician Liaison and Clinical Champion for the NYC DOH Primary Care Information Project and NYC REACH (Regional Extension Center).

Kim Benjamin Woods, MD, has been practicing Internal Medicine in New York City's South Bronx since 1994. He received his Bachelor's Degree in Natural Science at Hampshire College in Amherst, Mass., and received his MD degree from the State University of New York, School of Medicine at Buffalo. Dr. Woods' Internship and Residency training in Internal Medicine was completed at New York City's Harlem Hospital Center, a teaching institution affiliated with Columbia University College of Physicians and Surgeons. He has consistently worked in medically underserved communities and is a co-founder of Uptown Medical, a successful private practice in an African American/Hispanic community.

Dedication

To Kimberly and Ryan for inspiring us to believe in a better tomorrow and to Donna, Jo, Fawn and Edwin for making today possible.

Acknowledgments

Thanks to Donna, my wife, for her unending support for not only this particular project but for letting me pursue this field when it was less well appreciated than it is today. My special thanks to all the chapter authors who were generous enough to take time out of their busy schedules to share their expertise and knowledge. Thanks to Nancy Vitucci, Manager of Publications at HIMSS—our publisher, whose enduring patience and commitment made this project a reality.

Contents

Foreword

On March 23, 2010, President Barack Obama signed into law the Patient Protection and Affordable Care Act of 2010 (PPACA). The law is the most comprehensive and ambitious healthcare legislation in more than 40 years. It seeks to provide insurance coverage to more than 30 million persons who now lack such coverage. It seeks to reorganize and improve the nation's healthcare delivery system. It seeks to slow the rising cost of the nation's healthcare bill. Given its comprehensive scope, it is hardly surprising that the PPACA has generated sharp partisan debate and vigorous political opposition. These political battles will play out over the next several years, in Congress, in the courts and in the statehouses. Interestingly, however, one of the very few things that health policy analysts on all sides agree about is that the nation needs to dramatically increase the utilization of health information technology (IT). Health IT is critically important to any effort to improve coverage, reform delivery systems, improve quality or control costs—regardless of the specific nature of the proposal itself.

Medical Informatics: An Executive Primer, Second Edition provides an informative and invaluable primer on the state of the nation's health information technologies; the options for improvement; and the organizational, political and economic challenges to an improved system. Ken Ong, MD, MPH, the volume's editor, is a national expert in medical informatics with years of experience in both designing and implementing health information systems. Dr. Ong is also a longstanding member of the Mailman School's Department of Health Policy and Management. This volume, which grew out of Dr. Ong's highly-rated course in health information technology, provides a comprehensive tutorial to health policymakers and healthcare managers on the opportunities and the obstacles to effectively implementing the new technological advances.

The first few chapters provide an overview of key legislative and regulatory provisions. In Chapter 1, for example, Dr. Ong reviews the American Recovery and Reinvestment Act of 2009 (ARRA), which appropriates over $2 billion to the Office of the National Coordinator for Health Information Technology, and billions more in financial incentives for the "meaningful use" of electronic health records. What is the money designed to do? How likely is it to be used effectively? What are the key issues and obstacles?

Following this overview, the next several chapters examine the policy and management environment more in depth. What is "meaningful use"? What are the certification requirements for health information technologies? How do state and regional health information exchanges work? What do we know about personal health records, identity management, clinical decision support, project management, software selection, and so on? The book next provides a series of case studies that examine what worked and what did not in efforts to implement new information technologies in various clinical settings, from large academic medical centers to small primary care practices.

Taken together, this edited volume provides an extraordinary view of both the policy options and the management challenges that lie at the heart of the new information revolution. If we succeed over time in harnessing the enormous potential of these new technologies, it will be because experts like Dr. Ong and his colleagues have provided us with the managerial capacity to match the technical advances. This book is an important part of that mission.

Michael Sparer, PhD, JD
Professor and Chair, Department of Health Policy and Management
Mailman School of Public Health, Columbia University
New York, NY

Introduction

Ken Ong, MD, MPH

"A crisis is a terrible thing to waste."

—*Paul Romer*[1]

We face an unprecedented opportunity in healthcare.

On the heels of the nation's worst recession since the Great Depression of the 1930s, the American Recovery and Reinvestment Act of 2009/Health Information Technology for Economic and Clinical Health Act of 2009 (ARRA/HITECH) was enacted to promote the "meaningful use" of electronic health records (EHRs) and related technologies.

Significant funding and resources are now available for eligible professionals and hospitals to improve patient outcomes, efficiency of care and coordination with health information technology. In particular, HITECH funds regional extension centers and workforce training to implement EHRs; Medicare and Medicaid incentives and penalties to promote meaningful use; and standards for health information exchange, privacy and security (see Figure 1).

A transformation of this magnitude will require between 45,000 and 50,000 net new jobs in health IT over the next five years to develop, install and maintain this technology.[3]

A recent HIMSS survey indicates the initial top three opportunities will be for implementation support specialists, implementation managers and technical support. While implementation support specialists will have to know more about clinical workflows and technical support staff more about technology, each must have a working knowledge about both. This primer and the graduate school course of the same name that inspired it serve as a bridge between the worlds of healthcare and IT.[4]

The book's chapters are designed to be read either in sequence or individually by topic:

- *ARRA/HITECH: An Executive Summary.* The chapter offers a high-level overview of the legislation.
- *Meaningful Use,* co-authored by Robin Raiford, BSN, RN-BC, CPHIMS, FHIMSS. This introduction to CMS' Final Rule explores how physician practices and hospitals can achieve meaningful use of EHRs.
- *Certification in Health Information Technology* by Abha Agrawal, MD, FACP. CCHIT is an Office of the National Coordinator - Authorized Testing and Certification Body (ONC-ATCB). The ONC-ATCBs certify EHRs required for meaningful use.
- *Meaningful Usability: Health Information Technology for the Rest of Us* by Joseph Kannry, MD, Andre Kushniruk, PhD, MSc, and Ross Koppel, PhD.

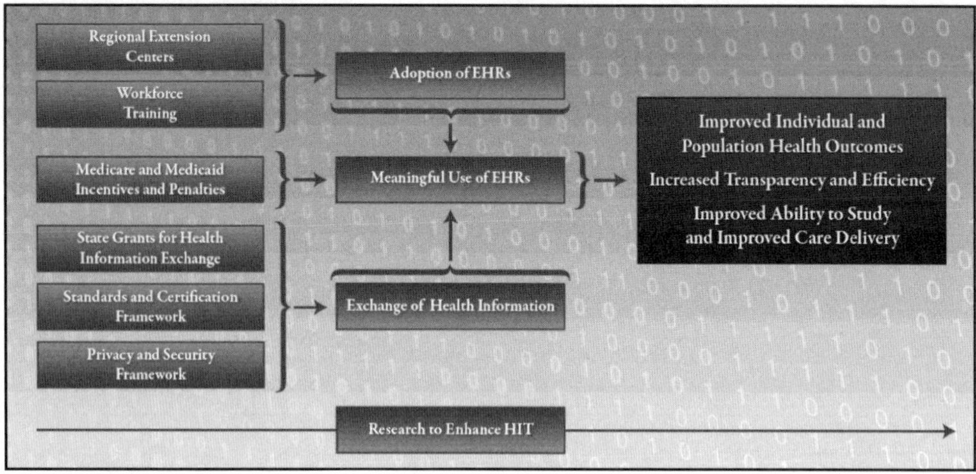

Figure 1: HITECH's Framework for Meaningful Use of EHRs[2]

Usability is not yet a requirement for EHR certification but should be in the future. Doing the right thing has to be easy to do. As one of the physicians in my hospital recently opined: "It's all about the clicks."

- *State and Regional Health Information Exchange Activities: Current Status and Future Direction* by Rachel Block. New York State has been a leader in health IT advancement nationally. Ms. Block offers her vision for transforming healthcare with health IT.
- *Ambulatory Systems* by Curtis L. Cole, MD, and Adam Cheriff, MD. For too long, the ambulatory EHR has stood in the shadow of its sibling—the hospital EHR. The national focus on the patient-centered medical home and accountable care organizations has placed the ambulatory EHR in the spotlight of health IT.
- *The Personal Health Record* by Glenn Martin, MD. If you have little familiarity with the PHR, Dr. Martin's chapter is the perfect place to learn about this technology from someone who has implemented it.
- *Health Information Exchange* by Jason S. Shapiro, MD, and Gilad Kuperman MD, PhD. Drs. Shapiro and Kuperman are co-founders of one of New York's leading regional health information exchanges—the New York Clinical Information Exchange (NYCLIX).
- *Identity Management* by Jonathan Leviss, MD. There is much more to identity management than just remembering your various logins.

- *Clinical Decision Support.* And clinical decision support is more than just alerts.
- *Project Management: Lessons from the Primary Care Information Project* by Mytri Pritam Singh, MPH. To date, PCIP has successfully installed the ambulatory EHR for 2,300 physicians, with no more than a one percent failure rate. Ms. Singh tells how they did it.
- *Quality and Health IT* by Joseph Conte, MPH. It is really all about quality. Unless health IT betters quality care, what is the point? Performance improvement is a discipline and an evidence-proven body of knowledge. Mr. Conte discusses its history and offers a basic toolkit.
- *Software Selection.* I am often asked to suggest what the best EHR is for an office practice or what the best emergency department system is. Find out why I usually answer: "It depends…".
- *The Patient Centered Medical Home Model* by Salvatore Volpe, MD, FAAP, FACP, CHCQM. Dr. Volpe is the first and, as of this writing, only physician in solo practice in the state of New York to acquire NCQA Level 3 Patient-Centered Medical Home Recognition. You have read about it in the newspapers and journals. Find out from Dr. Volpe what it really means to put this care delivery model into practice.
- *Nursing Informatics: Perspective for Healthcare Executives* by Leanne M. Currie, RN, DNSc. Nurse informaticists are essential members of any health IT team. Dr. Currie describes the current state of this growing specialty.
- *Case Study: Primary Care Information Project—The Evolution to an Extension Center* by Amanda Parsons, MD, MBA. PCIP has helped transform public health by making meaningful use a reality before it became the watchword it has become today. Dr. Parsons describes the natural progression to becoming New York City's regional extension center.
- *Case Study: A Small Primary Care Practice's Experience in Assessing Quality with Data Obtained from an Electronic Health Record* by Deborah Johnson-Ingram; Yvette A. Ortiz, MD; Kim Benjamin Woods, MD, and Alan L. Silver, MD, MPH. An early adopter of the EHR, the authors describe their quest for quality data from their EHR.

Imagine a hospital that is entirely electronic—without paper charts. A small but growing number of hospitals have done exactly that. HIMSS Analytics developed the EMR Adoption Model^{SM} (EMRAM) to track the hospital adoption of health IT.[5] In the EMRAM model, the Stage 7 hospital is paperless (see Figure 2). Needed patient information flows seamlessly between the emergency department and inpatient. Physicians access imaging studies digitally. Health information is exchanged in a secure fashion with other healthcare organizations, providers, payers and regulatory agencies.

In this book, five Stage 7 hospitals detail their EHR journey in informative case studies:

- *Citizens Memorial Healthcare* by Denni McColm, MBA
- *Sentara Healthcare* by Bertram S. Reese
- *NorthShore University HealthSystem* by Thomas W. Smith

FIGURE EMRAM1 | EMR Adoption Model^{SM}, Final 2009 – Q3 2010		2009 Final	2010 Q3
STAGE 7	Complete EMR; CCD transactions to share data; Data warehousing; Data continuity with ED, ambulatory, OP	0.7%	1.0%
STAGE 6	Physician documentation (structured templates), full CDSS (variance & compliance), full R-PACS	1.6%	2.8%
STAGE 5	Closed loop medication administration	3.8%	3.7%
STAGE 4	CPOE, Clinical Decision Support (clinical protocols)	7.4%	10.3%
STAGE 3	Nursing/clinical documentation (flow sheets), CDSS (error checking), PACS available outside Radiology	50.9%	49.7%
STAGE 2	CDR, Controlled Medical Vocabulary, CDS, may have Document Imaging; HIE capable	16.9%	15.4%
STAGE 1	Ancillaries - Lab, Rad, Pharmacy - All Installed	7.2%	6.7%
STAGE 0	All Three Ancillaries Not Installed	11.5%	10.5%

Figure 2: Stages of HIMSS Analytics Electronic Medical Record Adoption Model^{SM} (EMRAM)

- *Stanford Hospital and Clinics* by Pravene Nath, MD, MSE, FACEP
- *University of Pittsburgh Medical Center* by G. Daniel Martich, MD, FACP

Ultimately, this book aims to offer a look into how medical informatics is evolving and affecting today's healthcare delivery system and the role incentives, such as those from the federal government, are playing in transforming healthcare through IT.

REFERENCES

1. Available at www.nytimes.com/2009/08/02/magazine/02FOB-onlanguage-t.html. Accessed November 28, 2010.
2. Celebrating the First Anniversary of the HITECH Act and Looking to the Future – Health Information Technology for Economic and Clinical Health. Department of Health and Human Services. February 2010. Available at http://healthit.hhs.gov/portal/server.pt/gateway/PTARGS_0_11673_911674_0_0_18/FINAL_ONC-HITECH-Anniversary.pdf. Accessed Feb. 4, 2011.
3. Health IT funding to create 50,000 jobs: Sixty regional IT help centers will help health care facilities implement electronic medical records By Lucas Mearian. *ComputerWorld*, April 30, 2010.
4. HIMSS Vantage Point: Industry Staffing Needs. HIMSS Foundation, Volume 7; Issue 6, March 2010.
5. 2010 Annual Report of the U.S. Hospital IT Market: An industry report provided by HIMSS Analytics and HIMSS. ©2010 by the Healthcare Information and Management Systems Society and HIMSS Analytics.

CHAPTER 1

ARRA/HITECH: An Executive Summary

Ken Ong, MD, MPH

INTRODUCTION

In 2000, the Institute of Medicine (IOM) sounded the tocsin on medical errors in their report "To Err is Human: Building a Safer Health System," which disclosed that 44,000 to 98,000 Americans die each year as a result of medical errors.

The report recommended computerized practitioner order entry (CPOE), pharmaceutical decision support, relevant patient information at point of care, and other reforms to create safety systems.[1]

Despite agreement among healthcare professionals and even bipartisan support, nearly a decade later adoption of the electronic health record (EHR) was marginal.

According to one survey, only 1.5 percent of U.S. hospitals had a comprehensive electronic records system, and no more than an additional 7.6 percent had a basic system. Further, CPOE for medications was implemented in only 17 percent of hospitals.[2] Survey respondents cited capital requirements and high maintenance costs as the primary barriers to implementation.

A survey by the Centers for Disease Control and Prevention (CDC) found that office-based physician adoption was no less challenging. No more than 20.5 percent had a basic system, and only 6.3 percent had a fully functional system.[3]

In response to the economic crisis, the U.S. Congress passed, and President Obama signed, the American Recovery and Reinvestment Act of 2009 (ARRA) in February 2009.

A portion of ARRA is critical to the nation's efforts to adopt the EHR—the Health Information Technology for Economic and Clinical Health Act (HITECH). This act provides funding to promote the adoption of health IT.[4]

Although former president George W. Bush first established the Office of the National Coordinator for Health Information Technology (ONC) in 2004, funding for the agency was meager at $32.8 million.[5]

In contrast, HITECH appropriates $2 billion to that office and up to $27 billion in Medicare and Medicaid incentives for "meaningful use" of the EHR.[6]

Where Is That Money Going?

As shown in Table 1-1 and Figure 1-1, HITECH funding to ONC covers the spectrum of programs, from policy to standards, office-based physicians and hospitals, implementation and maintenance, training and health information exchange (HIE).

OFFICE OF THE NATIONAL COORDINATOR FOR HEALTH INFORMATION TECHNOLOGY

HITECH empowers the ONC in collaboration with advisory committees to develop policy and standards.[7]

The HIT Policy Committee is charged with recommending a policy framework for the development and adoption of a nationwide health IT infrastructure that permits the electronic exchange and use of health information. The HIT Standards Committee's purview is to recommend standards, implementation specifications, and certification criteria for the electronic exchange and use of health information.

RECs and HIE

The two programs that account for two-thirds of ONC's funding are (1) Health Information Technology Research Center and Regional Extension Center Cooperative Agreements, and (2) State Health Information Exchange Cooperative Agreements.

Table 1-1: HITECH Funding for ONC (Dollars in Millions)[6]

Program/Project/Activity	Total Appropriated	FY 2009 Actual Obligations	FY 2010 Estimated Obligations	FY 2011 Estimated Obligations	FY 2012 Estimated Obligations
NIST (National Institute of Standards and Technology)	20.00	0	16.371	3.525	1.04
Privacy and Security – Enforcement	16.16	0.57	15.59	0	0
Privacy and Security – Regulations, Guidelines and Studies	8.13	0	8.13	0	0
State Health Information Exchange Cooperative Agreements	564.00	0	564.00	0	0
Health Information Technology Research Center and Regional Extension Center Cooperative Agreements	774.00	0	726.20	0	47.80
Health IT Workforce Cooperative Agreements	118.00	0	83.73	34.27	0
Beacon Communities Cooperative Agreements	265.38	0	265.38	0	0
Other Initiatives/Omnibus	203.77	0	201.77	2	0
Public Health	30.58	0	30.58	0	0
Totals	**2,000.00**	**0.57**	**1911.75**	**39.79**	**48.84**

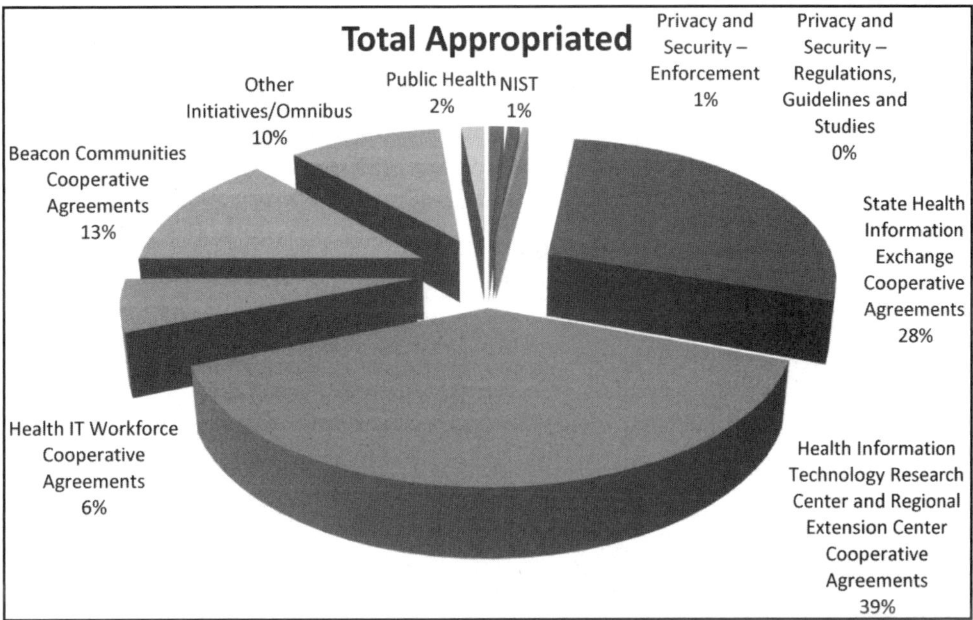

Figure 1-1: HITECH Funding for ONC[6]

Health IT Regional Extension Centers (RECs) are similar to their predecessors in agriculture, the National Institute of Food and Agriculture (NIFA). NIFA was formerly known as the Extension Service. NIFA is an agency within the U.S. Department of Agriculture which provides federal leadership in creating and disseminating knowledge spanning the biological, physical and social sciences related to agricultural research, economic analysis, statistics, extension and higher education.[8]

The mission of the RECs is to provide technical assistance, guidance and information to support and accelerate healthcare providers' efforts to become meaningful users of EHRs and promote participation in HIE. They collaborate with the health IT industry, universities and state governments, disseminating best practices and research on implementation, effective use, upgrading and ongoing maintenance.

Given the relatively lower adoption rates of primary care providers in solo and small group practices (fewer than 10 licensed independent practitioners), the RECs prioritize those providers who provide primary care services in public and critical access hospitals, community health centers, rural health clinics, and in other settings that mainly serve uninsured, underinsured and medically underserved populations.

The goal of the program is to cover outreach and implementation services to at least 100,000 priority primary care providers within two years.

The Health Information Technology Research Center (HITRC), funded at $53 million, will provide technical assistance, guidance and information on best practices to healthcare providers to become meaningful users of EHRs. Under the HITECH legislation, financial support to any REC must be matched by the state and is not to exceed four years.

For a case study of the REC, see Chapter 16 in this volume on New York City Reach, the REC of New York City.[9]

The second largest HITECH allocation funds determine initiatives to build governance, policies, technical infrastructure and financing for HIE across each state and territory during a four-year period. HIE among physicians and healthcare organizations will be organized regionally, by state and nationally. For the individual patient, this nationwide health information network will enable sharing of relevant portions of a patient's health record in one state with a healthcare provider in another state when needed.

For a case study of a regional health information organization (RHIO), see the chapter in this book on the New York Clinical Information Exchange (NYCLIX).

Training

Implementing and maintaining EHRs and an HIE for physician offices and healthcare organizations will require more than 50,000 new health IT professionals. The Health IT Workforce Cooperative Agreements have awarded $84 million to 16 universities and 70 junior colleges to support training and development. Another $34 million is available for two-year funding to participating community colleges after successful completion of a mid-project evaluation. Programs will permit (a) healthcare providers to learn skills and competencies in IT and (b) IT professionals to learn about healthcare.

A Competency Examination Program will develop standards for "basic competency for individuals trained in short-term, non-degree health IT programs and for members of the workforce seeking to demonstrate their competency in certain health IT workforce roles."[6]

Beacon Communities Lighting the Way

Adoption of new technology is complex. Physicians, patients, and hospitals getting to meaningful use of EHRs and exchanging health information will be a dramatic change for many. What should all the pieces look like when they are put together?

HITECH assigns an approximate $250 million to fund demonstration communities—Beacon Communities that will show how the meaningful use of EHRs can improve quality, safety, efficiency and population health in selected areas.

Testing Standards

The National Institute of Standards and Technology (NIST), an agency of the U.S. Department of Commerce, was founded in 1901 as the nation's first federal physical science research laboratory. To sustain ongoing work on developing and coordinating standards through collaboration with the American National Standards Institute (ANSI), Healthcare Information Technology Standards Panel (HITSP), standards developing organizations, federal agencies, professional societies and industry. NIST will also take part in testing standards for certification; developing security technologies and guidance, and conducting research on usability.

Public Health

Meaningful use of the EHR includes immunization registries and electronic laboratory reporting from office-based physicians and hospitals to public health agencies. HITECH devotes approximately $30.5 million to public health agencies to enable these technologies.

PRIVACY AND SECURITY

Privacy leaks make the headlines more often than most consumers would like. Whether it is stolen laptops with protected health information, burgled back-up tapes with Social Security numbers or a hacker engaged in identity theft, these crimes raise justifiable concerns about the privacy and security of health information.[10]

The Health Insurance Portability and Accountability Act of 1996 (HIPAA) took steps to protect patient privacy and security. HITECH extends that protection further and requires that a covered healthcare organization respond to a breach in the following manner:

- Notify each individual whose unsecured protected health information has been, or is reasonably believed by the covered entity to have been, accessed, acquired or disclosed as a result of such breach.
- Notify prominent media outlets serving a state or jurisdiction following the discovery of a breach if the unsecured protected health information is of more than 500 residents of such state or jurisdiction.
- If the breach involves 500 or more individuals, notify the U.S. Department of Health & Human Services (HHS) immediately.
- If the breach involves fewer than 500 individuals, maintain a log of any such breach and annually submit such a log to HHS.

HITECH also prohibits a covered entity or business associate from receiving remuneration in exchange for any protected health information of an individual unless authorized by an individual.

As of this writing, the Office for Civil Rights (OCR) is working on a notice of proposed rulemaking to implement the privacy section (Subtitle D) of the HITECH Act such as business associate liability; new limitations on the sale of protected health information (PHI), marketing, and fundraising communications; and stronger individual rights to access EHRs and restricting the disclosure of certain information.

A Disclaimer

Despite the national interest in the Medical Home Model and the Chronic Care Model, HITECH does not fund adoption of Aging Services Technology. Instead, it makes funding available to study methods for identifying current and future Aging Services Technology, technology in other countries that may be applied in the United States and barriers to innovation and adoption.

TO BE CONTINUED...

Will all this money spent on EHR adoption lead to better healthcare?

Linder et al. analyzed ambulatory visits in the 2003 and 2004 National Ambulatory Medical Care Survey. They examined the association of EHR use with 17 ambulatory quality indicators. For 14 of the 17 quality indicators, there was no significant difference in performance between visits with EHR use versus without EHR use. The indicators included medical management of common diseases, recommended antibiotic prescribing, preventive counseling, screening tests and avoiding potentially inappropriate medication prescribing in elderly patients. For two quality indicators, visits to medical practices using EHRs had significantly better performance: avoiding benzodiazepine use for patients with depression and avoiding routine urinalysis during general medical examinations. The authors concluded that "As implemented, EHRs were not associated with better quality ambulatory care."[11]

HITECH seeks not just EHR adoption but the *meaningful use* of the EHR to improve quality, safety, and efficiency. It provisions implementation services, best practice research, standard development, health information exchange, training, and privacy and security.

After this brief overview of the HITECH, a reasonable next question might be this: "What exactly is *meaningful use*?"

To answer that question, read on.

REFERENCES

1. To Err Is Human: Building a Safer Health System. Committee on Quality of Health Care in America, Institute of Medicine 2000; Washington, DC: The National Academies Press.

2. Jha AK, DesRoches CM, Campbell EG et al. Use of electronic health records in U.S. hospitals. *N Engl J Med.* 2009; 16;360(16):1628-38.

3. Hsiao CJ, Burt CW, Rechtsteiner E et al. Preliminary estimates of electronic medical records use by office-based physicians: United States, 2008. Health E-Stat. National Center for Health Statistics. 2008. Available online at: www.cdc.gov/nchs/products/pubs/pubd/hestats/hestats.htm. Last accessed July 2010.

4. HITECH and Funding Opportunities. Available online at: http://healthit.hhs.gov/portal/server.pt/community/healthit_hhs_gov__hitech_and_funding_opportunities/1310. Last accessed July 2010.

5. Brode C. Congress restores $32.8 million to healthcare IT czar. *HealthCare IT News,* May 06, 2005. Available online at: www.healthcareitnews.com/news/congress-restores-328-million-healthcare-it-czar. Last accessed July 2010.

6. American Recovery and Reinvestment Act Implementation Plans. U.S. Department of Health & Human Services, June 2010. Available online at: www.recovery.gov/Transparency/agency/Recovery%20Plans/HHS%20Recovery%20Act%20Plan%20-%20June%202010.pdf. Last accessed July 2010.

7. American Recovery and Reinvestment Act of 2009. Available online at: http://frwebgate.access.gpo.gov/cgi-bin/getdoc.cgi?dbname=111_cong_bills&docid=f:h1enr.pdf. Last accessed July 2010.

8. National Institute of Food and Agriculture (NIFA). Available online at: www.csrees.usda.gov/about/background.html. Last accessed July 2010.

9. Available online at: www.nycreach.org/. Last accessed November 2010.

10. Marsan CD. Is your health privacy at risk? *Network World,* September 02, 2009. Available online at: www.networkworld.com/news/2009/090209-health-breach.html. Last accessed July 2010.

11. Linder JA, Ma J, Bates DW et al. Electronic health record use and the quality of ambulatory care in the United States. *Arch Intern Med.* 2007;167(13):1400-05.

CHAPTER 2

Meaningful Use

Ken Ong, MD, MPH, and Robin Raiford, BSN, RN-BC, CPHIMS, FHIMSS

> "Like an escalator, HITECH attempts to move the health system upward toward improved quality and effectiveness in healthcare. But the speed of ascent must be calibrated to reflect both the capacities of providers who face a multitude of real-world challenges and the maturity of the technology itself."
>
> —*David Blumenthal, MD*
> *National Coordinator of*
> *Health Information Technology*[1]

INTRODUCTION

The passengers on the Health Information Technology for Economic and Clinical Health Act of 2009 (HITECH) escalator are the healthcare professionals and hospitals that HITECH defines as "eligible." CMS estimates there are about 477,500 non-hospital based eligible professionals and 5,011 eligible hospitals.[2]

Up to $27 billion in incentives over the next 10 years will be available to eligible providers and hospitals for "Meaningful Use" of the electronic health record (EHR). A provider can accrue as much as $44,000 (through Medicare) and $63,750 (through Medicaid). Eligible hospitals (EHs) can garner $2 million and more.

Aetna has also announced it will offer financial incentives to physicians who achieve meaningful use of the EHR and who make investments in technology for implementation of an EHR.[3] Other payers are sure to follow with similar pay-for-performance incentives.

As much a motivator, if not more, are the penalties that will result in 2015 if eligible providers and hospitals fail to demonstrate meaningful use.

This chapter summarizes the 864-page final rule on "Meaningful Use" from the Centers for Medicare & Medicaid Services (CMS). Links to the final rule in its entirety, the official meaningful use sites by CMS and the Office of the National Coordinator for Health Information Technology (ONC), and other useful links are listed at the end of this chapter.

Who's Eligible?

The devil is indeed in the details. In this case, it is actually the incentives that are in the details.

The Medicare Fee For Service (FFS), Medicare Advantage, and Medicaid EHR Incentive Programs each define eligible professionals differently (see Tables 2-1, 2-2, and 2-3). Physicians and dentists are eligible for both Medicare FFS and Medicaid incentives. Yet, the same is not true for all health professionals. Chiropractors, podiatrists and optometrists are eligible for Medicare FFS incentives but not Medicaid incentives. In contrast, nurse practitioners, certified nurse-midwives, and certain physician assistants are eligible for Medicaid incentives but not Medicare.

Even the details have details. In order for any of the professionals just listed to qualify for Medicaid, at least 30 percent of their patients must have Medicaid. The threshold is lower for pediatricians, i.e., 20 percent.[4] Also, eligible professionals can only apply for either Medicare or Medicaid incentives, while hospitals can apply for both.

Table 2-1: Eligible Providers in Medicare FFS[5]

Eligible Professionals (EPs)
• Doctor of Medicine or Osteopathy
• Doctor of Dental Surgery or Dental Medicine
• Doctor of Podiatric Medicine
• Doctor of Optometry
• Chiropractor
Eligible Hospitals
• Acute Care Hospitals*
• Critical Access Hospitals (CAHs)

* Subsection (d) hospitals that are paid under the PPS and are located in the 50 States or Washington, DC (including Maryland). This excludes hospitals that are not paid under the IPPS in accordance with section 1886(d)(1)(B) of the Act, such as psychiatric, rehabilitation, long-term care, children's, and cancer hospitals (CMS EHR incentive program final rule page 44450).

Adapted from: Medicare & Medicaid EHR Incentive Program Final Rule Training Presentation. CMS EHR Incentive Program, July 20, 2010.

Table 2-2: Medicare Advantage (MA) Eligible Provider

MA Eligible Professionals (EPs)
• Must furnish, on average, at least 20 hours/week of patient-care services and be employed by the qualifying MA organization; or,
• Must be employed by, or be a partner of, an entity that through contract with the qualifying MA organization furnishes at least 80% of the entity's Medicare patient care services to enrollees of the qualifying MA organization
MA-Affiliated Eligible Hospitals
• Will be paid under the Medicare fee-for-service EHR incentive program

Adapted from: Medicare & Medicaid EHR Incentive Program Final Rule Training Presentation. CMS EHR Incentive Program, July 20, 2010.

Table 2-3: Medicaid Eligible Provider

Eligible Professionals (EPs)
• Physicians • Nurse Practitioners (NPs) • Certified Nurse-Midwives (CNMs) • Dentists • Physician Assistants (PAs) working in a Federally Qualified Health Center (FQHC) or rural health clinic (RHC) that is so led by a PA • Medicaid share 30% for all EPs except 20% for pediatricians[5]
Eligible Hospitals
• Acute Care Hospitals (now including CAHs) • Children's Hospitals

Adapted from: Medicare & Medicaid EHR Incentive Program Final Rule Training Presentation. CMS EHR Incentive Program, July 20, 2010.

Altogether, approximately 44,100 non-Medicare eligible professionals (such as dentists, pediatricians, and eligible non-physicians such as CNMs, NPs, and PAs) will be eligible to receive the Medicaid incentive payments.[6]

Not all professionals employed by hospitals qualify for Medicare or Medicaid EHR incentive payments. Hospital-based professionals who provide 90 percent or more of their services in either the inpatient (place of service code 21) or emergency department (place of service code 23) of a hospital are not eligible. Conversely, clinicians who serve in hospital outpatient clinics (place of service code 22) are eligible to receive Eligible Professionals (EPs) Incentives under Medicare FFS.

There are 5,011 EHs. They comprise the following:

- 3,620 acute care hospitals
- 1,302 CAHs
- 78 children's hospitals (Medicaid only)
- 11 cancer hospitals (Medicaid only)

At time of this writing, neither behavioral health hospitals nor continuing care facilities are eligible for incentives.

WHAT IS MEANINGFUL USE?

Okay, you have read the fine print and figured out you are either an EP or EH. You now must achieve Meaningful Use of the EHR to get the incentives. Where did the Meaningful Use goals come from, and what exactly are they?

The health outcome priorities for Stage 1 of Meaningful Use were derived from the National Quality Forum (NQF)-sponsored National Priorities Partnership:[7]

- Improve quality, safety, efficiency, and reduce health disparities
- Engage patients and families in their healthcare
- Improve care coordination
- Improve population and public health
- Ensure adequate privacy and security protections for personal health information

The HITECH Act defines three components of "Meaningful Use:"

- Use of a certified EHR in a meaningful manner (e.g., electronic prescribing)
- Use of certified-EHR technology for electronic exchange of health information to improve quality of healthcare
- Use of certified-EHR technology to submit clinical quality measures (CQM) and other such measures selected by HHS

Having a "certified" EHR is an absolute requirement. Even if you have an EHR that meets all the Stage-1 objectives, you will not qualify for the meaningful use incentives unless the EHR is CMS-certified. If you are an eligible professional (or hospital) who has built your own EHR from scratch, you will need to submit your EHR to CMS for certification.

The Office of the National Coordinator (ONC) has authorized the Certification Commission for Healthcare Information Technology, Drummond Group, and Info-Gard Laboratories to temporarily certify EHR products on CMS's behalf in 2011 and 2012.[8] All EHR products will subsequently have to be approved for permanent certification in 2013. EHR certification is discussed in another chapter in this volume.

ONC-authorized certification means the EHR technology has the capacity to accomplish the objectives of Meaningful Use.

The "Certified EHR" must be either a "Complete EHR" or a combination of certified "EHR modules" that make up a complete EHR.

Listed next are the definitions for Qualified EHR, Complete EHR, EHR Module, and Certified-EHR Technology. Each module or complete EHR must have a certification ID that is issued upon completion of certification by the CMS Authorized Testing and Certification Body. Those official certification sections are also listed. All applications for EHR and EHR-module certification must pass the same certification process regardless of whether the software was developed by an EHR vendor or by the provider. Hospitals and eligible professionals will be required to have certification numbers of each of the modules whether or not they are ever implemented to achieve meaningful use. For example, if a hospital has different EHRs in its emergency department (ED), outpatient, and inpatient, the certification for each must be available upon request.

Definition "Qualified EHR"[9]

An electronic record of health-related information on an individual that:

- Includes patient demographic and clinical health information, such as medical history and problem lists; and
- Has the capacity:
  - To provide clinical decision support;
  - To support physician order entry;
  - To capture and query information relevant to healthcare quality; and
  - To exchange electronic health information with, and integrate such information from, other sources.

Definition of "Complete EHR"[10]

> The term Complete EHR is used to mean EHR technology that has been developed to meet all applicable certification criteria adopted by the Secretary. We believe this definition helps to create a clear distinction between a Complete EHR, an EHR Module, and Certified EHR Technology. The term Complete EHR is not meant to limit the capabilities that a Complete EHR can include. Rather, it is meant to encompass EHR technology that can perform all of the applicable capabilities required by certification criteria adopted by the Secretary and distinguish it from EHR technology that cannot perform those capabilities. We fully expect some Complete EHRs to have capabilities beyond those addressed by certification criteria adopted by the Secretary.

Definition of "EHR Module"[10]

> We have defined the term EHR Module to mean any service, component, or combination thereof that can meet the requirements of at least one certification criterion adopted by the Secretary. Examples of EHR Modules include, but are not limited to, the following:
>
> - An interface or other software program that provides the capability to exchange electronic health information;
> - An open source software program that enables individuals online access to certain health information maintained by EHR technology;
> - A clinical decision support rules engine;
> - A software program used to submit public health information to public health authorities; and
> - A quality measure reporting service or software program.

Definition of "Certified EHR Technology"[10]

> Certified EHR Technology is defined at section 3000(1) of the PHSA as "a qualified electronic health record that is certified pursuant to section 3001(c)(5) as meeting standards adopted under section 3004 that are applicable to the type of record involved.

What follows is a broad overview of the Meaningful Use objectives. For details, visit the CMS EHR Incentives website.[11]

Whether you are an EP or an EH, the tables that follow can be modified to create a Pronovost-style checklist of Meaningful Use objectives and clinical quality measures. A sample gap analysis and action plan from New York Hospital Queens is described later in this chapter.

During Stage 1 (2011 and 2012), EPs have to report on 20 of 25 Meaningful Use objectives and EHs have to report on 19 of 24 Meaningful Use objectives. The reporting period for Stage 1 is 90 days for the first year but one year thereafter (see Table 2-4).

Table 2-4: What Are the Requirements of Stage 1 Meaningful Use?[12]

- **Eligible Professionals must complete:**
  - 15 core objectives
  - 5 objectives out of 10 from menu set
  - 6 total Clinical Quality Measures (3 core or alternate core, and 3 out of 38 from alternate set)
- Hospitals must complete:
  - 14 core objectives
  - 5 objectives out of 10 from menu set
  - 15 Clinical Quality Measures

The Meaningful Use objectives and associated measures core and menu sets are described in Tables 2-5 and 2-6.

Table 2-5: Stage 1 Meaningful Use Core Set[2]

- Computerized Practitioner Order Entry (CPOE)
- Drug-drug and drug-allergy interaction checks
- Electronic prescribing (for eligible professionals)
- Record demographics
- Problem list
- Medication list
- Medication allergy list
- Record and chart changes in vital signs
- Smoking status for patients 13 years old or older
- Implement one clinical decision support rule relevant to specialty or high clinical priority along with the ability to track compliance with that rule
- Report clinical quality measures to CMS or the states
- Provide patients with an electronic copy of their health information upon request
- Provide patients with an electronic copy of their discharge instructions at time of discharge, upon request (for hospitals)
- Provide clinical summaries for patients for each office visit
- Capability to exchange key clinical information (for example, problem list, medication list, medication allergies, diagnostic test results) among providers of care and patient authorized entities electronically
- Protect electronic health information created or maintained by the certified EHR technology through the implementation of appropriate technical capabilities

All core set measures must be reported, and five measures from the menu set must be reported. In particular, EPs must report all 15 measures from the core set and 5 selected measures from the menu set. EHs must report all 14 measures from the core set and 5 selected measures from the menu set.

At least one public health objective must be selected from the menu set measures:

- Capability to provide electronic submission of reportable lab results to public health agencies (EHs only)
- Capability to submit electronic data to immunization registries/systems

Table 2-6: Stage 1 Meaningful Use Menu Set[2]

• Drug-formulary checks • Record advance directives for patients 65 years old or older (for hospitals) • Incorporate clinical lab test results into certified EHR technology as structured data • Generate lists of patients by specific conditions to use for quality improvement, reduction of disparities, research or outreach • Send reminders to patients per patient preference for preventive/ follow-up care (for eligible professionals) • Provide patients with timely electronic access to their health information (for eligible professionals) • Use certified EHR technology to identify patient-specific education resources and provide those resources to the patient, if appropriate • Medication reconciliation • Summary of care record for each transition of care or referral • Capability to submit electronic data to immunization registries or Immunization Information Systems • Capability to submit electronic data on reportable (as required by state or local law) lab results to public health agencies and actual submission in accordance with applicable law and practice (for hospitals) • Capability to submit electronic syndromic surveillance data to public health agencies and actual submission in accordance with applicable law and practice

- Capability to provide electronic syndromic surveillance data to public health agencies

More than a few of the measures include specifications that impact their compliance:

- Certified EHRs will be required to calculate each measure's numerator, denominator and exclusions.
- Measures are collected for all patients regardless of payer.
- Eligible professionals and hospitals can report the Stage 1 measures (2011) by attestation. Electronic submission of measures will start in 2012.
- The measure calculation may have a denominator based on counting actions for patients:
  - Denominator of unique patients regardless of whether patient's records are maintained using certified EHR technology
  - Whose records are maintained using certified EHR technology
  - May require only a yes/no attestation
- Computerized practitioner order entry (CPOE) only pertains to medications in Stage 1, not laboratory, imaging, nursing or ancillary orders
- All EHR technology must be CMS certified. CMS will certify EHRs that can generate the meaningful use measures.
- Hospital measures include inpatient and emergency department (ED).
- The patients in the ED included in the measure calculations are those who are either admitted to inpatient or treated in an observation service.[13]
- Some measures require structured data (e.g., record demographics, problem and medication lists, clinical lab test results) to enable reporting and clinical decision support, which at this time cannot be performed with free text.
- Electronic copies of health information and discharge instructions must be made upon patient request. If a patient does not request electronic copies of

health information or discharge instructions, they are not included in the relevant measure's denominator.

- Some measures only require attestation that a test was performed of particular EHR technology, e.g. exchanging health information electronically, submitting data to immunization registries or reportable lab results, or for syndromic surveillance. If the local public health agency does not have the capacity to accept electronic submissions, the measure is excluded.
- Patients' electronic access to their health information is subject to the EP's discretion to withhold certain information.
- Unlike The Joint Commission's requirement for medication reconciliation within levels of care in a hospital, the meaningful use measure stipulates that medication reconciliation only need be recorded between transitions from one setting of care to another.
- Patient-specific education resources do not have to reside in nor be generated by the certified EHR.
- The preliminary cause of death need not be updated if a final cause of death is determined at a later date.
- If patients are too ill to have their height or weight measured safely, they can be self-reported or estimated.
- CPOE can be performed by any professional licensed by their state to enter orders, e.g. physician assistant or nurse practitioner.
- At time of this writing, each eligible professional must register individually.

There is no provision for groups of EPs to register together.

The Frequently Asked Questions section of the CMS EHR Incentives Program website is a treasure trove of information.[14]

For those circumstances when the measure is out of scope of an eligible professional's practice, there are named exclusions in the CMS final rule. These exclusions are noted in the CMS final rule.[15]

For example, if an eligible professional writes less than 100 prescriptions during the reporting period, the electronic prescribing and CPOE measures are not required for the EP to qualify for incentives.[16]

CLINICAL QUALITY MEASURES FOR ELIGIBLE PROFESSIONALS

Reporting the Meaningful Use objectives alone is not enough to qualify for the incentives. Clinical quality measures (CQMs) are required, as well.

EPs must report on a total of six measures: three required core measures and three additional measures. If the denominator of one or more required core measures is zero, EPs must substitute up to three alternate core measures (see Tables 2-7 and 2-8). The 3 additional CQM can be selected from a set of 38 CQM (other than the core/alternate core measures). These 38 CQM are the proposed core measures for 2012 and 2013 (see Table 2-9).

Table 2-7: Core Set for EPs[12]

• Hypertension: Blood Pressure Measurement • Preventive Care and Screening Measure Pair: (a) Tobacco Use Assessment (b) Tobacco Cessation Intervention • Adult Weight Screening and Follow-up

Table 2-8: Alternate Core Set for EPs[12]

• Weight Assessment and Counseling for Children and Adolescents • Preventive Care and Screening: Influenza Immunization for Patients 50 Years Old or Older • Childhood Immunization Status

The CQMs for EPs are being aligned with CMS's existing quality programs for physicians:

- CMS's Physician Quality Reporting Initiative (PQRI)
- Children's Health Insurance Program Reauthorization Act of 2007 (CHIPRA)

The CQMs for Meaningful Use and CHIPRA share four measures:

1. Childhood Immunization Status
2. Weight Assessment Counseling for Children and Adolescents
3. Chlamydia Screening for Women
4. Appropriate Testing for Children with Pharyngitis

CLINICAL QUALITY MEASURES FOR ELIGIBLE HOSPITALS AND CRITICAL ACCESS HOSPITALS

EHs and CAHs must report data on all 15 quality measures, which are related to (see Table 2-10):[17]

- Stroke care
- Prevention and treatment of blood clots (venous thromboembolism)
- ED throughput measures

The CQMs for EHs are being aligned with Reporting Hospital Quality Data for Annual Payment Update (RHQDAPU), the pre-existing CMS quality reporting program for hospitals.

The inherent nuances and complexities of collecting and reporting quality measures are the domain of the nurse managers and others who work in quality and performance improvement. Not only does the GIGO principle ("garbage in, garbage out") pertain, but its often underappreciated correlate—the NINO principle ("nothing in, nothing out") can be equally problematic. The EHR by itself does not capture all the data elements required to report quality measures. People and their workflows populate allergy histories, problem lists, and the numerous other data elements that define meaningful use now and in the future. In Chapter 12, our friends from the Upper Manhattan Group describe their journey reporting quality measures from an EHR before the HITECH era.

Table 2-9: Additional Set for EPs[12]

1. Diabetes: Hemoglobin A1c Poor Control
2. Diabetes: Low Density Lipoprotein (LDL) Management and Control
3. Diabetes: Blood Pressure Management
4. Heart Failure (HF): Angiotensin-Converting Enzyme (ACE) Inhibitor or Angiotensin Receptor Blocker (ARB) Therapy for Left Ventricular Systolic Dysfunction (LVSD)
5. Coronary Artery Disease (CAD): Beta-Blocker Therapy for CAD Patients with Prior Myocardial Infarction (MI)
6. Pneumonia Vaccination Status for Older Adults
7. Breast Cancer Screening
8. Colorectal Cancer Screening
9. Coronary Artery Disease (CAD): Oral Antiplatelet Therapy Prescribed for Patients with CAD
10. Heart Failure (HF): Beta-Blocker Therapy for Left Ventricular Systolic Dysfunction (LVSD)
11. Anti-depressant medication management: (a) Effective Acute Phase Treatment, (b) Effective Continuation Phase Treatment
12. Primary Open Angle Glaucoma (POAG): Optic Nerve Evaluation
13. Diabetic Retinopathy: Documentation of Presence or Absence of Macular Edema and Level of Severity of Retinopathy
14. Diabetic Retinopathy: Communication with the Physician Managing Ongoing Diabetes Care
15. Asthma Pharmacologic Therapy
16. Asthma Assessment
17. Appropriate Testing for Children with Pharyngitis
18. Oncology Breast Cancer: Hormonal Therapy for Stage IC-IIIC Estrogen Receptor/Progesterone Receptor (ER/PR) Positive Breast Cancer
19. Oncology Colon Cancer: Chemotherapy for Stage III Colon Cancer Patients
20. Prostate Cancer: Avoidance of Overuse of Bone Scan for Staging Low Risk Prostate Cancer Patients
21. Smoking and Tobacco Use Cessation, Medical Assistance: (a) Advising Smokers and Tobacco Users to Quit, (b) Discussing Smoking and Tobacco Use Cessation Medications, (c) Discussing Smoking and Tobacco Use Cessation Strategies
22. Diabetes: Eye Exam
23. Diabetes: Urine Screening
24. Diabetes: Foot Exam
25. Coronary Artery Disease (CAD): Drug Therapy for Lowering LDL Cholesterol
26. Heart Failure (HF): Warfarin Therapy Patients with Atrial Fibrillation
27. Ischemic Vascular Disease (IVD): Blood Pressure Management
28. Ischemic Vascular Disease (IVD): Use of Aspirin or Another Antithrombotic
29. Initiation and Engagement of Alcohol and Other Drug Dependence Treatment: (a) Initiation, (b) Engagement
30. Prenatal Care: Screening for Human Immunodeficiency Virus (HIV)
31. Prenatal Care: Anti-D Immune Globulin
32. Controlling High Blood Pressure
33. Cervical Cancer Screening
34. Chlamydia Screening for Women
35. Use of Appropriate Medications for Asthma
36. Low Back Pain: Use of Imaging Studies
37. Ischemic Vascular Disease (IVD): Complete Lipid Panel and LDL Control
38. Diabetes: Hemoglobin A1c Control (<8.0%)

Table 2-10: CQMs for Eligible Hospitals and CAHs[12]

1.	Emergency Department Throughput – admitted patients – Median time from ED arrival to ED departure for admitted patients
2.	Emergency Department Throughput – admitted patients – Admission decision time to ED departure time for admitted patients
3.	Ischemic stroke – Discharge on anti-thrombotics
4.	Ischemic stroke – Anticoagulation for A-fib/flutter
5.	Ischemic stroke – Thrombolytic therapy for patients arriving within 2 hours of symptom onset
6.	Ischemic or hemorrhagic stroke – Antithrombotic therapy by day 2
7.	Ischemic stroke – Discharge on statins
8.	Ischemic or hemorrhagic stroke – Stroke education
9.	Ischemic or hemorrhagic stroke – Rehabilitation assessment
10.	VTE prophylaxis within 24 hours of arrival
11.	Intensive Care Unit Venous Thromboembolism (VTE) prophylaxis
12.	Anticoagulation overlap therapy
13.	Platelet monitoring on unfractionated heparin
14.	VTE discharge instructions
15.	Incidence of potentially preventable VTE

Changes from the Interim to Final Rule and Clarification of Terms

CMS received more than 2,000 comments on the proposed rule for meaningful use.

In response, CMS made the following significant changes to the final rule:[18]

- CMS lowered the number of required measures and made many measures selectable.
- CMS lowered thresholds for compliance, e.g., from 75 to 40 percent for electronic prescribing by EPs
- Hospital-based physicians are permitted to be EPs
- Critical access hospitals were made eligible for EHR incentives under Medicaid
- Patient-specific educational resources were added as a measure
- Recording advance directives was made a measure for hospitals

Whether or not you have read all of the 276 pages that comprise the Meaningful Use Final Rule, it will come as no surprise that after the final rule was released, more questions were asked and clarifications made. The public comment period elicited 43 clarifications of terms in the final rule.[19]

We will mention three of particular note in CMS's own words:

- **Up-to-date:** "The term 'up-to-date' means the list is populated with the most recent diagnosis known by the EP, EH, or CAH. This knowledge could be ascertained from previous records, transfer of information from other providers, or querying the patient. However, not every EP has direct contact with the patient and therefore has the opportunity to update the list. Nor do we believe that an EP, EH, or CAH should be required through meaningful use to update the list at every contact with the patient."[20]
- **Transition of Care:** "The term 'transition of care' means a transfer of a patient from one clinical setting (inpatient, outpatient, physician office, home health, rehab, long-term care facility, etc.) to another or from one EP, EH, or CAH (as

defined by CMS Certification Number [CCN] to another."[21] In addition, in the absence of interoperable certified electronic healthcare records within organizations, and within the industry at large, The Joint Commission addresses transition of care as transitions within an organization as in ED, to ICU, to Med Surg units. Without interoperable certified EHRs, there is an issue of accuracy on medication reconciliation between units, and will become part of The Joint Commission survey as a violation if not done starting 2011.[22]

- **Key Clinical Information:** "By 'clinical information,' we mean all data needed to diagnose and treat disease, such as blood tests, microbiology, urinalysis, pathology tests, radiology, cardiac imaging, nuclear medicine tests, and pulmonary function tests. We leave it to the provider's clinical judgment as to identifying what clinical information is considered key clinical information for purposes of exchanging clinical information about a patient at a particular time with other providers of care."[9]

One stipulation that did not change limits the incentives to hospitals in health systems. Individual hospitals of systems that share a single CCN, or Medicare provider number will *not* be able to qualify for meaningful use payments.

For example, in New York state a total of 46 hospitals are represented by only 20 Medicare provider numbers. The final rule would prevent hospitals across New York state from receiving more than $80 million in EHR incentive payments.[23] As this book goes to press, a bill is making its way through Congress that will provide incentives to each hospital in a health system if it meets meaningful use.[23]

MEANINGFUL USE GAP ANALYSIS

If you have made it through the chapter this far, you have seen more tables than you have ever seen in any flea market or street fair.

Those tables do have a purpose. Let us put them to work.

Ken Ong, MD, MPH, has made a gap analysis of his own hospital, New York Hospital Queens (NYHQ). NYHQ is a 519-bed teaching hospital of Weill-Cornell Medical College and a member of the New York Presbyterian Health System. It serves the most linguistically and ethnically diverse county in the nation. NYHQ deployed CPOE for medications, laboratory, imaging, nursing and all other orders in 2006. The hospital's EHR is Allscripts' Sunrise Clinical Manager (SCM), version 5.0. Version 5.0 is not CMS-certified but its upgrade, Version 5.5, will be.

The high-level Meaningful Use gap analysis is a simple table with the following format (see Tables 2-11, 2-12 and 2-13):

- Rows:
  - Meaningful use objectives (core and menu)
  - Clinical quality measures
- Columns:
  - Current state
  - Action plan
  - Owner

In the actual NYHQ Meaningful Use gap analysis, familiar traffic light colors indicate current state compliance by color. Green indicates that minimal to no change is

Table 2-11: NYHQ–14 Core Objectives: Must Meet All 14

#	Core Measures	Current State	Action Plan	Owner
1	Computerized provider order entry (CPOE) > 30% unique patients with at least 1 medication	Green: 100% Meds, Lab, & Rad		
2	Drug-drug and drug-allergy interaction checks	Green: All medication orders require allergy documentation		
3	Record demographics			
	• Preferred language	Red: Captured in Registration	Capture in nursing clinical documentation	Nurse informaticists, CNO, & CMIO
	• Gender	Green: Yes		
	• Race	Green: Yes		
	• Ethnicity	Green: Yes		
	• Date of birth	Green: Yes		
	• Date and preliminary cause of death in the event of mortality in the eligible hospital or CAH	Red: Date of death captured	Preliminary cause of death as type in Health Issue Manager in SCM 5.0 Upgrade to SCM 5.5 (Problem List Manager)	CIO & CMIO
4	Maintain up-to-date problem list of current and active diagnoses	Red: Registration capture reason for admission	Develop Medical Logic Modules that send diagnosis from diagnosis-specific order sets and clinical documentation to Health Issues Manager in SCM 5.0 Upgrade to SCM 5.5 (Problem List Manager)	CIO & CMIO
5	Maintain active medication list	Green: Yes		
6	Maintain active medication allergy list	Green: Yes		
7	Record and chart changes in vital signs			
	• Height	Green: Yes		
	• Weight	Green: Yes		
	• Blood pressure	Green: Yes		
	• Calculate and display	Green: Yes		
	• BMI (body mass index)	Green: Yes		
	• Plot and display growth charts for children 2–20 years, including BMI > 50% unique patients 2–20 years old	Red: Height & weight captured	Start performance improvement project with Pediatrics Department to train staff to enter height and weight simultaneously to enable the growth chart	Pediatrics & CMIO
8	Record smoking status for patients 13 years old or older > 50% unique patients 13 years old or older	Red: Captured on paper	Revise nursing clinical documentation	CMIO & Informatics work group

Table 2-11: *(Continued)*

#	Core Measures	Current State	Action Plan	Owner
9	Implement one clinical decision support rule related to a high priority hospital condition along with the ability to track compliance with that rule	Yellow: CPOE order sets active but not tracked	Upgrade to SCM 5.5 (Clinical Analytics)	CIO , CMIO, & VP, Quality
10	Report hospital clinical quality measures to CMS or States	Red: Paper chart review	Upgrade to SCM 5.5 (Clinical Analytics)	CIO , CMIO, & VP, Quality
11	Provide patients with an electronic copy of their health information, upon request	Red: Copy of paper chart upon request	Upgrade to SCM 5.5 (Patient Portal & ExitCare)	CIO , CMIO, & CNO
12	Provide patients with an electronic copy of their discharge instructions at time of discharge, upon request	Red: Paper but not electronic copies given	Upgrade to SCM 5.5 (Patient Portal & ExitCare)	CIO , CMIO, & CNO
13	Capability to exchange key clinical information among providers of care and patient-authorized entities electronically	Green: Testing with regional health information organization in progress		CIO
14	Protect electronic health information	Yellow: Conduct or review a security risk analysis	Track CMS and ONC specifications for performing security risk analysis	CIO

needed; yellow, moderate change needed; and red, major change in workflow or technology needed.

Each action plan item is a placeholder for more detailed project plans that may have dozens or hundreds of tasks.

Clinical Informatics Committee (CIC) is chaired by the CMIO and comprises the CMO, CIO, representatives of all clinical departments, quality, nursing, chief medical and surgical residents, and manager of the core clinical applications team in IT. Other hospitals have similar committees with names such as physician advisory or clinical decision support.

Another tool you may find helpful is available from HIMSS—an ARRA requirements self-assessment tool for EPs and hospitals online.[24]

No matter how costly or resource intensive it is to install a CMS-certified EHR, it will not by itself get you to meaningful use. Whether it is a matter of improving workflows or optimizing the scope of practice for each member of the care team, it really comes down to people. While the technology enables better care, patient and family engagement and better care coordination, it is our nurses, physicians, dentists, front desk staff and others who make it happen.

FINANCIAL INCENTIVES

Eligible Professionals

Medicare incentives will be available from calendar year 2011 through 2014. Medicaid incentives will end 2016.

The "payment year" for EPs will be any calendar year beginning in 2011. Medicare providers must report on 90 consecutive days for Year 1 (2011) and a full 12-month

Table 2-12: NYHQ–10 Menu Objectives: May Defer 5 of 10

#	Menu Set	Current State	Action Plan	Owner
1	Drug-formulary checks	Green: Yes		
2	Record advance directives for patients 65 years or older	Red: Paper	Revise electronic nursing clinical documentation	Nurse informaticists, CNO, & CMIO
3	Incorporate clinical lab test results as structured data	Green: Yes		
4	Generate lists of patients by specific conditions	Red: No	Upgrade to SCM 5.5 (Problem List Manager & Clinical Analytics)	CMIO & Clinical Informatics Committee
5	Use certified EHR technology to identify patient-specific education resources and provide to patient, if appropriate	Red: No	Upgrade to SCM 5.5 (Patient Portal & ExitCare)	Nurse informaticists, CNO, & CMIO
6	Medication reconciliation	Red: No	Upgrade to SCM 5.5 (Orders Reconciliation)	CMIO & Clinical Informatics Committee
7	Summary of care record for each transition of care/referrals	Red: No	Develop discharge summary notes for ED and inpatient	CMIO & Clinical Informatics Committee
8	Capability to submit electronic data to immunization registries/systems	Red: No	Upgrade to SCM 5.5 (Immunization Manager)	Nurse informaticists, CNO, & CMIO
9	Capability to provide electronic submission of reportable lab results to public health agencies	Green: Yes		Chair of Pathology, CIO, & CMIO
10	Capability to provide electronic syndromic surveillance data to public health agencies	Green: Yes	ED system	Chair of ED, CIO, ID, & CMIO

period thereafter. Medicaid providers will not have to report until 2012.[25] Penalties for not having achieved meaningful use will then follow in 2015.

Incentives differ for Medicare (Table 2-14), Medicare in Health Professional Shortage Areas (HPSAs) (Table 2-15) and Medicaid (Table 2-16). The maximum incentive for EPs in the Medicare EHR Incentive Program is $44,000. The maximum in the Medicaid program is $63,750 per EP. EPs can apply for either Medicare or Medicaid incentives but not both. Other differences are listed in Table 2-17.[5]

EPs who practice in a HPSA can receive additional incentives.

The sooner an EP achieves Meaningful Use, the more incentives are accrued.

EPs can participate in other CMS pay-for-performance programs, such as the Medicare Physician Quality Reporting Initiative (PQRI), Medicare Electronic Health Record Demonstration (EHR Demo), and the Medicare Care Management Performance Demonstration.

However, if EPs participate in the Medicare EHR Incentive Program, they cannot participate in the Medicare eRx Incentive Program. This restriction does not apply to EPs who participate in the Medicaid EHR Incentive Program.

Table 2-13: NYHQ Clinical Quality Measures: Report All 15

#	Clinical Quality Measures	Current State Validation	Action Plan	Owner
1	Emergency Department Throughput – admitted patients – Median time from ED arrival to ED departure for admitted patients	Yellow: Monthly reports from old ED system now; Eclipsys ED will report in future.	Upgrade to SCM 5.5 (Clinical Analytics)	CIO, VP of Quality, & CMIO
2	Emergency Department Throughput – admitted patients – Admission decision time to ED departure time for admitted patients			
3	Ischemic stroke – Discharge on anti-thrombotics	Yellow: Measures are manually abstracted from paper and electronic medical record and manually entered into state health department data system.		
4	Ischemic stroke – Anticoagulation for A-fib/flutter	Yellow: Stroke order set in SCM 5.0 & utilization is monitored.		
5	Ischemic stroke – Thrombolytic therapy for patients arriving within 2 hours of symptom onset			
6	Ischemic or hemorrhagic stroke – Antithrombotic therapy by day 2			
7	Ischemic stroke – Discharge on statins			
8	Ischemic or hemorrhagic stroke – Stroke education			
9	Ischemic or hemorrhagic stroke – Rehabilitation assessment			
10	VTE prophylaxis within 24 hours of arrival	Yellow: VTE order sets are built in SCM 5.0. Post-discharge reporting available.		
11	Intensive Care Unit VTE prophylaxis			
12	Anticoagulation overlap therapy			
13	Platelet monitoring on unfractionated heparin			
14	VTE discharge instructions	Yellow: VTE discharge instructions are in paper only, not electronic.	Upgrade to SCM 5.5 (Patient Portal & ExitCare)	CIO, VP of Quality, & CMIO
15	Incidence of potentially preventable VTE	Green: Crystal reports are generated then validated by medical record review. Reported to state health department using their criteria.	Upgrade to SCM 5.5 (Clinical Analytics)	CIO, VP of Quality, & CMIO

Table 2-14: Incentive Payments for Medicare EPs by First Calendar Year for Which EP Receives Incentive Payment[5]

	CY 2011	CY 2012	CY 2013	CY2014	CY 2015 and later
CY 2011	$18,000				
CY 2012	$12,000	$18,000			
CY 2013	$8,000	$12,000	$15,000		
CY 2014	$4,000	$8,000	$12,000	$12,000	
CY 2015	$2,000	$4,000	$8,000	$8,000	$0
CY 2016		$2,000	$4,000	$4,000	$0
TOTAL	$44,000	$44,000	$39,000	$24,000	$0

Table 2-15: Additional Incentive Payments for Medicare EPs Practicing in HPSAs[5]

	CY 2011	CY 2012	CY 2013	CY2014	CY 2015 and later
CY 2011	$1,800				
CY 2012	$1,200	$1,800			
CY 2013	$800	$1,200	$1,500		
CY 2014	$400	$800	$1,200	$1,200	
CY 2015	$200	$400	$800	$800	$0
CY 2016		$200	$400	$400	$0
TOTAL	$4,400	$4,400	$3,900	$2,400	$0

The American Board of Medical Specialties (ABMS) has announced plans to promote the meaningful use of health IT by incorporating health IT into its certification programs. The ABMS Maintenance of Certification® (ABMS MOC®) promotes lifelong learning and self-assessment for physician specialists. "Over 750,000 U.S. physicians are certified by an ABMS Member Board, so it is readily apparent that building meaningful use of health IT into MOC will benefit patients," said Kevin B. Weiss, MD, ABMS president and CEO. "Aligning MOC and meaningful use of health IT will help to facilitate physicians' knowledge, skill and use of health IT, and in turn can improve physician performance and patient outcomes."[26]

Eligible Hospitals

Unlike EPs, EHs can receive both Medicare and Medicaid incentives. A "payment year" for EHs and CAHs will be any federal fiscal year beginning in fiscal year 2011 (after

Table 2-16: Incentive Payments for Medicaid EPs by First Calendar Year for Which EP Receives Incentive Payment[5]

	CY 2011	CY 2012	CY 2013	CY 2014	CY 2015	CY 2016
CY 2011	$21,250					
CY 2012	$8,500	$21,250				
CY 2013	$8,500	$8,500	$21,250			
CY 2014	$8,500	$8,500	$8,500	$21,250		
CY 2015	$8,500	$8,500	$8,500	$8,500	$21,250	
CY 2016	$8,500	$8,500	$8,500	$8,500	$8,500	$21,250
CY 2017		$8,500	$8,500	$8,500	$8,500	$8,500
CY 2018			$8,500	$8,500	$8,500	$8,500
CY 2019				$8,500	$8,500	$8,500
CY 2020					$8,500	$8,500
CY 2021						$8,500
TOTAL	$63,750	$63,750	$63,750	$63,750	$63,750	$63,750

Table 2-17: Notable Differences Between the Medicare and Medicaid EHR Programs[5]

Medicare	Medicaid
Federal Government will implement (will be an option nationally)	Voluntary for States to implement (may not be an option in every State)
Payment reductions begin in 2015 for providers that do not demonstrate Meaningful Use	No Medicaid payment reductions
Must demonstrate MU in Year 1	A/I/U option for 1st participation year
Maximum incentive is $44,000 for EPs (bonus for EPs in HPSAs)	Maximum incentive is $63,750 for EPs
MU definition is common for Medicare	States can adopt certain additional requirements for MU
Last year a provider may initiate program is 2014; Last year to register is 2016; Payment adjustments begin in 2015	Last year a provider may initiate program is 2016; Last year to register is 2016
Only physicians, subsection (d) hospitals and CAHs	5 types of EPs, acute care hospitals (including CAHs) and children's hospitals

October 1, 2010).[25] Each EH receives $2 million base plus a per-discharge amount (based on Medicare/Medicaid share).

The Medicare incentive payment calculation for EHs is given in Figure 2-1.

If an EH or CAH gets meaningful use with one stage but not the subsequent stage, the year missed is counted in the maximum number of incentive program years allowed,

Incentive Amount = [Initial Amount] x [Medicare Share] x [Transition Factor]

Initial Amount = $2,000,000 + [$200 per discharge for the 1,150th – 23,000th discharge]
Medicare Share = *Medicare/(Total*Charity Care) = [M/(T*C)]*
M = [# of Inpatient Bed Days for Part A Beneficiaries] + [# of Inpatient Bed Days for MA Beneficiaries]
T = [# of Total Inpatient Bed Days]
C = [Total Charges – Charges for Charity Care*]/[Total Charges]

Consecutive Payment Year	Transition Factor
1	1
2	¾
3	½
4	¼

*If data on charity care is not available, then the Secretary would use data on uncompensated care as a proxy. If the proxy data is not also available, then "*C*" would be equal to 1.

Figure 2-1: Medicare Incentive Payment Calculation for Eligible Hospitals[27]

e.g., four years. Thus, if an EH reaches Stage 1 in 2011, it must achieve Stage 2 in 2013 to receive the incentive.

Operationally, this means that EHs and CAHs should be preparing to achieve the menu set measures by 2012.

After 2015, EPs and EHs that have failed to meet meaningful use of the EHR will have their Medicare "market basket" payments reduced by 1 percent in 2015, 2 percent in 2016, and 3 percent in 2017 and later.

REGISTER FOR THE INCENTIVE PROGRAMS

Registration for the Medicare EHR Incentive Program became available January 3, 2011. Registration for the Medicaid program will start in 2011, but the actual date will vary by state.

Before making Medicare EHR incentive program payments, CMS will verify Medicare enrollment by the registrant's National Provider Identifier (NPI) and enrollment in the Provider Enrollment, Chain and Ownership System (PECOS) and National Plan and Provider Enumeration System (NPPES).

Medicaid EPs who are only participating in the Medicaid EHR incentive program do not have to be enrolled in PECOS.

Data required for registration will include:

1. Name of the EP, EH or qualifying CAH
2. National Provider Identifier (NPI)
3. Business address and business phone
4. Taxpayer Identification Number (TIN) to which the provider would like his or her incentive payment made
5. CMS Certification Number (CCN) for EHs
6. Medicare or Medicaid program selection (may only switch once after receiving an incentive payment before 2015) for EPs
7. State selection for Medicaid providers

Registration information is available (e.g., to register for Meaningful Use online or how to acquire a NPI or enroll in PECOS or NPPES).[11]

BARRIERS TO ADOPTION

While the Association for the Advancement of Retired Persons (AARP) and National Partnership for Women & Families advocated for keeping the higher standards in the proposed rule, the American Medical Association (AMA) and American Hospital Association expressed concern that the final rule was still unreachable for the nation's physicians and hospitals.

Eligible Professionals

According to the AMA, barriers remain for physicians on the path to meaningful use of the EHR[28]:

- **Timing:** Physicians will have had only have a couple of months to purchase, implement and assess the usability of certified EHR technology prior to January 2011 (the start data of the program);
- **Volume of measures:** The volume of measures that physicians must meet totals 20, which is still too high;
- **Hospital-based professionals:** Hospital-based physicians are not eligible for incentives if they provide 90 percent or more of their services in an inpatient or emergency room setting;
- **Time frames for furnishing patient information electronically:** The measures that require physicians to electronically produce, within several days, health information contained in EHRs conflict with HIPAA requirements that allow for a longer period of time for the production of medical records;
- **Threshold requirements still too high:** Some of the threshold requirements are still too high and some of the measures have narrow exclusions, which will be burdensome for physicians to meet;
- **No appeals process:** There is no mechanism for physicians to appeal any aspect of the incentive program;
- **Usability:** The certification process does not take into account whether a product will meet a physician's unique workflow and practice needs, rather, it will only provide the means for meeting the meaningful use criteria;
- **Early adopters:** Physicians who are EHR early adopters must upgrade their systems to meet certification criteria in order to be eligible for incentives; and
- **Testing of re-tooled measures:** There is no guarantee that the e-specifications imbedded in EHR vendor products are accurate and operational.

Each of these points has some value.

One would always prefer to have more time to deploy a costly and complex product like an EHR. Nonetheless, EPs who want to collect the maximum incentives for Medicare can start no later than 2012. For those taking the Medicaid track, the latest year to start is 2016.

The volume of measures may be high from the AMA's perspective, but AARP and other consumer groups have argued for more measures, not less. Not surprisingly, the resulting compromise from CMS has not completely satisfied either. EPs should take advantage of the expertise the regional extension centers (REC) offer to aid software selection, installation and optimizing practice to achieve meaningful use. Some RECs also offer software discounts for selected EHR vendors. More on ARRA/HITECH funded RECs can be found in Chapter 16 in this volume by Amanda Parsons, MD.

Hospital-based professionals, defined as those who provide 90 percent or more of their services in an inpatient or emergency department setting, are not eligible for incentives, the rationale being that the hospitals they work for will buy the EHR technology and accrue hospital incentives (if they meet meaningful use). That said, outpatient physicians who are hospital employees and work more than 10 percent of their time in an ambulatory setting are eligible for incentives.

Time frames for furnishing patient information and education electronically can be mitigated by a personal health record (PHR) tethered to the EP's EHR. Dr. Ong's mother is a patient at Kaiser-Permanente and is a frequent user of her PHR for her test results, medication refills, appointment requests and secure health messaging.[29] Sal Volpe, MD, author of Chapter 14 in this volume on the patient-centered medical home (PCMH), is the first physician in solo practice in New York State to receive NCQA Level 3 recognition for the PCMH.[30] Leveraging MedlinePlus and the PHR from his EHR vendor, his patients have access similar to those of much larger organizations, such as Kaiser-Permanente.[31]

What is usability? For health IT, it is making it easy to do the right thing. A recent Agency for Healthcare Research and Quality (AHRQ) report recommends that ONC and CMS address usability as part of the certification process.[32] Few standards for usability for health IT exist yet, and those that exist are not enforced. The Certification Commission for Health Information Technology provides usability ratings for ambulatory EHRs, which is a welcome start.[33] Joseph Kannry, MD, et al. has contributed a chapter (see Chapter 4) on usability in this volume.

Hospitals

A HIMSS Analytics survey reports 9.61 percent of the 687 hospitals that responded were able to meet at least 12 of 14 of the core objectives and 8 of 10 of the menu objectives. John P. Hoyt, FACHE, FHIMSS, Executive Vice President, HIMSS, concluded: "Our data indicate that hospitals have the capability now to meet some of the requirements for meaningful use, which is significant in the lead up to the Medicare and Medicaid EHR Incentive Programs because they indicate that healthcare organizations continue to move toward implementation of health IT."

In a survey of some 3,000 hospitals, Jha et al. found that the proportion of hospitals that had either basic or comprehensive electronic records rose 'modestly' from 8.7 percent in 2008 to 11.9 percent in 2009 (see Figure 2-2).[34] Only 2 percent of the hospitals with electronic records thought they would meet the meaningful use criteria. The primary barriers to adoption cited were capital requirements and high maintenance. The study concluded: "Critical strategies for policymakers hoping to promote the adoption of electronic health records by U.S. hospitals should focus on financial support, interoperability, and training of information technology support staff." (See Figure 2-3.)

Rich Umbdenstock, president and CEO of the American Hospital Association, conceded that the final rule includes "some important improvements." Yet the AHA "remains concerned that the requirements may be out of reach for many of America's

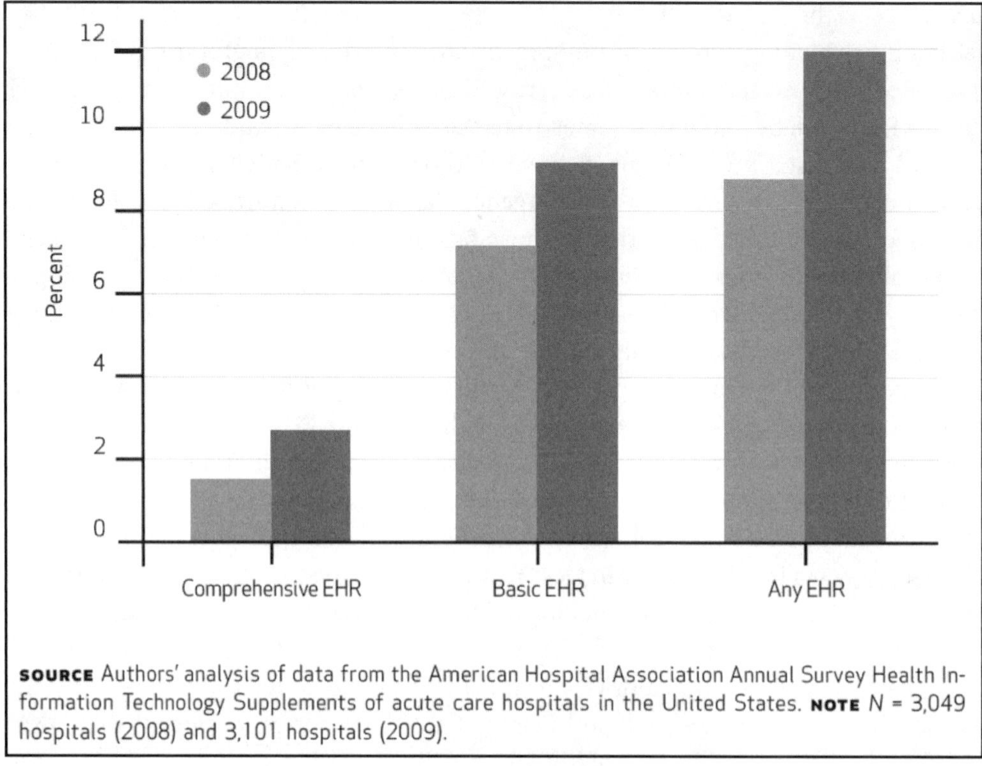

Figure 2-2: Changes in EHR Adoption Rate from 2008 to 2009

Copyrighted and published by Project HOPE/*Health Affairs* as Ashish K. Jha, Catherine M. DesRoches, Peter D. Kralovec, Maulik S. Joshi, A Progress Report on Electronic Health Records in U.S. Hospitals, *Health Affairs*, Volume 29, No. 10, October 2010, pp. 1951–1957. Used by permission.

hospitals" and is "concerned this rule may adversely impact rural hospitals and the patients they serve and exacerbate the digital divide in healthcare."[18,35]

Despite the different methodologies and conclusions of the HIMSS Analytics and AHA surveys, the data from both studies suggest that many of the nation's hospitals face challenges achieving meaningful use. Funding, interoperability, and training IT staff are significant barriers. The federal incentives are rewards given after the EHR has already been purchased and installed. While these rewards may be sufficient to justify capital expenditures by many hospitals, others may not have the available capital to invest.

Engaging trained IT staff is an obstacle for hospitals, EHR vendors and other sectors of the health IT industry. Experts estimate we need 51,000 new health IT professionals to implement EHR technology. The U.S. Department of Health & Human Services has allocated $144 million in American Recovery and Reinvestment Act of 2009 (ARRA) funds to institutions of higher education and research.[36] Training 51,000 people does take time and will not happen instantaneously. Until then, the hospital EHR vendors do not have enough staff to accommodate every hospital that wants to achieve meaningful use in 2011 and soon after.

Many questions remain, yet one thing is certain: HITECH is a work in progress. Further changes by Congress and CMS will surely follow.

Criterion	Overall	Size				Ownership			Location	
		Critical access	Small	Medium	Large	For-profit	Public	Private nonprofit	Urban	Rural
CORE MEASURES										
Record key demographics	86%	72%	82%	94%	97%	82%	78%	90%	91%	78%
Maintain up-to-date problem list	46	32	43	53	61	43	42	48	52	39
Maintain active medication list	66	46	63	77	87	68	55	71	75	55
Give patients, upon request, electronic copy of their health information, including discharge summary	62	44	56	74	78	60	67	52	70	53
Use CPOE	30	19	27	33	53	27	27	32	35	23
Implement drug-drug, drug-allergy checks[a]	14	8	12	15	33	13	13	15	18	10
Have capability to exchange key clinical information	11	8	9	12	18	4	9	13	12	9
Implement at least 1 of 4 clinical decision rules	61	40	59	71	80	61	51	64	69	50
Report hospital quality measures to state or CMS	26	16	24	31	35	26	22	27	30	21
All 9 core criteria except clinical data exchange[a]	**3.9**	**1.8**	**3.4**	**4.1**	**10.0**	**2.6**	**4.0**	**4.2**	**5.3**	**2.1**
All nine core criteria[a]	**2.1**	**1.0**	**1.2**	**2.0**	**7.5**	**0.0**	**2.0**	**2.7**	**3.0**	**1.0**
MENU MEASURES										
Incorporate clinical lab-test results into EHR as structured data	84	66	81	95	97	83	74	89	92	74
Perform medication reconciliation	53	39	48	63	67	47	47	58	60	45
Record advanced directives	49	34	42	58	66	39	54	42	54	41
All 3 menu criteria	**34**	**22**	**27**	**42**	**50**	**25**	**29**	**38**	**39**	**27**
All 9 core and all 3 menu criteria, except clinical data exchange[a]	**3.4**	**1.7**	**2.9**	**3.2**	**9.4**	**2.6**	**3.4**	**3.5**	**4.7**	**1.6**
All 9 core and all 3 menu criteria[a]	**1.6**	**0.9**	**1.0**	**1.2**	**6.7**	**0.0**	**1.7**	**2.0**	**2.4**	**0.6**

SOURCE Authors' analysis of data from the American Hospital Association Annual Survey and the American Hospital Association Annual Survey Health Information Technology Supplement of acute care hospitals in the United States. **NOTES** N = 3,101 hospitals. All results were statistically significant ($p < 0.05$). CPOE is computerized physician order entry. CMS is Centers for Medicare and Medicaid Services. EHR is electronic health record. [a]Statistically significant for hospital size and location.

Figure 2-3: Percentage of U.S. Hospitals That Could Meet Certain Criteria of Meaningful Use, 2009

Copyrighted and published by Project HOPE/*Health Affairs* as Ashish K. Jha, Catherine M. DesRoches, Peter D. Kralovec, Maulik S. Joshi, A Progress Report On Electronic Health Records In U.S. Hospitals, *Health Affairs*, Volume 29, No. 10, October 2010, pp. 1951–1957. Used by permission.

NEXT STEPS

It is time to get on the HITECH's meaningful use escalator. EPs and hospitals have already queued up, and the line only grows longer as the weeks pass. The time line is indeed short and achieving meaningful use requires money, resources, and planning (see Figure 2-4 and Table 2-17).

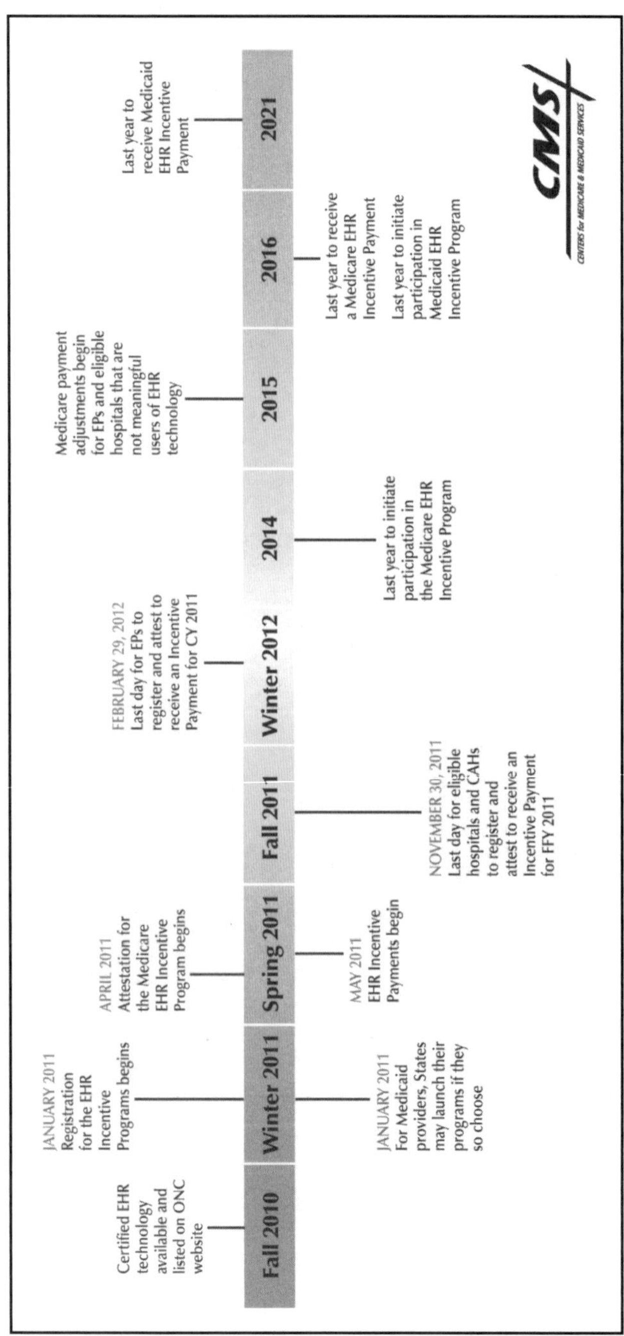

Figure 2-4: CMS Medicare and Medicaid EHR Incentive Programs: Milestone Time Line[37]

Table 2-17: Important Dates[11]

- October 1, 2010 – Reporting year begins for eligible hospitals and CAHs.
- January 1, 2011 – Reporting year begins for eligible professionals.
- January 3, 2011 – Registration for the Medicare EHR Incentive Program begins.
- January 3, 2011 – For Medicaid providers, states may launch their programs if they so choose.
- April 2011 – Attestation for the Medicare EHR Incentive Program begins.
- May 2011 – EHR Incentive Payments expected to begin.
- July 3, 2011 – Last day for eligible hospitals to begin their 90-day reporting period to demonstrate meaningful use for the Medicare EHR Incentive Program.
- September 30, 2011 – Last day of the federal fiscal year. Reporting year ends for eligible hospitals and critical access hospitals.
- October 1, 2011 – Last day for eligible professionals to begin their 90-day reporting period for calendar year 2011 for the Medicare EHR Incentive Program.
- November 30, 2011 – Last day for eligible hospitals and critical access hospitals to register and attest to receive an Incentive Payment for federal fiscal year (FY) 2011.
- December 31, 2011 – Reporting year ends for eligible professionals.
- February 29, 2012 – Last day for eligible professionals to register and attest to receive an Incentive Payment for calendar year (CY) 2011.

The tasks outlined next should help EPs, EHs and CAHs plan for achieving meaningful use:[38]

1. Attend webinars and other educational opportunities from HIMSS, your local medical society, or hospital association to educate your organization on all aspects of the HITECH Act.
2. Review your organization's strategic health IT plan.
3. Perform a Gap Analysis.
4. Estimate future capital requirements.
5. Estimate your organization's financial, operational and clinical ramifications of not moving forward at this time.
6. Establish a Governance Committee, Program Office, Project Management team and required staffing resources.
7. Define Project Charters and time lines.
8. Begin projects.
9. Monitor progress and continue to seek updates and education.

Nearly two decades have passed since the Institute of Medicine described the EHR (formerly known as the computer-based patient record) as an essential technology for healthcare.[39]

One of the authors, Dr. Ong, saw firsthand the value of this technology in his very first ambulatory EHR install in 1999, in an HIV/AIDS clinic in Manhattan where they implemented health maintenance reminders; CPOE; structured lab results; and problem, allergy, and medication lists. As a result, prophylaxis for opportunistic infections, tuberculosis, syphilis and dental screening improved dramatically.[40]

No matter how real the barriers to EHR adoption are, the resources allocated nationally to promote adoption of this essential technology among clinicians and hospitals are unprecedented. The path to get to today has been long and we are not yet finished.

But make no mistake. The EHR is an idea whose time has finally come.

Sidebar 2-1: Get the Latest Updates from CMS

For details and the latest updates on EHR incentives, visit the CMS site.[11]

A sample of some of the information on the CMS Website follows:

- Some providers may have no eligible patients for some measures, e.g., dentists do not perform immunizations and chiropractors do not e-prescribe. These providers will be exempted from reporting these measures.
- For those eligible professionals who work at multiple sites, only those patient encounters that occurred at those sites with a certified EHR need be counted.
- States can ask CMS to require four Meaningful Use objectives of Medicaid eligible professionals.

Sidebar 2-2: Meaningful Links

Legislation and regulation are dynamic. Check the following sources for the latest, up-to-date information about meaningful use:

- CMS Final Rule Posted on Federal Register (July 13, 2010)[41]
  www.ofr.gov/OFRUpload/OFRData/2010-17207_PI.pdf
- Official CMS Website for the Medicare and Medicaid EHR Incentive Programs[11]
  www.cms.gov/EHRIncentivePrograms/
- Office of the National Coordinator of Health IT & 'Meaningful Use'[8]
  http://healthit.hhs.gov/portal/server.pt?open=512&objID=2996&mode=2
- Healthcare Information Management & Systems Society & 'Meaningful Use'[42]
  www.himss.org/EconomicStimulus/
- American Hospital Association & 'Meaningful Use'[43]
  www.aha.org/aha/issues/HIT/100226-hit-meaningful.html
- Center for Health IT at the American Academy of Family Practice[44]
  www.centerforhit.org/online/chit/home/project-ctr/meaningful_use.html
- American College of Physicians & 'Meaningful Use'[45]
  www.americanehr.com/
- Child Health Informatics Center of the American Academy of Pediatrics[46]
  www.aap.org/ehr/
- Greater New York Hospital Association Health I.T. resources[47]
  www.gnyha.org/2984/Default.aspx
- Hospital Association of New York State Health I.T. resources (requires login)[48]
  www.hanys.org/technology/legislation/

REFERENCES

1. Blumenthal D, Tavenner M. The "Meaningful Use" regulation for electronic health records. *New Engl J Med.* 2010;13.
2. Final Rule on Meaningful Use: Medicare and Medicaid Programs; Electronic Health Record Incentive Program, 42 CFR Parts 412, 413, 422, and 495, CMS-0033-F Available at: http://edocket.access.gpo.gov/2010/pdf/2010-17207.pdf. Last accessed July 2010.
3. Aetna to Offer Incentives for Physicians to Achieve Meaningful Use. Healthcare Informatics, August 6, 2010. Available at: www.google.com/url?sa=t&source=web&cd=1&sqi=2&ved=0CBIQFjAA&url=http%3A%2F%2Fwww.healthcare-informatics.com%2FME2%2Fdirmod.asp%3Ftype%3Dnews%26mod%3DNews%26mid%3D9A02E3B96F2A415ABC72CB5F516B4C10%26tier%3D3%26nid%

3D28261783FDDF47B4A2780A094CDEAFC4&ei=hxNrTKOGLMaqlAfqvrxi&usg=AFQjCNEJBLrC3qzRNl154yZKKNC6KFulXg&sig2=kekFVzx_vu2oRDsr-ckulw. Last accessed August 2010.

4. *The Medicare and Medicaid EHR Incentive Program.* Greater New York Hospital Association Webinar, August 13, 2010.

5. Medicare & Medicaid EHR Incentive Program Final Rule: Implementing the American Recovery & Reinvestment Act of 2009. CMS, July 20, 2010. Available at: www.cms.gov/EHRIncentivePrograms/Downloads/EHR_Incentive_Program_Agency_Training_v8-20.pdf. Last accessed July 2010.

6. Pages 44548 of the CMS Final Rule on Meaningful Use. Available at: http://edocket.access.gpo.gov/2010/pdf/2010-17207.pdf. Last accessed August 2010.

7. National Priorities Partnership. National Priorities and Goals: Aligning Our Efforts to Transform America's Healthcare. Washington, DC: National Quality Forum; 2008. Available at: www.google.com/url?sa=t&source=web&cd=1&ved=0CBIQFjAA&url=http%3A%2F%2Fwww.nationalprioritiespartnership.org%2FuploadedFiles%2FNPP%2F08-253-NQF%2520ReportLo%255B6%255D.pdf&ei=kzhSTLeZH4SBlAe41ZiPBQ&usg=AFQjCNGnDCHttXqfDbqziIelVuf8D-JKRg. Last accessed July 2010)

8. *ONC-Authorized Testing and Certification Bodies.* Available at: http://healthit.hhs.gov/portal/server.pt?open=512&mode=2&objID=3120. Last accessed on November 2010.

9. Page 44360 of the CMS EHR Incentive Program Final Rule. *Federal Register*; Vol. 75, No. 144; July 28, 2010.

10. Page 2022. *Federal Register.* Vol. 75, No. 8; January 13, 2010 / Rules and Regulations.

11. Official Web Site for the Medicare and Medicaid EHR Incentive Programs. Available at: www.cms.gov/ehrincentiveprograms/. Last accessed November 2010.

12. Medicare & Medicaid EHR Incentive Program Meaningful Use Stage 1 Requirements Summary, August 24, 2010. Available at: www.google.com/url?sa=t&source=web&cd=1&ved=0CBIQFjAA&url=https%3A%2F%2Fwww.cms.gov%2FEHRIncentivePrograms%2FDownloads%2FMU_Stage1_ReqSummary.pdf&ei=HWWVTIbEFsSBlAfu5PyjCg&usg=AFQjCNFfyGGZWDMiftl3QdyxdN4mephIiQ&sig2=TxRXooaEQc8pNiIGbYR9_g. Last accessed September 2010.

13. Available at: http://questions.cms.hhs.gov/app/answers/detail/a_id/10126. Last accessed September 2010.

14. Frequently Asked Questions (FAQs). Available at: www.cms.gov/EHRIncentivePrograms/99j_Frequently_Asked_Questions.asp. Accessed November 2010.

15. Final Rule. *Federal Register;* Vol. 75, No. 144; July 28, 2010; Rules and Regulations.

16. Dolan PL. HHS spreads the word about how specialists can meet meaningful use. *Am Med News.* Posted November 15, 2010. Available at: www.ama-assn.org/amednews/2010/11/15/bisc1115.htm. Accessed November 2010.

17. The Medicare and Medicaid EHR Incentive Payment Program. HANYS presentation. July 29, 2010.

18. Ackerman K. Long-awaited Final Rule on 'Meaningful Use' strikes compromise. *iHealthBeat.* July 15, 2010. Available at: www.ihealthbeat.org/features/2010/longawaited-final-rule-on-meaningful-use-strikes-compromise.aspx#ixzz0vJToWZHy. Last accessed July 2010.

19. Available at: www.google.com/url?sa=t&source=web&cd=1&ved=0CDEQFjAA&url=https%3A%2F%2Fwww.cms.gov%2FEHRIncentivePrograms%2FDownloads%2FEHR_Incentive_Program_Agency_Training_v8-20.pdf&ei=Lad6TImfF8P78AbF_OSYBg&usg=AFQjCNG2_0y_jC7p8aG-sb7TWvnEjD6piw&sig2=3CvDCzwzDf_zjLk1aiKzdA. Last accessed August 2010.

20. From page 44336 of the CMS EHR Incentive Program Final rule.

21. From page 44363 of the CMS EHR Incentive Program Final rule.

22. *National Patient Safety Goals.* March 05, 2010. Medication reconciliation National Patient Safety Goal to be reviewed, refined. Available at: www.jointcommission.org/PatientSafety/NationalPatientSafetyGoals/npsg8_review.htm. Last accessed August 24, 2010.

23. Final Meaningful Use Rule Allows Limited Flexibility; Overall Bar Still Set Too High. HANYS e-Alert, July 13, 2010.

24. Available at: www.himss.org/ASP/ContentRedirector.asp?ContentID=72885. Last accessed September 2010.

25. Highlights of the Medicare and Medicaid EHR Incentive Programs (Meaningful Use) Final Rule. ©2010 HIMSS.

26. News Release: *ABMS to Develop Physician Assessments Related to Health Information Technology as Part of its ABMS Maintenance of Certification® Program.* American Board of Medical Specialties News Release August 5, 2010. Available at: www.google.com/url?sa=t&source=web&cd=1&ved=0CBIQFjAA&url=http%3A%2F%2Fwww.abms.org%2FNews_and_Events%2FMedia_Newsroom%2FReleases%2Frelease_ABMSAligns_MOC_MUHIT_08052010.aspx&ei=ZxJrTJncIoP58AaBkNWBBQ&usg=AFQjCNE1CK1OkbETP8zKcEscjQSu44rBNg&sig2=NP7jHfPi7cdFqDYCyg_0WA. Last accessed August 2010.

27. Final Rule on Meaningful Use: Medicare and Medicaid Programs; Electronic Health Record Incentive Program, 42 CFR Parts 412, 413, 422, and 495, CMS-0033-F; page 428 Available at: http://edocket.access.gpo.gov/2010/pdf/2010-17207.pdf. Last accessed July 2010.

28. American Medical Association. EHRs Don't Meet All Stage 1 Meaningful Use Criteria. *CMIO.* July 21, 2010. Available at: www.cmio.net/index.php?option=com_articles&view=article&id=23295&division=cmio. Last accessed July 2010.

29. Kaiser-Permanente. Available at: www.kaiserpermanente.org/. Last accessed November 21, 2010.

30. Volpe S. Available at: http://svolpemd.com/. Last accessed November 2010.

31. *MedlinePlus.* Available at: www.nlm.nih.gov/medlineplus/. Last accessed November 2010.

32. Mosquera M. *AHRQ says usability should be part of EHR certification.* Government Health IT. June 02, 2010. Available on www.healthcareitnews.com/news/ahrq-says-usability-should-be-part-ehr-certification. Last accessed November 2010.

33. *Certification Commission for Health Information Technology.* Available at: www.cchit.org. Last accessed November 2010.

34. Jha AK, DesRoches CM, Kralovec PD et al. A progress report on electronic health records in U.S. hospitals. *Health Aff.* 2010;29(10):1-7.

35. CMS Releases Final Rule on HIT Incentive Payments to Hospitals – ML77. Greater New York Hospital Association, July 14, 2010.

36. *HHS Awards $144 Million in Recovery Act Funds to Institutions of Higher Education and Research to Address Critical Needs for the Widespread Adoption and Meaningful Use of Health Information Technology.* HHS Press Release. Available at: www.hhs.gov/news/press/2010pres/04/20100402a.html. Last accessed November 2010.

37. Medicare & Medicaid EHR Incentive Program: Meaningful Use Stage 1 Requirements Overview. Centers for Medicare & Medicaid Services. August 24, 2010. Available at: www.cms.gov/EHRIncentivePrograms/Downloads/MU_Stage1_ReqOverview.pdf. Last accessed September 2010.

38. *Implications of Meaningful Use for Hospitals:* An HIMSS Webinar. Amy Thorpe and Edna Boone. HIMSS, July 28, 2010. Available at: www.himss.org/EconomicStimulus/mu_webinars.asp#archive. Last accessed December 2010.

39. *The Computer-Based Patient Record: An Essential Technology for Health Care.* 1st Edition. Institute of Medicine. Washington, DC: The National Academies Press; 1991.

40. Johnston BE, Leon RW, Ong K. *Using an Electronic Medical Record to Improve HIV Care:* KR. 2002 - XIV International AIDS Conference, Barcelona, Spain.

41. Available at: www.ofr.gov/OFRUpload/OFRData/2010-17207_PI.pdf. Last accessed December 2010.

42. Available at: www.himss.org/EconomicStimulus/. Last accessed December 2010.

43. Available at: www.aha.org/aha/issues/HIT/100226-hit-meaningful.html. Last accessed December 2010.

44. Available at: www.centerforhit.org/online/chit/home/project-ctr/meaningful_use.html. Last accessed December 2010.

45. Available at: www.americanehr.com. Last accessed December 2010.

46. Available at: www.aap.org/ehr. Last accessed December 2010.

47. Available at: www.gnyha.org/2984/Default.aspx. Last accessed December 2010.

48. Available at: www.hanys.org/technology/legislation. Last accessed December 2010.

CHAPTER 3

Certification in Healthcare Information Technology

Abha Agrawal, MD, FACP

> "A surgeon can't operate without the proper equipment. A clinician can't achieve meaningful use of electronic health records without an EHR that is designed to improve patient care and practice efficiency."
>
> —*David Blumenthal, Health IT Buzz blog, June 18, 2010*

INTRODUCTION

Americans have enjoyed the benefits of tremendous advances in modern medicine over the past several decades. Physicians can now visualize internal body structures with astonishing clarity and speed, prescribe "miracle" pharmaceuticals that precisely target abnormal cells or molecules, and perform surgery to repair and replace organs with minimal invasion. However, there remains an appalling gap between the healthcare industry's adoption of modern technology pertaining to new diagnostics and therapeutics and its adoption of modern IT pertaining to delivery and management of healthcare information.

Health IT, such as electronic health records (EHRs), holds the promise of transforming our healthcare system by improving quality and safety, enhancing care coordination and reducing costs.[1-5] However, adoption of EHRs remains low, especially in small group practices. A national survey of 2,758 physicians in ambulatory care practices published in 2008 revealed that fewer than 10 percent of physicians who practice in small groups of one to three have adopted EHRs.[6] Of note, 46 percent of physicians in the United States practice in such small groups. Another study estimated that only 1.5 percent of U.S. hospitals have a comprehensive EHR system (i.e., present in all clinical units), and an additional 7.6 percent have a basic system (i.e., present in at least one clinical unit). Further, computerized practitioner order entry (CPOE) for medications has only been implemented in 17 percent of hospitals.[7] Although slowly rising, health IT adoption remains at a low level compared with other information-intense industries.

The most commonly cited barriers to adoption of EHRs are capital costs involved, not finding a system that meets the needs, uncertainty about the return on investment (ROI), and concern that a system would become obsolete. The most important facilitator of adoption was cited to be the financial incentives for purchase of an EHR.[6]

Over the years, various national initiatives have been launched with the objective of facilitating adoption of EHRs. In 2001, the landmark Institute of Medicine report *Crossing the Quality Chasm* recommended that "Congress, the executive branch, leaders of health care organizations, public and private purchasers, and health informatics associations and vendors should make a renewed national commitment to building an information infrastructure to support health care delivery, consumer health, quality measurement and improvement, public accountability, clinical and health services research, and clinical education. This commitment should lead to the elimination of most handwritten clinical data by the end of the decade."[8] In April 2004, then-President George W. Bush announced a bold vision to provide most Americans with interoperable EHRs within the next 10 years and set in motion a chain of events leading to transformation of healthcare with IT.

Shortly thereafter, the Office of the National Coordinator for Health Information Technology (ONC) was created under the U.S. Department of Health & Human Services (HHS) with David Brailer, MD, serving as its first National Coordinator. In July 2004, Dr. Brailer released a *Framework for Strategic Action* outlining four goals and 12 corresponding strategies for improving healthcare.[9] One of the key actions listed in the strategic framework was the private sector certification of health IT products to "develop minimal products standards for EHR functionality, interoperability and security." In response to this call for action, the Certification Commission for Healthcare Information Technology (CCHIT) was founded as the first organization in the United States with the goal to create credible certification mechanisms for various health IT products.[10]

These initiatives aimed to facilitate adoption of EHR through advocacy, certification and standardization. More recent initiatives have aimed at providing financial incentives for using health IT. Medicare Improvements for Patients and Providers Act of 2008 (MIPPA) authorized a new incentive program for eligible professionals for successful use of electronic prescribing.[11] The most recent and profoundly transformative action is the Health Information Technology for Economic and Clinical Health (HITECH) Act, part of the American Recovery and Reinvestment Act of 2009 (discussed next).[12]

Since passage of HITECH, the health IT certification landscape has altered dramatically with clear and specific regulations and guidance regarding EHR certification criteria and process. This chapter focuses on health IT certification primarily from the perspective of HITECH.

THE HITECH ACT

On February 17, 2009, President Barack Obama signed the American Recovery and Reinvestment Act (ARRA).[13] The bill included provisions, known as HITECH, for transforming quality, safety, efficiency and coordination of healthcare through financial incentives for providers (eligible professionals, hospitals and critical access hospitals) to become "meaningful users of certified EHR technology." The HITECH bill lays the foundation for the Patient Protection and Affordable Care Act (PPACA), colloquially called the "health care reform" bill, by providing the much-needed digital infrastructure built on EHRs and health information exchange (HIE). HITECH and ARRA together stand to reshape the delivery of healthcare in America in the most fundamental ways with a focus on reducing costs and improving quality.

The lynchpin of HITECH is to promote *meaningful use of certified EHR technology*. To this end, ONC and the Centers for Medicare & Medicaid Services (CMS) have implemented the following programs:

(A) Regulations and Guidance to Promote Meaningful Use of Certified EHR (see Figure 3-1)

Under HITECH, eligible healthcare professionals and hospitals can qualify for Medicare and Medicaid incentive payments when they adopt certified EHR technology and use it to achieve specified objectives. These regulations consist of:

- **Incentive Program for Meaningful Use:** Issued by CMS, this final rule released in July 2010 defines the minimum meaningful use requirements that providers must meet in order to qualify for the payments. Through HITECH, the federal government will make available incentive payments totaling up to $27 billion over 10 years, or as much as $44,000 (through Medicare) and $63,750 (through Medicaid) per clinician.

  Since the meaningful use is to be achieved through the use of certified EHR technology, the following two rules specify elements of certified EHR and the process of achieving certification.
- **Standards and Certification Criteria for Electronic Health Records:** Issued by ONC, this rule identifies the standards and certification criteria for the certification of EHR technology, so eligible professionals and hospitals may be assured that the systems they adopt are capable of performing the required functions to support meaningful use objectives. The details of the certification criteria are in the Meaningful Use chapter (see Chapter 2); a summary is provided in the Meaningful Use section of this chapter.
- **Certification Programs:** Issued by ONC, certification programs prescribe a rigorous process to ensure that EHRs meet the adopted standards, certification criteria, and other technical requirements.

(B) Programs to Promote Adoption of EHRs

It is acknowledged that merely providing incentives for EHR adoption may not be enough. Many providers also lack the technical expertise to select, implement, and use an EHR. Therefore, HITECH provides approximately $2 billion in additional funds for programs that support EHR adoption and HIE. These include the following:[14]

- Establishment of up to 70 regional extension centers (RECs) to support providers in adopting and becoming meaningful users of health IT ($643 million).
- Support of state HIE programs ($564 million).
- Creation of workforce training programs that aim to support the education of health IT professionals, including curriculum development, competency exam-

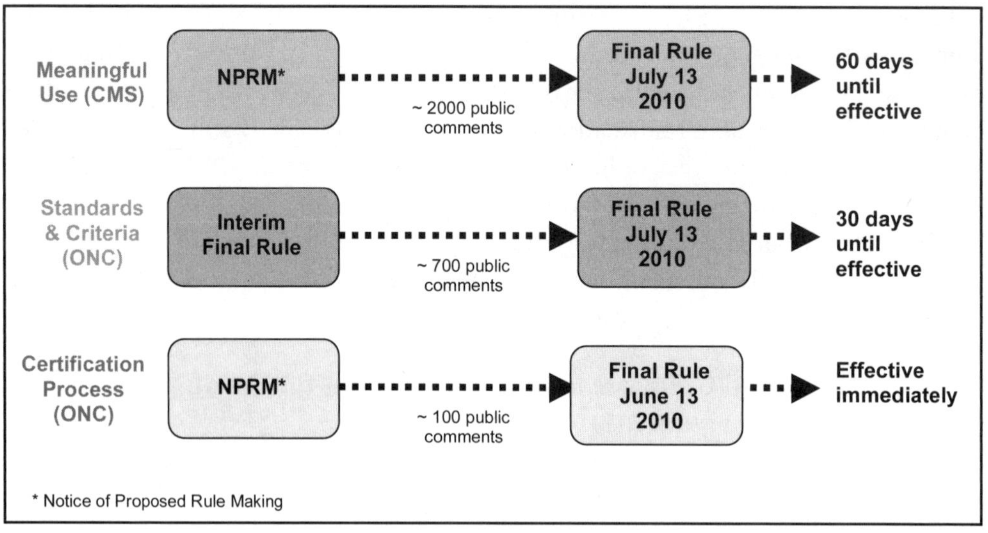

Figure 3-1: Rules Supporting HITECH

inations, and training ($118 million). The goal is to train up to 45,000 new health IT workers to assist providers in becoming meaningful users of EHRs.

- Creation of up to 15 demonstration projects, called Beacon Communities, in which clinicians, hospitals and consumers show how the meaningful use of EHRs can achieve measurable improvement in the quality and efficiency of health services or public health outcomes in a given geographic area ($235 million).
- Funding of strategic health IT advanced research projects (SHARP) focused on achieving breakthrough advances to address well-documented problems that have impeded adoption of health IT, including the security, patient-centered cognitive support, healthcare application and network-platform architectures and secondary use of EHR data ($60 million).
- Creation of a nationwide health information network as a common platform for HIE across diverse entities to promote a more effective marketplace, greater competition, and increased choice through accessibility to accurate information on healthcare costs, quality and outcomes ($64 million to include a nationwide health information network and standards and certification programs).

MEANINGFUL USE

HITECH provisions incentive payments for "meaningful use" and not just adoption of health IT. This approach is sensible and strikes the right balance. It recognizes that adoption of technology is not enough for care improvement—it must be used in a meaningful manner by clinicians. At the same time it acknowledges that improvement in outcomes will take time and is dependent on many factors in addition to EHRs. Therefore, it stops short of basing incentive payments on improved outcomes, at least initially. While reporting quality measures is required in stage 1 of meaningful use (see

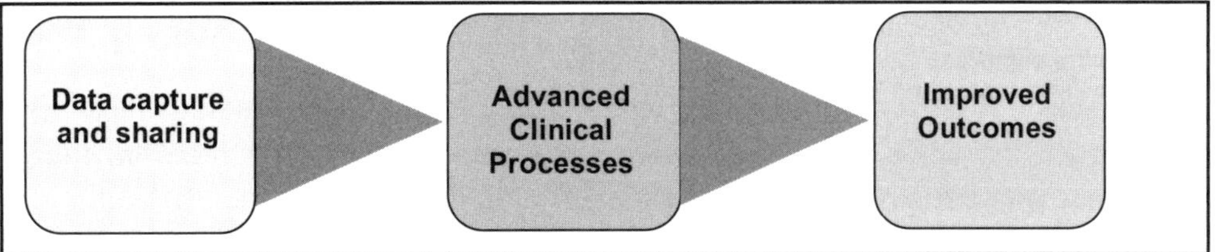

Figure 3-2: Conceptual Approach to Meaningful Use

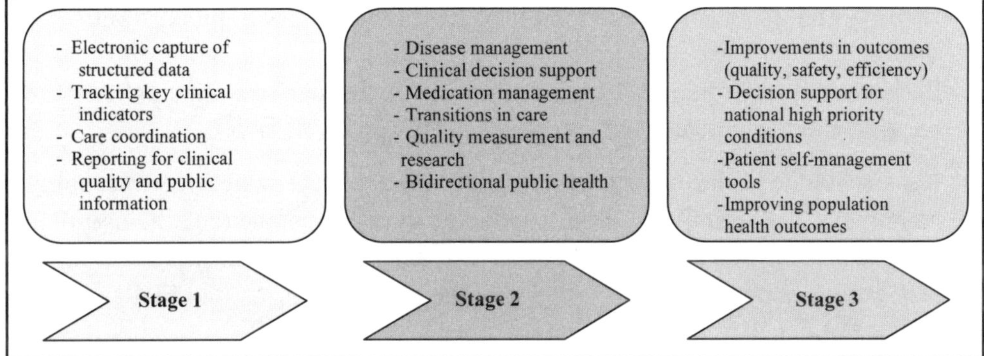

Figure 3-3: Policy Objectives of the Three Stages of Meaningful Use

next discussion), the incentives are based on quality reporting and not on improvement in outcomes.

The meaningful use criteria are planned to be rolled out in three stages, each with a distinct set of objectives that build on the anticipated success in the earlier stage. Figure 3-2 depicts the conceptual approach to incremental stages of meaningful use. Figure 3-3 describes various policy objectives underpinning the certification criteria for each stage.

Stage 1 Meaningful Use Objectives and Criteria

In the final regulation released in July 2010, stage 1 meaningful use criteria have been divided into two groups: a set of core objectives that are required to be met by all eligible professionals, hospitals, and critical access hospitals to receive incentive payment, and a separate menu set of additional objectives from which providers will choose several for implementation. The full list of all meaningful use criteria is available in the Meaningful Use chapter in this book (see Chapter 2). The entire meaningful use rule from the *Federal Register*[15] and a summary by Blumenthal and Tavenner[16] are both available, as well. Basically, eligible providers need to meet 15 criteria from the core set, and five from a menu set of 10, including at least one public health measure. Hospitals need to meet 15 criteria from the core set, and five from a menu set of 10, including at least one public health measure. This approach ensures that everyone is using, at minimum, the essential elements that constitute a functional EHR and at the same time provides some flexibility in choosing additional criteria. The new set of criteria are lenient compared with the interim final rule released in January 2010, as there was an outpouring of public comments calling them "too ambitious," "too aggressive," and expected to be done in "too short a time-frame."[17]

The stage 1 criteria can be mapped to five concepts and corresponding objectives:

1. Improve quality, safety, efficiency and reduce health disparities by requiring the use of computerized practitioner order entry (CPOE), patient access to health data, clinical decision support, and quality reporting.
2. Engage families and patients in healthcare by requiring the use of patient access to health data.
3. Improve care coordination by requiring the use of health information exchange.
4. Improve population and public health by communicating with public health agencies.
5. Ensure adequate privacy and security protections through operating policies, procedures, and technologies and compliance with applicable laws.

It is essential to understand that meaningful use is not the same as certification.

Meaningful use is not only about products but about people (i.e., the users) and processes as well. Certification only ensures that certain functionality is available in a product, but meaningful use "takes a village"; therefore, certification of EHRs is necessary but not sufficient to achieve meaningful use.

CERTIFICATION OF HEALTH IT

Since 2004, CCHIT, a non-profit non-governmental organization, has been the only credible organization offering voluntary EHR certification with the objective of facilitating adoption of EHRs. With the passage of HITECH, the certification landscape has altered dramatically with ONC now responsible for certification of EHR technology for the purpose of receiving meaningful use incentive payments. This does not preclude CCHIT or any other organization from offering additional EHR certification services; in fact, CCHIT continues to offer voluntary certification of EHRs separate and independent from the ONC-required certification.

The Need for Certification in Health IT

In general, certification is a mechanism for enhancing the confidence, orderliness and transparency of a product or service in the marketplace. Certification may encompass functionality, safety, compatibility or other aspects of products and services. The inspection and testing process performed when certifying products and services must be based on consensus-driven standards, unbiased inspection and testing, or both.

According to a study by the Gartner Group, the private sector spends over $2.2. trillion on IT annually. Notwithstanding this spending, 50–70 percent of the major software products fail due to software quality and interoperability problems.[18] Testing and certification of software to ensure that it meets the requirement detailed in the specification can improve the quality of software, the likelihood of achieving interoperability and the success of the implementation. For healthcare providers, certification ensures that the EHR technology they adopt is capable of enabling their participation in the incentive programs. For EHR developers, certification criteria provide a blueprint for development, and certification provides the official "seal of approval" to their prospective customers that their product is capable of supporting meaningful use.

ONC Certification Programs

Currently, ONC has established two certification programs—the temporary program expected to be operational in fall 2010 and a permanent program expected to be available by the end of 2011. It was considered necessary and urgent to establish a temporary program so that certified EHR technology could be made available to eligible providers at the earliest possible to qualify for stage 1 meaningful use incentive payments scheduled to start in fall 2010.

On June 18, 2010, ONC issued the final rule to establish a temporary certification program for the voluntary certification of health IT.[19] Under the temporary program, ONC is responsible for establishing ONC-Authorized Testing and Certification Bodies (ONC-ATCBs) that will conduct both testing and certification of EHRs. ONC has a rigorous process in place to evaluate and grant ONC-ATCB status to prospective applicant organizations. An up-to-date list of ONC-ATCBs is available on the ONC website (http://healthit.hhs.gov/portal/server.pt?open=512&mode=2&objID=3120).[20]

Under the temporary certification program, while ONC-ATCB will conduct the testing and certification, actual testing methodology, tools and data set are to be developed by the National Institute of Standards and Technology (NIST) for every certification criterion. NIST may establish these tools and procedures based on multiple sources, such as NIST-developed tools, industry-developed tools, or open source tools. NIST will submit these to ONC for approval. Once approved by ONC, ONC-ATCBs will have the responsibility and flexibility to configure their own test scripts, i.e., specific scenarios using the test tools and test procedures.

Figure 3-4 provides an overview of the temporary certification program.

The temporary program also outlines the details of the testing and certification process for EHRs and EHR modules, principles of proper conduct for ONC-ATCBs, and the mechanisms to share the list of certified health IT products with eligible healthcare providers and the public in an open and transparent manner.

The permanent program has a more complex structure. For testing, NIST would accredit one or more NIST-Accredited Testing Labs (NIST-ATL) through the National

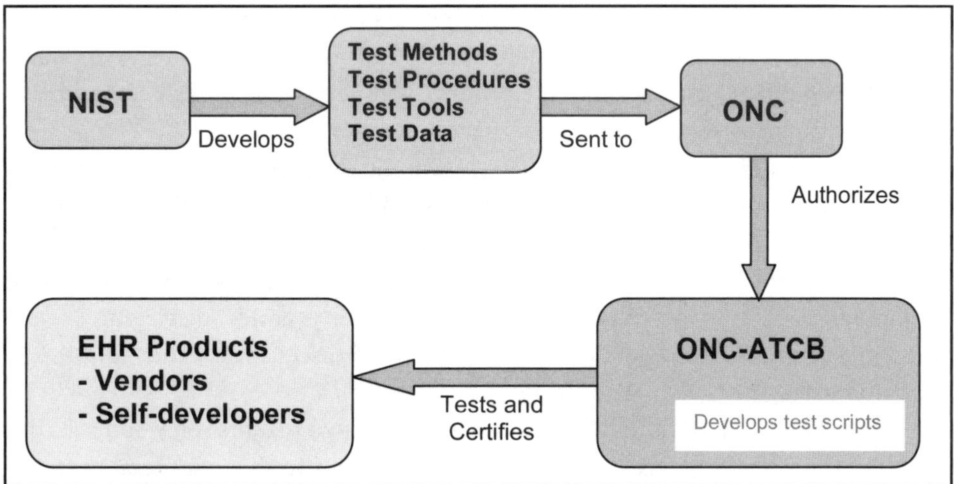

Figure 3-4: Overview of the Temporary Certification Program

Voluntary Laboratory Accreditation Program (NVLAP). For the certification part, ONC would recognize one—and only one—Approved Accreditor (ONC-AA) and one or more ONC-Authorized Certification Bodies (ONC-ACB). An entity applying for ONC-ACB will need to be accredited first by ONC-AA. Under the permanent program, both testing and certification may be performed by the same organization by becoming both an NIST-ATL and ONC-ACB respectively or by two separate entities. ONC-ACBs may only use NIST-ATLs for their testing. The temporary program would end when the first ONC-ACB is accredited by the permanent program.

Complete EHR and EHR Module

The current certification process recognizes two types of EHR technology. *Complete EHR* refers to EHR technology that has been developed to meet, at a minimum, all applicable certification criteria. These certification criteria represent the minimum capabilities EHRs need to include and have properly implemented in order to achieve certification. The program does not preclude Complete EHR developers from including additional capabilities that are not required for the purposes of certification. The second type, *EHR Module,* refers to any service, component, or combination thereof that meets at least one certification criterion. Therefore, if an EHR Module does not provide a capability that can be tested and certified, it would not meet the definition of an EHR Module. An EHR Module could provide a single capability required by one certification criterion, or it could provide all capabilities but one required by the certification criteria for a Complete EHR. In other words, if 10 certification criteria are required for a complete EHR, a product certified against 9 criteria will still be called an EHR Module.

The Testing and Certification Process

These are two separate and distinct processes. *Testing* is the process used to determine the degree to which a Complete EHR or EHR Module can meet specific, predefined, measurable and quantitative requirements. In contrast, *certification* is the process of the assessment and subsequent assertion made by analyzing the quantitative results rendered by testing along with other qualitative factors. These qualitative factors could include whether a product has a quality management system in place or whether a developer has agreed to the policies and conditions associated with being certified (e.g., proper logo usage). The act of certification typically promotes confidence in the quality of a product, offers assurance that the product will perform as described and helps consumers to differentiate which products have met specific criteria.

Consider a developer submitting an E-prescribing module to an ONC-ATCB. To pass testing, the module, among other functions, will need to transmit an electronic prescription using mock patient data according to the specified standards. Once testing is successful, the certification phase could require that the E-prescribing module developer agree to a number of provisions, including, for example, displaying its version and revision number, so potential purchasers could discern when the module was last updated or certified.

All EHRs and EHR modules will be tested and certified to all privacy and security certification criteria set by ONC. There are two exceptions to this requirement in the case of EHR modules. First, if a set of EHR modules is presented as a pre-coordinated, integrated bundle which would otherwise constitute a complete EHR, then only the module(s) responsible for providing all of the privacy and security capabilities for the entire bundle will be tested. Second, if it is demonstrated that a privacy and security certification criterion is inapplicable or that it would be technically infeasible for a module to be tested, then testing is not required.

The current certification program does not prescribe the testing to determine whether various EHR modules can integrate with one another due to understandable technical, logistical and financial costs of testing integration among each of the modules, even though such testing would make it easier for purchasers to be reassured that the various EHR modules are compatible and could be used together to achieve meaningful use objectives. Although the certification rule does not require such integration testing, nothing precludes an ONC-ATCB or other entity from offering a service to test and certify EHR module-to-module integration.

An ONC-ATCB must have the capacity to perform testing and certification at its facility. Additionally, testing and certification may be performed at the site where the EHR or EHR module has been developed, at the site where the EHR or EHR module has been implemented or remotely, such as using Web-based tools.

The program also establishes principles of proper conduct for ONC-ATCBs, including the requirement to maintain an effective quality management system, the use of NIST test tools and test procedures, allowing ONC or its authorized agent to periodically observe and demonstrate compliance and providing at least weekly a list of EHRs and EHR modules that have been tested and certified.

ONC compiles, publishes, and updates the Certified HIT Products List (CHPL) on its website (http://onc-chpl.force.com/ehrcert).[21] The list will include, at a minimum, the vendor name (if applicable), the date certified, product version, the unique certification number and the clinical quality measures to which the product has been tested and certified. In addition, the information will include any additional software the product relied upon to demonstrate its compliance with certification criteria. The last requirement is an important consideration for purchasers of technology. For example, if an EHR relied upon an operating system's automatic log-off functionality to demonstrate its compliance with a certification criterion, it would be expected that the operating system be reported. However, if an EHR included its own automatic log-off capability, even though it was tested and certified on a particular operating system, there is no need to report on the operating system.

Conformance Testing

NIST plans to use the conformance testing (testing whether a product faithfully implements a standard or specification) method to develop testing material including test assertions, test procedures, test methods, test tools, and test data. Figure 3-5 illustrates the methodology used by NIST[22] (adapted from http://healthcare.nist.gov/use_testing/index.html).

Table 3-1 illustrates the elements of conformance testing for a sample certification criterion, "Maintain up-to-date problem list."

Further details about conformance testing and testing methodology for all certification criteria are available at the NIST website (www.nist.gov).[23]

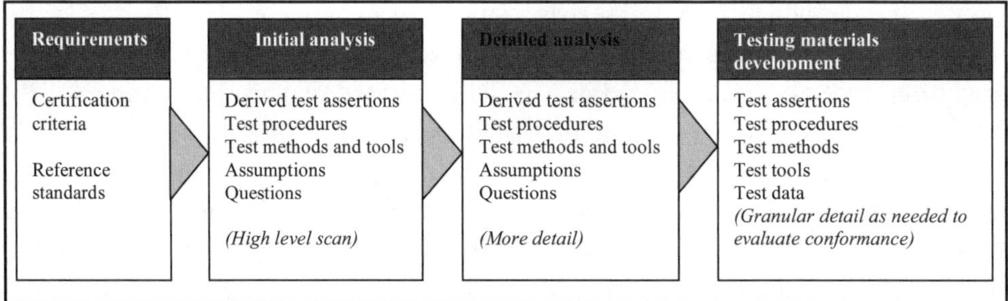

Figure 3-5: Overview of Conformance Testing Methodology for EHR Certification
Adapted from http://healthcare.nist.gov/use_testing/index.html.

Table 3-1: Elements of Conformance Testing for Sample Certification Criterion, "Maintain Up-to-date Problem List"

Certification Criteria	Maintain up-to-date problem list: enable a user to electronically record, modify and retrieve a patient's problem list for longitudinal care in accordance with the referenced standard.
Referenced Standard	ICD-9; alternative standard: SNOMED CT® July 2009 version.
Informative Test Description	This is a description of how the test procedure is organized and conducted. This test procedure has three sections: (1) Record: evaluates the capability to enter patient health problems into EHR to create the patient problem list, (2) Modify: evaluates the capability to edit patient problem list data which have been previously entered into EHR, and (3) Retrieve: evaluates the capability to display and view the patient problem list data which have been previously entered into the EHR, including the capability to display the patient problem list spanning multiple visits.
Normative Test Procedures	These specify the actual testing and inspection procedure and include (a) derived test requirements (DTRs), (b) required test procedure, and (c) inspection test guide for each of the three items in the above row.
Example Test Data	Test data supplied by NIST to testers such as: **Record:** ICD-9 code - 780.2; Problem – Syncope and collapse; Status – Active; Date diagnosed: 2/15/10 ICD-9 code – V13.02; Problem – UTI; Status – Active; Date diagnosed: 9/22/08 **Modify:** Modify the date diagnosed for syncope and collapse to 7/9/08 Resolve the problem UTI **Retrieve:** Active problems only – should not display UTI; should display the correct date for syncope and collapse

CCHIT Certification Programs

The primary focus of this chapter is the ONC certification process and programs. However, since CCHIT was the most mature and widely accepted certifying body prior to the new CMS certification process, an update on CCHIT is included.

CCHIT is an independent non-profit organization and has been offering voluntary certification of EHRs since 2005. It has certified more than 250 EHR products representing 85 percent of the installed market. At the time of this writing, CCHIT has applied to be an ONC-ATCB under ONC's temporary certification program while continuing to offer a separate and independent CCHIT certification to EHR vendors and self-developers.

CCHIT's main strengths include a long track record of successfully certifying EHR products and support from a diversity of stakeholders. It utilizes voluntary consensus-based development process for certification criteria subject to public comments and pilot testing. It has developed a robust, repeatable and efficient inspection process with demonstrated scalability. The inspection is based on an "open book" model, so that all criteria and test scripts are published in advance for all vendors to use in preparation.

Compared with the ONC program, CCHIT has a number of specialized programs (in addition to the ambulatory EHR and inpatient EHR certification) available that target various clinical settings and subspecialties such as cardiovascular medicine, child health, behavioral health, emergency department and long-term care. In addition, CCHIT also performs usability testing and provides EHR usability ratings on its website (more about usability in the next section), verifies live usage of the software, and publishes vendor characteristics for particular EHR products.

CCHIT has been granted ONC-ATCB status under the temporary program. It will be competing with other newly formed ONC-ATCBs to perform ONC testing and certification; a list of all ONC-ATCBs is available.[20] It is too early to know whether EHR product developers will seek a separate, more rigorous certification by CCHIT in addition to subjecting themselves to the required ONC certification. That will be determined by purchasers who may demand more assurance that an EHR product's capabilities are integrated well enough to support the achievement of meaningful use in the short term while also being able to meet their special practice needs in the longer term.

DISCUSSION

HITECH is widely expected to successfully transform the healthcare landscape by laying the foundation for a digital infrastructure for documentation and exchange of clinical information. There are several policy risks worth considering.

First, though the final stage 1 meaningful use criteria, released in July 2010, are more lenient than the original version released in January 2010,[17] they are still considered by many to be too ambitious and as requiring too much change in too short a time. Eligible healthcare providers, especially small and rural practices and certain community health centers, may find the process of adopting EHRs and demonstrating meaningful use too expensive, complicated and not worth the risk of even a temporary decline in productivity. The amount of funding available for health IT infrastructure support, such as RECs, is likely to be less than 10 percent of the actual expenditure on supporting the EHR and HIE implementation. Therefore, if a substantial number of small practices, for which the EHR adoption rate is lowest, perceive the financial costs and risks to be greater than the incentive payments, they may not adopt EHRs.

Further, even if EHR adoption improves, but the HIE programs do not take hold, this may lead to a scenario of a siloed paper system being replaced by siloed EHRs. A recent article that analyzed the experience of the Canadian EMR program revealed that despite an early start in initiatives to accelerate the adoption of EHRs, Canada ranked last in proportion of primary care doctors who have "advanced electronic health information capacity" conceptual equivalent of meaningful use.[24] Another report that analyzed the usage pattern of E-prescribing in the U.S. found that many physicians do not routinely use E-prescribing even after its implementation.[25]

Second, only the first of the three stages of meaningful use criteria have been released. Therefore, healthcare providers are not clear about what requirements they will have to meet in future years, and software developers are unsure of the features that will need to be built into their products in order to remain certified. The anxiety caused by this uncertainty may further erode the trust of physicians, leading to less than anticipated adoption rates.

Finally, the current HIE strategy in HITECH is fragmented, ill-defined and too heavily dependent on market forces that have not worked in the past. HITECH calls for the "development of a nationwide health information technology infrastructure that allows for the electronic use and exchange of information and that....promotes a more effective marketplace, greater competition....[and] increased consumer choice," among other goals.[13] The current approach relies heavily on point-to-point connections between individual providers or labs, based on the EHR products instead of an emphasis on multi-point interoperability based on state HIE programs or on a nationwide digital backbone. Since many benefits of the EHRs on improving healthcare are dependent on robust and secure information exchange, this poses the risk of undermining the policy objectives of HITECH.

When Congress enacted HITECH, President Obama touted it as a "down payment on health reform." EHRs and health IT infrastructure are necessary but not sufficient in achieving the goal of high-quality, patient-centric care. Realizing the full potential of HITECH depends on changing the overall payment incentives from fee-for-service payment for disaggregated, uncoordinated care to outcomes-based payment for coordinated and efficient care.

Usability

Current certification criteria from ONC focus on functionality, interoperability and security features of an EHR. This ignores one important aspect of the EHR products—usability. Usability or, more broadly, information design represents the art and science of preparing and conveying information so that it can be used by human beings with efficiency and effectiveness.[26] NIST defines usability as the "effectiveness, efficiency and satisfaction with which the intended users can achieve their tasks in the intended context of product use."[27] It will be oversimplification to equate usability with mere user satisfaction or ease of use; rather, usability is based on a science—a set of tangibles that can be reliably and reproducibly measured.

Usability is an important consideration for all information products, and it is even more relevant to EHRs used in clinical care where time is constrained, important decisions are made based on multiple data points, and concerted rather than fragmented thinking is important for good clinical decision making. Usability or information design of EHRs has implications for many aspects of clinical care, such as ergonomic (navigating, documenting) and cognitive (reading, thinking, deciding) workload, data awareness and comprehension, patient safety and efficiency of care delivery. Recent research and news articles have described poor information design of EHRs as contributing to low adoption by physicians and introduction of new types of errors in care.[7,28,29]

Usability has been difficult to evaluate, and the oft-cited reason is that it is too subjective and poorly understood by EHR developers as well as users. In addition to addressing the general concepts of usability, EHRs need to address two important issues: the "learn-ability without teaching" and standardization of user-interface (navigation, menus, etc.) across various EHRs. The former is important to ensure that the implementation of EHR does not cost physicians extra time. The latter is important because many physicians, including house officers, practice at several different locations at the same time. The differences in user-interface of various EHRs can be quite confusing and can contribute to poor decision making.

Significant progress is being made in regard to evaluation of usability of EHRs. A recently published report by the Agency of Healthcare Research and Quality (AHRQ) outlined the following principles for usability: simplicity, naturalness, consistency, minimizing cognitive load, effective interactions, forgiveness and feedback, effective use of language, effective information presentation comprising of appropriate density, meaningful use of color, and readability, and preservation of context.[30] For more on usability, see the chapter on that topic (see Chapter 4) in this book.

With the ARRA incentive payments program, the adoption of EHRs is expected to increase significantly in coming years. As EHRs become increasingly central to clinical practice, both positive and negative effects of usability on care will become more apparent. Research as well as the vendor community should invest more effort and resources toward improving the usability of EHRs and studying their impact on care and safety. As the certification program evolves, usability criteria should be incorporated in the testing and certification process.

EHR certification currently is a black-and-white pass-or-fail process, which works well for the functionality measures. An EHR either is capable of recording, editing and retrieving a problem list according to structured vocabulary or is not, and this can be tested and certified. However, usability is more likely to be a graded scale, say from 1 to 5.

There is precedence for mandating good design for national programs that must maintain high safety standards. The National Highway Traffic Safety Administration (NHTSA) mandates the evaluation of the usability of child seats and communicates it to the public via a 5-star rating system.[31] The U.S. Food and Drug Administration (FDA) requires medical device manufacturers to follow Human Factors regulation to minimize errors that may harm patients. The Human Factors regulation considers design input, design verification and design validation.[32]

In conclusion, HITECH of 2009 and the Patient Protection and Affordable Care Act of 2010 together are a transformational opportunity to finally achieve the six ideals of healthcare in the United States: safe, effective, patient-centered, timely, efficient and equitable.[8]

REFERENCES

1. Bates DW, Leape LL, Cullen DJ et al. Effect of computerized physician order entry and a team intervention on prevention of serious medication errors. *JAMA.* 1998;21;280(15):1311-6.

2. Tierney WM, Miller ME, McDonald CJ. The effect on test ordering of informing physicians of the charges for outpatient diagnostic tests. *N Engl J Med.* 1990;24;322(21):1499-504.

3. Johnston D, Pan E, Walker J. The value of CPOE in ambulatory settings. *J Healthc Inf Manag.* 2004;18(1):5-8.

4. Walker J, Pan E, Johnston D et al. The value of health care information exchange and interoperability. *Health Aff* (Millwood). 2005 Jan-Jun;Suppl Web Exclusives:W5-10-W5-8.

5. Jha AK, Kuperman GJ, Rittenberg E et al. Identifying hospital admissions due to adverse drug events using a computer-based monitor. *Pharmacoepidemiol Drug Saf.* 2001;10(2):113-9.

6. DesRoches CM, Campbell EG, Rao SR et al. Electronic health records in ambulatory care—a national survey of physicians. *N Engl J Med.* 2008;3;359(1):50-60.

7. Jha AK, DesRoches CM, Campbell EG et al. Use of electronic health records in U.S. hospitals. *N Engl J Med.* 2009;16;360(16):1628-38.

8. Institute of Medicine (US). Committee on Quality of Health Care in America. *Crossing the Quality Chasm: a New Health System for the 21st Century.* Washington, DC: The National Academies Press; 2001.

9. Office of the National Coordinator. Framework for strategic action. 2004. Available at: www.hhs.gov/healthit/executivesummary.html. Last accessed July 2010.

10. Available at: www.cchit.org. Last accessed December 2010.

11. Electronic prescribing (eRx) incentive program. Available at: www.cms.gov/ERXincentive/01_overview.asp. Last accessed July 2010.

12. Blumenthal D. Stimulating the adoption of health information technology. *N Engl J Med.* 2009; 9;360(15):1477-9.

13. The Recovery Act. Available at: www.recovery.gov/About/Pages/The_Act.aspx. Last accessed July 2010.

14. Blumenthal D. Launching HITECH. *N Engl J Med.* 2010;4;362(5):382-5.

15. Department of Health & Human Services. Medicare and Medicaid Programs; Electronic Health Record Incentive Program. *Federal Register.* 2010;75(144).

16. Blumenthal D, Tavenner M. The "Meaningful Use" regulation for electronic health records. *N Engl J Med.* 2010;5,363(6):561-4. Last accessed July 2010.

17. Doctors and hospitals say goals on computerized records are unrealistic. *The New York Times.* Available att: www.nytimes.com/2010/06/08/health/policy/08health.html. Last accessed July 2010.

18. National Institute of Standards and Technology. What is this thing called conformance? Available at: www.itl.nist.gov/div897/ctg/conformance/bulletin-conformance.htm. Last accessed August 2010.

19. Establishment of the temporary certification program for health information technology; final rule. Available at: http://edocket.access.gpo.gov/2010/2010-14999.htm. Last accessed July 2010.

20. Available at: http://healthit.hhs.gov/portal/server.pt?open=512&mode=2&objD=3120. Last accessed December 2010.

21. Available at: http://onc-chpl.force.com/ehrcert. Last accessed December 2010.

22. Available at: http://healthcare.nist.gov/use_testing/index.html. Last accessed December 2010.

23. Available at: www.nist.gov. Last accessed December 2010.

24. Dermer M, Hogan M. Certification of primary care electronic medical records. *Journal of Health Information Management.* 2010;24(3):49-55.

25. Center for Studying Health System Change. Even when physicians adopt e-prescribing, use of advanced features lags. Available at: www.hschange.com/CONTENT/1133/. Last accessed July 2010.

26. Armijo D, McDonnell C, Werner K. Electronic health record usability: Interface design considerations. Rockville, MD: Agency for Healthcare Research and Quality 2009 Contract No.: 09(10)-0091-2-EF.

27. Common industry specification for usability requirements. Gaithersburg, MD: National Institute of Standards and Technology 2007 Contract No.: NISTIR 7432.

28. Kuehn BM. IT vulnerabilities highlighted by errors, malfunctions at veterans' medical centers. *JAMA.* 2009;4;301(9):919-20.

29. Terhune C, Epstein K, Arnst C. The dubious promise of digital medicine. *Business Week*; 2009. Available at: www.businessweek.com/magazine/content/09_18/b4129030606214.htm. Last accessed July 2010.

30. HIMSS EHR Usability Task Force. Defining and testing EMR usability: Principles and proposed methods of EMR usability evaluation and rating. June 2009.

31. Smith CS, Rockwell TE, Collins LA et al. NHTSA's Child Safety Seat Usability Rating Program. Available at: www.lifesaversconference.org/handouts2009/Smith2.pdf. Last accessed July 2010.

32. Callan JR, Gwynne JW. Human factors principles for medical device labeling: Available at: www.fda.gov/downloads/MedicalDevices/DeviceRegulationandGuidance/GuidanceDocuments/UCM095300.pdf. Last accessed December 2010.

CHAPTER 4

Meaningful Usability: Health Information Technology for the Rest of Us

Joseph Kannry, MD; Andre Kushniruk, PhD, MSc; and Ross Koppel, PhD

INTRODUCTION

The Health Information Technology for Economic and Clinical Health Act (HITECH) portion of the American Recovery and Reinvestment Act of 2009 (ARRA) authorized the Centers for Medicare & Medicaid Services (CMS) to provide reimbursement incentives to both health professionals and hospitals who become "meaningful users" of certified EHR technology. Usability as a concept is the measure of how easy it is to use an information system, how efficiently the system performs, and how easy it is to learn. We applaud and support efforts to incorporate usability into electronic health record (EHR) certification and meaningful use but argue that each healthcare organization needs its own usability unit to adequately address all the issues that arise from each distinct implementation and optimization. Only when a strong basis for system usability and safety exists both nationally and locally within each healthcare organization will meaningful use become a reality. When the need for usability engineering by the vendor and usability testing and assessment by national standards is fully addressed, vendors and healthcare organizations will only grow.

Objectives:

- Appreciate the general role of usability in meaningful use of EHRs
- Review examples of poorly designed, unsafe and unusable health IT
- Define usability engineering and testing
- Understand usability testing and engineering methodology
- Become familiar with examples of the successful application of usability engineering in health IT
- Differentiate proposed usability certification from local usability testing
- Justify the need for organizational usability units

Since the earliest days of clinical informatics research, the promise of healthcare information technology was shown to be the ability to dramatically improve and streamline the delivery and safety of healthcare through IT.[1-10] Subsequently these systems demonstrated data sharing, interoperability, and advanced clinical decision support.[10-16] These internally developed systems, originally begun as research projects, have demonstrated an almost unlimited ability to transform healthcare. Over the past decade, we have seen the emergence of commercial EHR systems for offices and hospitals and of enterprises that allow not only for the electronic entry, storage and retrieval of patient data but also for advanced clinical decision support, public health surveillance and ultimately, the beginnings of interoperable and highly interconnected health data. The promise of these clinical informatics research systems and some limited work on commercial systems is the very cornerstone, if not the driving force, behind the HITECH Act section of ARRA, which authorized CMS to provide reimbursement incentives to both health professionals and hospitals who become "meaningful users" of certified EHR technology.[17,18] Despite the great potential demonstrated by informatics research and the advancement possible with the advent of commercial systems, the adoption and uptake of such technology in the United States has been much slower than expected. Some of this lack of adoption has been attributable to cost, which HITECH attempts to, in part, address.[19-23] However, some may be attributable to the fact that commercial development and implementation of health IT systems have significantly lagged behind informatics developed systems in terms of functionality and usability,[24-27] leading to significant user frustration and at times, user rebellion.[28-31]

To speed the development and diffusion of commercial health IT in the United States, ARRA specified meaningful use of the EHR. The concept of "meaningful" within "meaningful use" includes the measurement of how often key aspects of patient-provider interactions are recorded in the EHR, including aspects of communication, diagnostic studies performed, medications administered, allergies recorded and other selected "meaningful" uses of the EHR.[17] However, despite the importance of such programs and initiatives, in this chapter we will argue that truly meaningful use of healthcare IT will only become a reality when such technology is proven to be both "usable" and safe.

The usability of an information technology is a measure of its ease of use by human users.[32] Usability as a concept can be considered a measure of how easy it is to use an information system, how efficiently the system performs and how easy it is to learn. In addition, usability, broadly defined, also considers the safety of healthcare IT (i.e., how safe it is to use a healthcare information system) as well as the concept of enjoyability (i.e., how enjoyable it is to use a system).[32] In recent years, usability has come to the fore as a major issue in healthcare informatics, with a number of systems having been criticized for being difficult to use and to learn, potentially leading to inadvertent inefficiencies and changes in workflow.[33] In addition, a growing body of literature on commercial systems is indicating that some system features and functions may actually introduce medical errors and that without proper testing they may be dangerous to use.[34-37] Interestingly, one of the first—or at least the first *reported*—system-induced error was reported by Bates et al. in a study that examined the reduction of medication errors during implementation of an internally developed (i.e., informatics) computerized practitioner order entry (CPOE) system with clinical decision support (CDS).[38] Even systems that may be tested to ensure that they pass traditional software testing during their development may be found to "facilitate"[34] or "induce"[35] certain types of errors when used in real healthcare settings and under real work situations and conditions.

To highlight the need for formal and organized usability assessments, the chapter will first review specific examples of a range of usability and safety issues involving EHRs and related technologies, such as CPOE. These examples, provided by Ross Koppel, are based on observation of real users and their reports of problems encountered using systems in use today. Although the names of the commercial systems will not be given to protect the innocent, these are real cases with real commercial systems. After reviewing a number of issues that need to be addressed regarding both the usability and safety of commercial health IT, the next section will review a methodologic solution, usability testing, and assessment. This will be followed by examples of successful deployment of usability methodology in healthcare. Finally the chapter will conclude with a discussion of what can be done to improve the situation nationally (i.e., meaningful use) and locally (i.e., IT and operations) to ensure that systems we deploy in healthcare are both safe and usable.

WHEN BAD SYSTEM EVENTS HAPPEN TO GOOD PROVIDERS

The need to improve the safety and usability of commercial health IT systems can be seen in the examples provided by noted health IT errors scholar Ross Koppel, at the University of Pennsylvania. The origin and evolution of Ross's research provide a litany of examples of the need to improve these systems. Several years ago Koppel, a sociologist, was studying why physicians might make medication prescribing errors. He was examining the usual suspects: sleeplessness, dealing with death and dying, new resident rotations, hierarchical work relations, etc. The young physicians, however, insisted more errors were generated by the CPOE system than by any other cause. This claim was in absolute contrast to the existing peer reviewed literature at that time that viewed CPOE as a solution for and not a cause of medication errors. The first paper written by Koppel et al. in *The Journal of the American Medical Association*, indicating that a commercial health IT system could cause errors[34] created a firestorm[39] because it documented 22 types of errors enhanced by what was then perceived as a panacea to what ails healthcare. Several subsequent studies, reports and editorials confirmed his observations and analyses indicating that these problems may not have been new.[36,37,40-51] The health IT industry response centered around differences in implementation and optimization (i.e., somewhat supported by the literature),[52] which ironically would have been addressed by a then unvoiced need for attention to usability and usability assessment.[53] Unfortunately, it was during the implementations and optimizations that usability was directly addressed by the end users during usage. It is the premise of this chapter that meaningful usability could have addressed these issues and will do so in the future.

Subsequently, Koppel and colleagues have produced many papers on the hazards that result from inadequate attention to usability—including the implications of poor design,[54,55] the role of workarounds in automated barcoding medication administration,[56] the contractual relations between vendors and clinicians regarding safe and usable systems,[57] international comparisons of CPOE use[58] and use of health IT for discovering medication errors.[59]

Koppel's examples focus on the inadequate attention to usability that limits the value and utility of the commercial EHR, CPOE, and electronic medication administration record (eMAR) systems.

Random Dosing: Good Intentions Leading to Bad Outcome

We start with a seemingly simple example: the default arrangements for all doses of a specific medication (see Figure 4-1).[60] In the first exhibit, 5 mg is on top, followed by 4 mg, and by 1 mg, etc. Why were the dosages displayed in this way? Should users assume 5 mg was the usual dose, followed by 4 mg, etc.? And could new physicians, working in a new rotation and not familiar with the usual dosages, assume some logical clinical guideline implicit in the order? The answer is very unexpected. In English, the word "five" is earlier in the alphabet than the word "four" which, in turn, is earlier than the word "one," and so on. The vendor was asked to change the ordering to reflect clinically guided doses, but the vendor explained that it could not be done until the next version of the software. After repeated complaints, the vendor allowed it could be changed, but the change would be made for each individual medication and required the users to promise not to change dosages. Because pharmaceutical manufacturers issue new dosages frequently, the misleading doses remained. This example reflects a difficulty in the design of health IT, which is the inability to rapidly make iterative changes found in the trenches usability testing (i.e., the users pointing out that the system isn't useable).

Designed for Deception: Allergy Information and Misinformation

The next example is from a well-known EHR system and demonstrates how the system handles allergy information (Figure 4-2).[61] On the system's general EHR screen, there is small section that allows clinicians to enter and see allergy information (e.g., "Patient is allergic to penicillin"). The default image in that section is the statement "No Allergies." However, one can click on that statement and enter further information. For example, a clinician might type in "Penicillin allergy, with anaphylaxis as the outcome." Another clinician might add another allergy, such as "Latex allergy, with a slight rash as the outcome." However, the next time the screen is seen, in a search by a clinician checking for allergies, the "Allergy" box would only show the default "No Allergies." Physicians and others in the know would click on "No Allergies" to access the list of allergies. How-

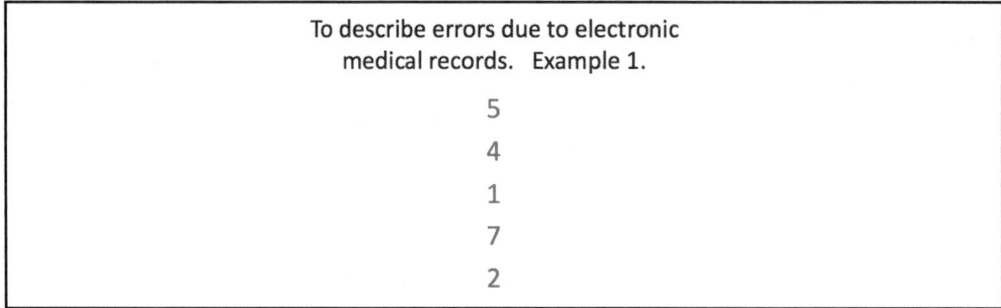

Figure 4-1: Default Arrangements for All Doses of a Specific Medication

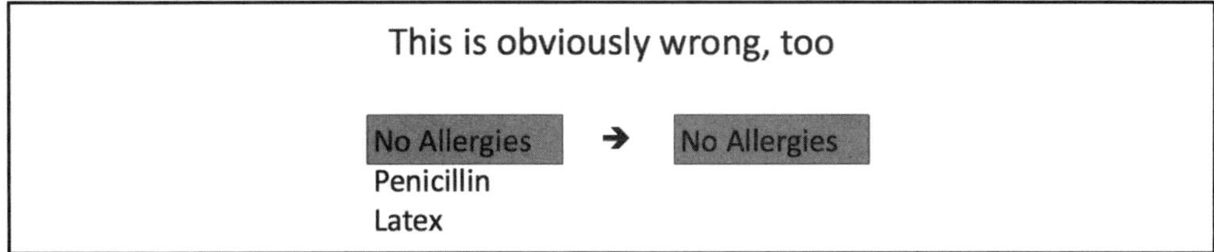

Figure 4-2: Example of How to Handle Allergy Information (from a well-known EHR system)

ever, even having clicked on it, the clinician in the know would then only see "'Latex allergy with a slight rash as the outcome"; only if he or she were to know to click on it again would it show "Penicillin allergy with anaphylaxis as the outcome." Clearly, the system is functioning in a way that is not useful. First, the default statement should not continue to read "No Allergy" after allergy information has been added. Second, clinicians should not have to "know" to continue clicking to find all possible allergies. In this example, if the user did not know to continue clicking past the latex allergy notice, he or she would miss the information about the deadly penicillin reaction.

Another allergy example shows how a key piece of medical information can be poorly captured when physicians select "Allergies" from a standard pull-down menu (Figure 4-3).[61] The first option may read: "No Allergies." But then the second option may read "No Known Allergies." Alas, if the doctor checked "No Allergies" and then saw the more epistemologically nuanced "No Known Allergies," he might well check that option, too. Unfortunately, the system displays those two choices as "Multiple Allergies," and, of course, everyone quickly learns that "Multiple Allergies" is the same as "No Allergies." Needless to say, there are many patients with multiple allergies. These patients would stand a good chance of not having their allergies identified or acted upon, because "Multiple Allergies" usually means "No Allergies."

Unlabeled Transformation of Weight Data

In the example shown in Figure 4-4, the first physician enters the child's weight in kilograms, which is the standard metric in the hospital. In another screen, seen by another physician and by a pharmacist, the weight has been transformed to pounds (undoubtedly for some legitimate reason, for example, in order to discuss related issues with parents in the USA). Unfortunately, the unit of measurement (pounds) is not indicated on the second screen, and the pharmacist or physician, assuming the usual measurement

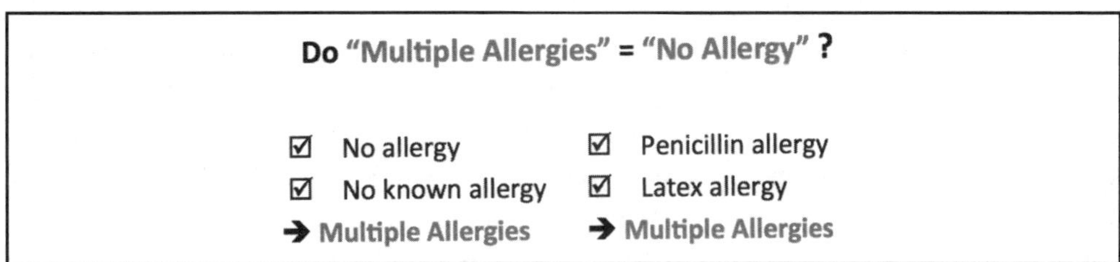

Figure 4-3: Selecting Allergies from a Standard Pull-down Menu

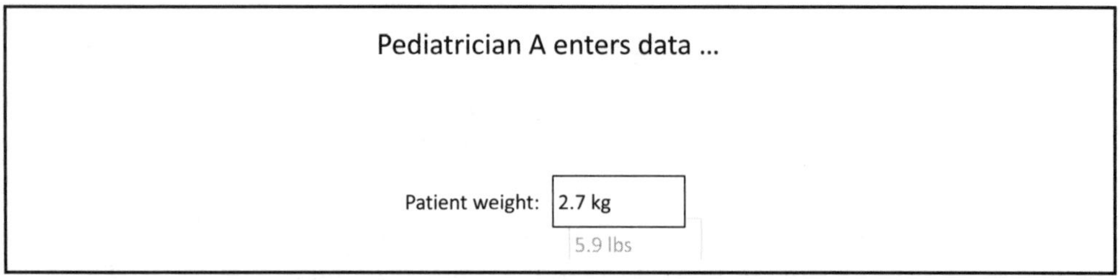

Pediatrician A enters data ...

Patient weight: 2.7 kg
5.9 lbs

Figure 4-4: Child's Weight Entered in Kilograms—Standard Hospital Metric

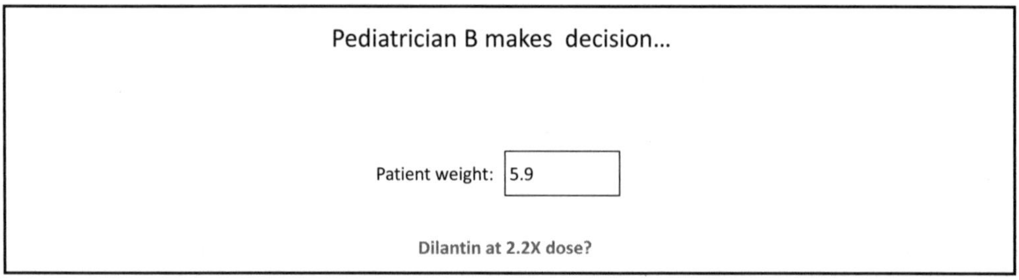

Pediatrician B makes decision...

Patient weight: 5.9

Dilantin at 2.2X dose?

Figure 4-5: Incorrectly Calculated Dosage for Child

units for the hospital, calculates a dosage in kilograms, thus more than double-dosing the child (shown in the next figure, Figure 4-5).

Obscured Information in the EHR

Sometimes partial information is as deceptive as no information.[60] In the next example (see Figure 4-6), essential information is obscured from the physician. It is only the physician's persistence and a memory of something not on the screen that saves the patient from a serious anticoagulation error.

In the first screen of the set of three, we see only the most recent clotting time (INR). Clotting times should be presented as trends, not isolated numbers. The effect of anticoagulation medicines takes a few days to be correctly observed, and trend data are needed to correctly adjust anticoagulation medications. Nevertheless, the trend information is not presented. Equally problematic, the medication dosage is not presented in parallel with the trend data.

In the second screen, the only visible dosage for the anticoagulation medication, Warfarin shows 2 mg (see Figure 4-7). However, the physician is quite sure her order for this patient was 7 mg and so she looks carefully at each cell but fails to find the dose she is sure was ordered. Finally, as the physician is moving the mouse around the screen, a small box suddenly emerges indicating that indeed she had ordered a 2 mg-dose and a 5 mg-dose, still not indicating the original prescribed dose of 7 mg. Luckily, she caught the popped up screen (shown in figure) out of the corner of her eye. Of course, the physician and all of us must wonder what would have happened if the mouse had not hovered above that spot on the screen. Why would essential information depend on what physicians call "mouse magic" when that information should be obviously stated in the electronic record (shown in the next figure, Figure 4-8)?

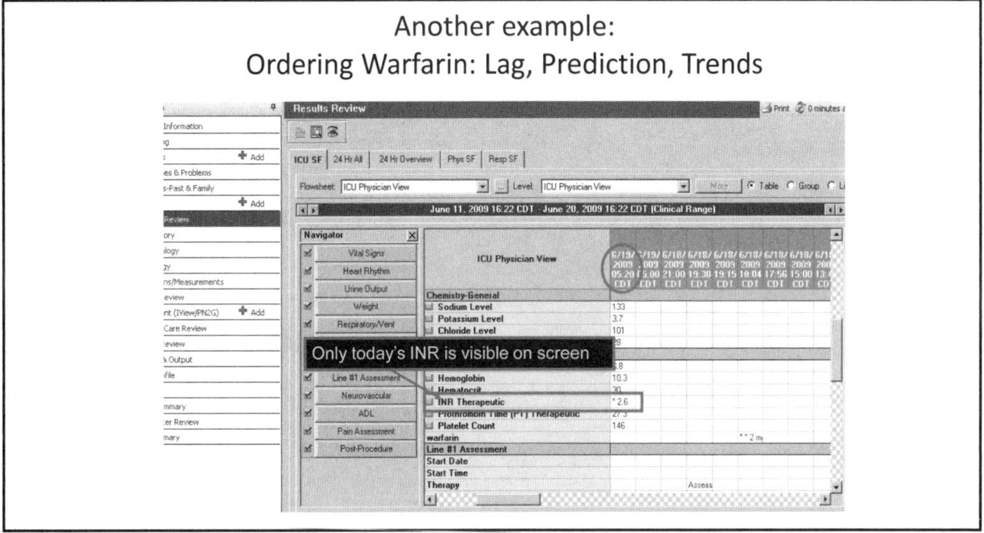

Figure 4-6: EHR with Essential Information Obscured from Physicians

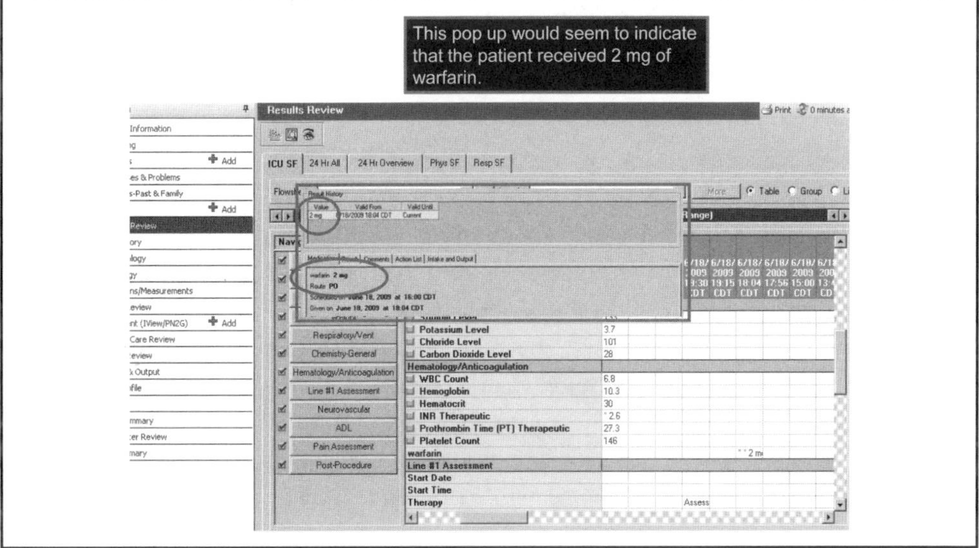

Figure 4-7: Visible Dosage for Anticoagulation Medication, Warfarin

Poor Engineering and Design

Koppel turned next to automated medication dispensing mechanisms. As an example, a power failure occurred in a very respected U.S. hospital, which shut down the automated dispensing system. Unfortunately, when the system came back online, the robotic mechanism that puts medications into the bottles started a fraction of a second before the mechanism that places (bar coded) labels on the bottles. The result was that 30,000 bottles were mislabeled and sent to both inpatients and outpatients. Nurses in the hospital quickly started calling the pharmacy with surreal stories of suppositories labeled as tablets and other errors that were far less obvious but therefore far more dangerous. The pharmacy was obliged to recall all of the medications.

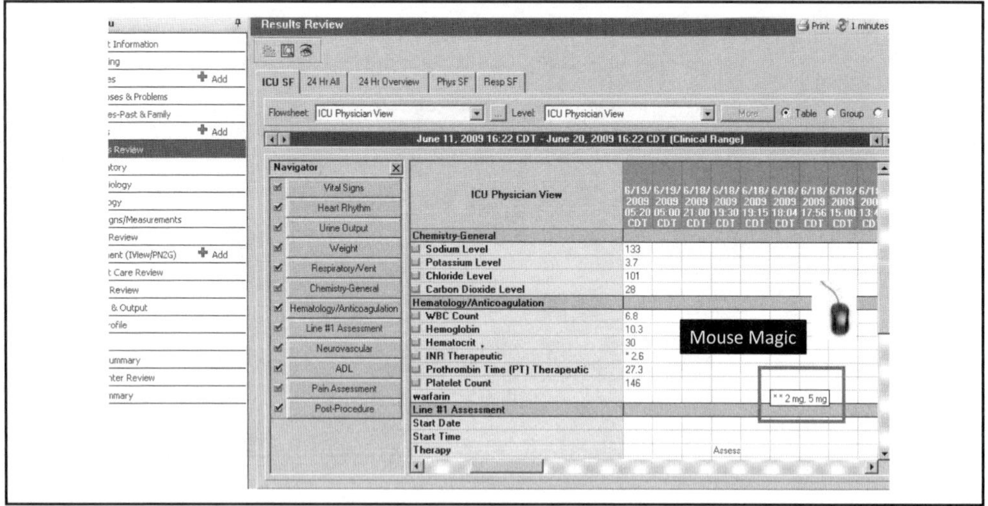

Figure 4-8: "Mouse Magic"

The problem was entirely predictable. Mechanical checks for failures of this type of coordination have been available for almost one hundred years, yet designers of the automated medication dispensing system, reliant on bar codes and other innovations, did not implement the simple checks that most soup companies have had for many decades.

What could have been done to anticipate this problem? Usability testing with scenarios could have picked this up.

Our last example is from what is supposed to be the latest panacea for reducing medication errors: bar code medication administration (BCMA) systems.[56] With these systems, the nurse scans the bar code on the medication and the bar code on the patient's wristband. As advertised, this method prevents medication administration errors. However, in a study by Koppel et al. conducted at five hospitals with BCMA systems, the authors found the reality of the BCMA systems differed dramatically from the error rates reported by vendors.[56] The study team, in which I was included, tested the medication bar codes in actual use, while the vendors tested their products as they came out of the pharmacy's printer.

We found, for example, that approximately 5 percent of the bar coded medication labels were torn, crinkled, missing, sodden, or (most ludicrous) covered by another label reminding the nurse to scan the bar code.

We also found that approximately 10 percent of patients' wristband bar codes were:

- Never provided.
- Invalid—because the patients had been transferred from one hospital unit to another or from a nursing home to the hospital.
- Sodden or covered in fluids (because patients in hospitals are often sick).
- Missing—because elderly individuals who are demented tear them off, children chew them off, those addicted to drugs remove them to obtain unscheduled

painkillers and neonates often have the bar codes attached to cribs which do not always move with the baby.

- Covered by sterile bandages and thus unreadable.

Moreover, to speed the process of scanning the patient bar codes, nurses often make extra copies of the bar codes. We have found extra copies of patient bar codes affixed to nurses' desks, supply room walls and cabinets, doorjambs in patient rooms, the scanning machine itself, the automated drug-dispensing machines, worn as bangles around the nurses arm (20 patients = 20 bar coded wristbands), worn on nurses' belt loops and affixed to the medication cart.

We also found that the system did not work in many parts of the hospital (i.e., no WiFi); that the same signal from the scanner could mean wrong patient, wrong medication, wrong time, wrong dose or wrong order from that expected by the software. Also, if the system was expecting a 20-mg dose but the pharmacy sent up 2 doses of 10 mg each, the scanning system would frequently define that as an error. Nurses overrode more than 14 percent of all attempted medication administration scanning system alerts.

Obviously, each of these nursing workarounds defeats the patient safety protections. As indicated, the initial problem is usually generated by insufficient attention to workflow, design frequently provided by a done-one-seen-them-all approach by commercial implementation specialists and organizational management stretched thin. However, the root cause is not the nurses' desire to avoid protocol or staff laziness.

How to Reduce or Eliminate Inadequate Design, Unanticipated Workflows, and Unsafe Computing: Usability

In addressing issues of usability in healthcare (such as those previously described), as well as other domains, the field of usability engineering has made significant advances. Usability engineering refers to a number of scientific methods that can be used for informing both the design and evaluation of information systems with the aim of producing usable systems.[62] Many of the approaches in this field have been developed from decades of research that has emerged from the study of human-computer interaction, but introduction into the design and testing of health IT has been slow. This work has led to the identification of the principles of good design that should be applied to ensure system usability—specifically, Shneiderman's eight "golden rules"[63] for guiding designers of information systems, which consist of the following:

- Strive for consistency in the user interface (e.g., do not confuse the user with many different ways to do the same operation).
- Enable frequent users to use shortcuts (e.g., offer menu options to new users but keystroke options for advanced users who want more efficient interactions).
- Offer informative feedback to users (e.g., when an error has occurred, provide informative error messages to users).
- Design system-user dialogs to yield closure (e.g., do not leave the user not knowing whether or not an operation has been completed).
- Offer simple error handling (e.g., provide the user with hints regarding what to fix if an error has occurred).

- Permit easy reversal of actions (e.g., support undo and redo operations).
- Support internal locus of control (e.g., make the user feel that he/she is "in control" when interacting with the system).
- Reduce the user's short-term memory load (e.g., do not make it necessary for the user to remember complex operations or command sequences).

Since these principles of design were defined, a wide variety of heuristics (or rules of thumb) have been developed for use in designing usable healthcare information systems. For example see Kushniruk and Patel[33] for heuristics that can be used in designing Web-based healthcare applications and Zhang et al.[64] for heuristics that have been used in assessing the safety of health systems. More recently, Carvalho and colleagues[65] have developed (based on systematic review) a set of heuristics specifically designed to identify and prevent technology-induced errors in CPOE systems.

USABILITY TESTING AND USABILITY INSPECTION METHODS FOR IMPROVING HEALTH IT

The field of usability engineering has emerged to improve the design and evaluation of interactive information systems from the perspective of the human user. The two main usability engineering methods are (1) usability testing and (2) usability inspection.

Usability testing refers to testing the usability of systems by observing (typically involving video recording) representative users of systems (e.g., in healthcare, this may be physicians or nurses) interacting with a system under study (e.g., an EHR system being developed) to carry out representative tasks (e.g., entering patient data into the system). In contrast, usability inspection does not involve observing real users of systems but rather a trained analyst evaluating a system or user interface in terms of how well the system conforms to a set of heuristics. The heuristics most widely adopted are Nielsen's heuristics, which consist of 14 heuristics that are similar to and are drawn from Shneiderman's eight golden rules. With the most popular form of usability inspection, violations of Nielsen's heuristics are noted and prioritized according to their severity. This information can be fed back to system designers to improve both the design of the system and the user interface.

A growing body of literature that developed in the field of health informatics since the 1990s has detailed how usability engineering methods can be applied to the design and evaluation of healthcare information systems. Kushniruk[66] has considered the application of these methods to what is known as the System Development Life Cycle (SDLC) of health IT. The SDLC provides a time line or lifecycle for considering when and where health IT may be evaluated and improved by applying usability engineering methods, beginning with the application of usability engineering methods from the early phases of a software product's development to the design, implementation and later deployment phases (e.g., deployment of systems in hospitals, clinics or medical offices). For example, to assess if a new user interface design would be acceptable to health professional users, representative users (e.g., nurses or physicians) could be asked to interact with a prototype system (employing the design), using artificial or in some cases real patient cases, while they are video recorded doing so.

This method also typically involves asking subjects (e.g., physicians or nurses) to "think aloud," or verbalize their thoughts, as they carry out the tasks.[33] The resulting video recordings (of computer screens and user actions) and audio (of subject verbalizations) provide a source of rich data that can be qualitatively analyzed to identify types of problems users may encounter (e.g., inability to navigate through a system, consistency problems, etc.) and the impact of the system on healthcare work processes. In addition, such testing can be taken into the real settings of clinical use to assess the impact of prototype or completed systems under realistic, simulated or even real healthcare conditions (e.g., within a ward, clinic or even the operating room).[67,68]

Other complementary methods have also been used to assess the impact of systems, including interviews and ethnographic observation of users of systems (e.g., Koppel et al.[34]). However, it can be argued that application of approaches to assessing potential usability problems or safety issues (whether they apply usability engineering or complementary methods) should ideally be conducted well before systems are ever released into clinical settings and used in real patient situations. This and related work has shown that the application of these methods prior to system release can significantly reduce the possibility of systems being developed and delivered that are highly unusable or unsafe. For example, the methods have been employed to evaluate the impact on health professionals' cognition and decision making of prototype and emerging EHR systems,[69,70] decision support systems and clinical guidelines[69-74] and CPOE.[37,75-81] This same methodology has been used to identify usability problems in both clinical and consumer information systems on healthcare workflow before they are ever released for widespread use.[67,82]

EXAMPLES OF SUCCESSFUL APPLICATION OF USABILITY ENGINEERING IN HEALTH IT

In this section of the chapter, we will describe a range of projects for which we have employed usability engineering methods to improve the usability of health IT, as well as decrease the chance of systems inadvertently creating medical error by introducing new systems.

Usability and Errors – A PDA Study

In an article published in 2005, Kushniruk, Kannry, Borycki and colleagues examined the relationship between usability problems and user errors—what they refer to as "technology-induced error" (similar to Koppel's "technology-facilitated error" category[34]). Technology-induced errors refer to medical errors that result from aspects of poor user interface design.[34]

These errors are not software errors in the traditional sense in that they are not necessarily software bugs that result from buggy programming and therefore are unlikely to be caught using traditional software testing approaches.[83] Rather technology-induced errors are related to poor design decisions leading to usability problems that may lead, or induce, the user to make medical errors at point of use. For example, placing a non-standard dosage at the top of menu as a default dose in CPOE will likely lead users to choose that dosage frequently, even it is not the most appropriate dosage in all situations (i.e., some physicians will assume that if it appears in the top of the list it may be a recommended dosage).

In their study of PDA (personal digital assistant) users, Kushniruk et al.[84] identified (1) usability problems associated with use of a handheld prescription writing application and (2) actual medication errors resulting from using the application to enter prescriptions. It was found that certain categories of usability problems (e.g., navigation problems, display visibility problems, and inappropriate default dosage displays) were highly associated with one or more medication errors (and hence identification and removal of those user interface aspects and features would result in a decreased medication error rate). It is worth noting that what led to both this study and a subsequent one was author Joseph Kannry's observation of a plethora of handheld E-prescribing tools which took a complex function (i.e., prescribing medications) and translated it to handhelds without rhyme or reason. This flood of handheld E-prescribing tools was more of the "we have the technology, so we can make it better" approach than any reasoned approach.[27] In subsequent work, the base rates obtained from this study (which involved video recording users of the prescription writing application as they used it to enter medications from a list) were input into a computer-based simulation to determine what the impact of specific usability problems would be in wide-scale release of this type of application. Given that usability problems are related to technology-induced errors, a number of initiatives have been taken in research and applied work to decrease their likelihood (and improve system usability), several of which will be described in the remainder of this chapter.

Customization of Health IT and Improvement of Training Processes

The relationship between usability, user training and system customization continues to be explored and systematically analyzed in order to not only identify technology-induced error but to make changes to mitigate potential errors. Implementations of complex healthcare information systems require careful consideration of both system design and customization, as well as an understanding of effective approaches for training new users. In one study, users of a new EHR system deployed at a large academic medical center were observed as they entered patient case information into the EHR. Approximately one month after receiving training on its use, details of the training process and cases used during training were collected and analyzed prior to user testing. From analysis of the video recordings of as few as five users as they interacted with the system, detailed information about their learning curve and learning issues (including areas for improvement) was collected, and potential problems were identified and documented. The results were fed back into iterative customization of both user interface features (e.g., improvements required of the terminology matching features and functions) and to the user training itself (e.g., recommendations made about including training on use of the system while conducting a patient interview). Although this type of usability testing was conducted late in the SDLC, it did result in some changes—ranging from slight to moderate in training and implementation, which improved user acceptance of the system being deployed.[85]

The issue of "catching" user and usability problems—and consequently the potential for a system to cause technology-induced error—earlier in the system design itself (i.e., prior to system implementation and deployment) has been discussed in Kushniruk[66] elsewhere and is closely related to the need for application and design guidelines and certifications tailored to health IT (to be discussed in a subsequent section of this chapter).

Improving Procurement of Health IT – Getting the Right System in the First Place

Perhaps, outside of providing input to design of systems, one of the most important leverage points for applying usability engineering methods to ensure system safety is at the point of selecting systems for use in healthcare institutions. Along these lines, a variety of evidence-based approaches have been applied to improve the selection process and ensure a better match between user and hospital needs with features and capabilities of candidate systems.[86] In a recent article, a framework for considering selection (i.e., procurement) processes has been developed that includes hands-on, in-depth usability testing of candidate systems (e.g., EHRs, CPOE, etc.) that can lead to better decisions and fewer "unpleasant surprises" regarding systems that may be error prone or may lead to a high level of technology-induced error.

Along these lines, Kushniruk et al.[85] and Kannry have argued for years that usability testing be a required part of the selection process to provide hospital, health authority and regional mangers of healthcare organizations with a much improved level of "evidence" regarding what systems best fit with organizational norms, socio-technical processes and work practices. The challenge has always been how to address commercial vendor concerns/reluctance to permit usability testing as part of vendor selection, citing user unfamiliarity with the system, as well as the stated difficulties in setting up sample cases for individual users to test in a "playground" system. For purposes of this chapter, we define playground system as a system loaded with test patients and data in which the user can play with or test most of the functionality. There seems to be little ability or interest in constructing playground system usability testing during selection. As a result, the best one can hope for, given vendor concerns about usability testing during selection, is an adequate and appropriate scripted representation of user workflow in demonstrations[86,87] though this is admittedly only a substitute for true usability testing.

In the case of sites with installed systems, this could be de-identified or scrambled data.

Success in integrating usability testing with the selection processes of large hospital organizations has been achieved at Lille University hospital in France.[87,88] This work has shown that in testing new possible systems and applications for purchase, candidate systems can be test installed and clinicians in the institution given the opportunity to try out the systems. Not only can this lead to improved system selection, in a number of cases, the resultant information about user needs, preferences, dislikes and potential problems were actually fed back into refinement and improvement of both the user interface and underlying architecture of the systems evaluated.

Need for Usability Standards, Guidelines, and Certification Processes

One of the issues in the development of health IT, in particular EHRs, is the lack of standards for user interfaces and user interactions. For example, a physician working in multiple institutions may be required to learn the idiosyncrasies of multiple systems (with each institution having its own EHR from different vendors and with their own different user interface designs). Many vendors feel their user interface is a selling point and therefore is proprietary and should not be standardized. This can lead to problems in learning how to use and master systems, confusion resulting from having to learn multiple systems and errors resulting from improper transfer of knowledge about how to use one system and another.[82] It is worth noting that this also increases the total training time for providers (e.g., housestaff) who rotate or see patients in multiple institutions.

There have been a number of projects aimed at developing standards that might lead to consistency of user interactions and safer systems. The largest project along these lines is the National Health Service's (NHS) Common User Interface (CUI) Project in the UK.[89] The project has led to a set of design guidelines and toolkit. The objective has been to provide improved safety by setting guidelines for a common look and feel for systems throughout the NHS. Issues have been encountered, however, in getting buy-in by system developers to adopt these standards. In addition to this work, the NHS has developed a series of guidelines for safe on-screen display of medication information.[90] These guidelines include information about possible sources of confusion to users and recommendations that would decrease the chance of technology-induced error. As one such example, based on research, it has been found that omitting leading zeros in front of displayed values (e.g., Volume .8 mL) introduces a high possibility of misreading errors if the decimal point in front of the number is not noticed by the user; hence the recommendation provided for this issue is to use leading zeros when a decimal point appears. The NHS document outlines a large number of such issues along with their associated recommendations.

The integration of usability criteria in the certification of health IT is another area of current focus in the attempt to decrease the possibility of technology-induced error and to provide some confidence in the usability and safety of products.[91] However, there are many challenges along these lines. In recent work in the United States, the Certification Commission for Health IT (CCHIT) has worked on developing scenarios and procedures used in the certification of EHR products (with system features and functions having to be demonstrated during the tests involving the scenarios). However, the process is currently undergoing a number of changes, and the usability component of the certification process currently involves only a very rapid assessment of a system's usability (during the testing for other system functions and capabilities using the scenarios). In addition, the process does not yet involve the use of formal usability engineering methods (e.g., usability testing as described in this chapter). It is expected that the inclusion of a stronger emphasis on key aspects of usability will need to be incorporated in future refinements of the certification process.

It is beyond the scope of this chapter to adequately explore the usability of personal health records (PHRs) for patients. It is of great concern that meaningful use has mandated the implementation and use of PHRs, though there is a limited knowledge on the usability of such systems by patients. The peer reviewed usability literature mainly focuses on internally developed systems.[70,92-102] The findings of these studies indicate that patients need to be educated on the use of such systems.[94,97,103-105] Some studies suggest usability issues related to healthcare providers who may think about healthcare differently than patients and whose concepts may not be adequately represented.[70,98] Meaningful use at the time of this publication does not specify patient education and training as part of meaningful use of a PHR.

The efforts previously described represent important steps toward improving the usability and safety of health IT. However, it is clear that more work along each of these lines will be needed. First, rigorous usability engineering methods will need to become used more widely in the design and customization of health IT. Second, the need is growing for evidence-based heuristics and guidelines for both the design and evaluation of health IT. Finally, although the concept of certification is an important step forward, more work needs to be done to ensure that certification processes developed really do provide strong evidence that systems will be safe to use and will effectively support user work activities in healthcare in a meaningful way.

DISCUSSION AND CONCLUSION

HITECH seeks to provide reimbursement incentives to both health professionals and hospitals who become "meaningful users" of certified EHR technology.[17,18] This will stress the ability of healthcare organizations, whether offices or medical centers, to select, implement and deploy certified EHRs, while at the same time have users utilize these systems in a way that complies with meaningful use, creating the perfect storm for potentially poorly designed, implemented and optimized systems. Anecdotally, Kannry has heard that multiple vendors are upgrading their systems to comply with meaningful use by adding screens for discrete data collection. This begs the question of how these multiple changes will be integrated into the workflow of daily system use and healthcare. Even if the vendors succeed, the race is to comply with the first stage of meaningful use, which is to demonstrate functionality, but the potential danger is meeting these requirements with bandaid solutions and then not being able to act on them (i.e., improve quality) in stage 2 of meaningful use without further changes. The examples of poor design and dysfunction provided by Koppel predated the HITECH era. The usability of these systems will be stretched to the limit in the era of rapid change that meaningful use/HITECH will engender.

Can CCHIT certification address these usability issues by incorporating usability testing into certification? One concern is the previously mentioned incorporation of usability engineering into the certification process. Author Kannry is aware of one vendor who has already incorporated this in their development in an effort that began a few years ago, while another vendor showed limited enthusiasm when it was broached by their physician leader. Both efforts are laudable, whether CCHIT mandates it or vendors incorporate usability testing on their own. However, in the case of the vendor that incorporated usability engineering, usability issues are still being experienced by one of the authors. In fairness, it is quite challenging to test everything when several thousand changes are being made to the system. However, the real problem lies with the fact that any customizable system will be implemented differently, sometimes with significant differences in each implementation and afterwards, during optimization.

Outcomes with the same health IT systems will be both variable and sometimes harmful.[40,106] For example, the successful Veterans Administration (VA) EHR system labeled the "Gold Standard" in the title of one article[1] is the same system contributing to medical errors in a study of a local implementation by Ammenworth et al.[52] The authors Kannry and Koppel had similar differing experiences with the same system, implemented during roughly the same time period. Koppel's experiences are well documented in peer-reviewed literature.[34] There are many possible factors that could have played a role, including an optimization effort[27] which was the result of a prior informatics study demonstrating overall significant user dissatisfaction that correlated with the ability to perform tasks efficiently in the subject system.[26]

National and vendor usability efforts would be challenged with ensuring usability at local implementations due to the sheer number of external factors that affect success and what we today call "meaningful use."[19,27,107,108] One approach would be to partner with local sites and make development more iterative with usability and iterative development, creating a sort of quality assurance feedback loop.[33,66] One challenge that will be a topic of discussion will involve sensitive and proprietary development and content, involving, at the very least, confidentiality agreements. Barriers will include the sheer number of sites, the lack of local usability professionals and infrastructure, playground systems with test cases and data and reimbursement for time and resources. A great deal of trust would be required, as there will be discussion of proprietary vendor content and development. If the local sites are academic with usability expertise, these sites will not be able to publish their work. Even if the academic barriers were overcome, published studies would be subject to the same scrutiny and skepticism that pharmaceutical-sponsored drug studies face today.

The solution to variable implementation and optimization is to set up local usability testing units that can examine new releases/upgrades before they are released to the user community at large, as well as study usage to identify issues that are being encountered by the vendor and the broader user community. Examining new releases/upgrades before release again depends on vendor ability to provide playground systems with test patients and data or scrambled data and patients. We are deliberately steering clear of the term *labs* because, while they can provide valuable information, such labs frequently employ costly equipment that cannot be brought to the point of care and perhaps sometimes rely too much on simulations. Local usability testing units would represent the interests of end users. This will be a challenging concept, as very few implementations and optimizations list testing as a budget line item or have funded such efforts. The hardware cost is actually relatively low, and it is possible to rapidly train existing personnel. However, IT methodology that would incorporate usability testing into project time lines and subsequent optimization is still quite rare, and while existing personnel can be employed, dedicated personnel would be preferred and would create greater efficiency.

Organizationally local usability testing units could reside in information technology, but there is an alternative. Kannry has made the argument for the development of operational departments (i.e., interventional informatics departments) to integrate the science of informatics into daily operations.[109] Usability testing units would fit neatly into such departments by employing usability testing to inform and improve an operational project. In short, locally sponsored usability testing is required to have usable meaningful use for the rest of us.

Only when there is strong basis for system usability and safety—nationally and locally—within healthcare organizations will meaningful use become a reality. When the need for usability engineering by the vendor and usability testing and assessment by national standards is fully addressed, vendors and healthcare organizations will only grow.

REFERENCES

1. Morgan MW. The VA advantage: the gold standard in clinical informatics. *Healthc Pap,* 2005. 5(4):26-9.
2. Kizer KW, Pane GA. The "New VA": Delivering health care value through integrated service networks. *Annals of Emergency Medicine,* 1997. 30(6):804-7.
3. Clayton PD et al. Building a comprehensive clinical information system from components. The approach at Intermountain Health Care. *Methods Inf Med,* 2003. 42(1):1-7.
4. Cimino JJ. The Columbia medical informatics story: from clinical system to major department. *MD Comput,* 1999. 16(2):31-4.
5. Safran C, Sands DZ, Rind DM. Online medical records: a decade of experience. *Methods Inf Med,* 1999. 38(4-5):308-12.
6. McDonald CJ et al. The Regenstrief Medical Record System: a quarter century experience. *Int J Med Inform,* 1999;54(3):225-53.
7. Slack WV, Bleich HL. The CCC system in two teaching hospitals: a progress report. *Int J Med Inf,* 1999. 54(3):183-96.
8. Teich JM et al. The Brigham integrated computing system (BICS): advanced clinical systems in an academic hospital environment. *Int J Med Inf,* 1999. 54(3):197-208.
9. Gardner RM, Pryor TA, Warner HR. The HELP hospital information system: update 1998. *Int J Med Inf,* 1999. 54(3): p. 169-82.
10. Miller RA et al. The anatomy of decision support during inpatient care provider order entry (CPOE): empirical observations from a decade of CPOE experience at Vanderbilt. *J Biomed Inform,* 2005. 38(6):469-85.
11. Bui AA et al. OpenSourcePACS: an extensible infrastructure for medical image management. *IEEE Trans Inf Technol Biomed,* 2007. 11(1):94-109.
12. Huff SM. Clinical Data Exchange Standards and Vocabularies for Messages. *Proc AMIA Symp,* 1998: 62-7.
13. McDonald CJ et al. The Indiana network for patient care: a working local health information infrastructure. An example of a working infrastructure collaboration that links data from five health systems and hundreds of millions of entries. *Health Aff.* (Millwood), 2005;24(5):1214-20.
14. Overhage JM, Tierney WM, McDonald CJ. Design and implementation of the Indianapolis Network for Patient Care and Research. *Bull Med Libr Assoc.* 1995. 83(1): 48-56.
15. Halamka JD, Osterland C, Safran C. CareWeb, a web-based medical record for an integrated health care delivery system. *Int J Med Inform,* 1999. 54(1): 1-8.
16. Friedlin J, Dexter PR, Overhage JM. Details of a Successful Clinical Decision Support System. *AMIA Annu Symp Proc,* 2007: 254-8.
17. Blumenthal D. Stimulating the adoption of health information technology. *N Engl J Med,* 2009. 360(15):1477-9.

18. Centers for Medicare & Medicaid Services (CMS), Health information technology: initial set of standards, implementation specifications, and certification criteria for electronic health record technology. Final rule. *Fed Register.* 2010. 75(144): 44589-654.

19. Overhage JM et al. Does national regulatory mandate of provider order entry portend greater benefit than risk for health care delivery? The 2001 ACMI debate. The American College of Medical Informatics. *JAMIA.* 2002. 9(3):199-208.

20. Bates DW et al. A proposal for electronic medical records in U.S. primary care. *J Am Med Inform Assoc,* 2003. 10(1):1-10.

21. Miller RH, Sim I. Physicians' Use Of Electronic Medical Records: Barriers And Solutions. *Health Aff,* 2004. 23(2):116-126.

22. Simon SR et al. Correlates of electronic health record adoption in office rractices: A statewide survey. *JAMIA.* 2007;14(1):110-117.

23. van Ginneken AM. The computerized patient record: balancing effort and benefit. *Int J Med Inf.* 2002;65(2):97-119.

24. Kuperman GJ et al. *Panel: Integrating Informatics into the Product: The CEO's Perspective.* in 1997 AMIA Annual Fall Symposium. 1997. Nashville, TN: Hanley & Belfus, Inc.

25. Weiner M et al. Contrasting views of physicians and nurses about an inpatient computer-based provider order-entry system. *JAMIA.* 1999;6(3): 234-44.

26. Murff HJ, Kannry J. Physician satisfaction with two order entry systems. *JAMIA.* 2001; 8(5):499-509.

27. Kannry J. *Computerized Physician Order Entry and Patient Safety: Panacea or Pandora's Box?* in Medical informatics: an executive primer. Ong KR, ed. 2007, HIMSS: Chicago, IL. p. xviii, 316.

28. Langberg M. Challenges to implementing CPOE: a case study of a work in progress at Cedars-Sinai. *Modern Physician.* 2003;7(2): 21-2.

29. Lawler F et al. Implementation and termination of a computerized medical information system. *J Fam Pract.* 1996;42(3):233-6.

30. Massaro TA. Introducing physician order entry at a major academic medical center: II. Impact on medical education. *Acad Med.* 1993;68(1):25-30.

31. Massaro TA. Introducing physician order entry at a major academic medical center: I. Impact on organizational culture and behavior. *Acad Med.* 1993;68(1):20-5.

32. Preece J. *Human-computer Interaction.* 1995, Wokingham, England; Reading, MA: Addison-Wesley Pub. Co. xxxviii, 775.

33. Kushniruk AW, Patel VL. Cognitive and usability engineering methods for the evaluation of clinical information systems. *J Biomed Inform.* 2004;37(1):56-76.

34. Koppel R et al. Role of computerized physician order entry systems in facilitating medication errors. *JAMA.* 2005;293(10):1197-203.

35. Kushniruk AW et al. Technology induced error and usability: the relationship between usability problems and prescription errors when using a handheld application. *Int J Med Inform* 2005;74(7-8): 519-26.

36. Han YY et al. Unexpected increased mortality after implementation of a commercially sold computerized physician order entry system. *Pediatrics.* 2005;116(6):1506-12.

37. Horsky J, Kuperman GJ, Patel VL. Comprehensive analysis of a medication dosing error related to CPOE. *JAMIA.* 2005;12(4):377-82.

38. Bates DW et al. The impact of computerized physician order entry on medication error prevention. *JAMIA.* 1999;6(4):313-21.

39. Koppel R et al. Neither panacea nor black box: responding to three Journal of Biomedical Informatics papers on computerized physician order entry systems. *J Biomed Inform.* 2005;38(4):267-9.

40. Aarts J, Berg M. Same systems, different outcomes—comparing the implementation of computerized physician order entry in two Dutch hospitals. *Methods Inf Med.* 2006; 45(1):53-61.

41. Campbell EM et al. Types of unintended consequences related to computerized provider order entry. *JAMIA.* 2006;13(5):547-56.

42. Chaudhry B et al. Systematic review: impact of health information technology on quality, efficiency, and costs of medical care. *Ann Intern Med.* 2006;144(10):742-52.

43. Davidson SM, Heineke J. Toward an effective strategy for the diffusion and use of clinical information systems. *J Am Med Inform Assoc.* 2007;14(3):361-7.

44. Palen TE et al. Evaluation of laboratory monitoring alerts within a computerized physician order entry system for medication orders. *Am J Manag Care.* 2006;12(7):389-95.

45. Shulman R et al. Medication errors: a prospective cohort study of hand-written and computerised physician order entry in the intensive care unit. *Critical Care.* 2005. 9(5): R516-21.

46. Wachter RM. Expected and unanticipated consequences of the quality and information technology revolutions. *JAMA.* 2006;295(23):2780-3.

47. Wears RL, Berg M. Computer technology and clinical work: still waiting for Godot. *JAMA.* 2005;293(10):1261-3.

48. Zhan C et al. Potential benefits and problems with computerized prescriber order entry: analysis of a voluntary medication error-reporting database. *Am J Health Syst Pharm.* 2006. 63(4):353-8.

49. Agency for Healthcare Research and Quality. Rockville, M.U.S.D.o.H.a.H.S., Agency for Healthcare Research and Quality; December 2006. *2006 National Healthcare Quality Report.* 2006.

50. Nemeth C, Cook R. Hiding in plain sight: what Koppel et al. tell us about healthcare IT. *J Biomed Inform.* 2005;38(4):262-3.

51. Silverstein S. *Contemporary Issues in Medical Informatics: Common Examples of Healthcare IT Failure.* [cited 2010 Sept. 3]; Available at: www.ischool.drexel.edu/faculty/ssilverstein/cases/?loc=cases&sloc=workshop. Last accessed October 2010.

52. Ammenwerth E et al. Impact of CPOE on mortality rates—contradictory findings, important messages. *Methods Inf Med.* 2006;45(6):586-93.

53. Miller-Jacobs H, Smelcer J. *Usability of Electronic Medical Record System: An Application in Its Infancy with a Crying Need.* Human Interface and the Management of Information. Interacting in Information Environments. 2007;4558: 759-765.

54. Harrison M, Koppel R. Interactive sociotechnical analysis –Identifying and coping with unintended consequences of IT implementation, in Khoumbati K. (Ed). *Handbook of Research on Advances in Health Informatics and Electronic Healthcare Applications: global adoption and impact of information communication technologies.* 2010, Medical Information Science Reference: Hershey PA. p. 595.

55. Harrison MI, Koppel R, Bar-Lev S. Unintended consequences of information technologies in health care—an interactive sociotechnical analysis. *J Am Med Inform Assoc.* 2007;14(5):542-9.

56. Koppel R et al. Workarounds to barcode medication administration systems: their occurrences, causes, and threats to patient safety. *JAMIA.* 2008:15(4): 408-23.

57. Koppel R, Kreda D. Health care information technology vendors' "hold harmless" clause: implications for patients and clinicians. *JAMA.* 2009;301(12):1276-8.

58. Aarts J, Koppel R. Implementation of computerized physician order entry in seven countries. *Health Aff.* (Millwood) 2009;28(2):404-14.

59. Koppel R et al. Identifying and quantifying medication errors: evaluation of rapidly discontinued medication orders submitted to a computerized physician order entry system. *JAMIA.* 2008;15(4):461-5.

60. Koppel R. *From the Front: Adventures in Healthcare Information Technology-Enhanced Clinical Errors,* Johns Hopkins School of Medicine. Grand Rounds, Editor. 2009.

61. Koppel R, Kreda D. Healthcare IT usability and suitability for clinical needs: challenges of design,workflow, and contractual relations, in Nehr C, Aarts J, (eds). *Information technology in health care: socio-technical approaches 2010.* 2010, IOS Press: Washington, DC.

62. Nielsen J. *Usability Engineering.* 1993, Boston: Academic Press. xiv, 358.

63. Shneiderman B. *Designing the User Interface : Strategies for Effective Human-Computer-Interaction.* 3rd ed. 1998, Reading, Mass: Addison Wesley Longman. xiv, 639.

64. Zhang J et al. Using usability heuristics to evaluate patient safety of medical devices. *J Biomed Inform.* 2003;36(1-2):23-30.

65. Carvalho CJ, Borycki EM, Kushniruk A. Ensuring the safety of health information systems: using heuristics for patient safety. *Healthc Q,* 2009;12:Spec No Patient: 49-54.

66. Kushniruk A. Evaluation in the design of health information systems: application of approaches emerging from usability engineering. *Comput Biol Med.* 2002;32(3):141-9.

67. Borycki E, Kushniruk A. Identifying and preventing technology-induced error using simulations: application of usability engineering techniques. *Healthc Q,* 2005;8 Spec No:99-105.

68. Kushniruk A et al. Predicting changes in workflow resulting from healthcare information systems: ensuring the safety of healthcare. *Healthc Q,* 2006;9 Spec No:114-8.

69. Kushniruk AW et al. Assessment of a computerized patient record system: a cognitive approach to evaluating medical technology. *MD Comput.* 1996;13(5):06-15.

70. Patel VL, Arocha JF, Kushniruk AW. Patients' and physicians' understanding of health and biomedical concepts: relationship to the design of EMR systems. *J Biomed Inform.* 2002;35(1):8-16.

71. Horsky J, Kaufman DR, Patel VL. Computer-based drug ordering: evaluation of interaction with a decision-support system. *Stud Health Technol Inform.* 2004;107(Pt 2): 1063-7.

72. Patel VL et al. Methods of cognitive analysis to support the design and evaluation of biomedical systems: the case of clinical practice guidelines. *J Biomed Inform.* 2001;34(1):52-66.

73. Peleg M et al. Interpreting procedures from descriptive guidelines. *J Biomed Inform.* 2006; 39(2):184-95.

74. Peleg M et al. The InterMed approach to sharable computer-interpretable guidelines: a review. *JAMIA.* 2004;11(1):1-10.

75. Beuscart-Zephir MC et al. A usability study of CPOE's medication administration functions: impact on physician-nurse cooperation. *Stud Health Technol Inform.* 2004;107(Pt 2):1018-22.

76. Beuscart-Zephir MC et al. Impact of CPOE on doctor-nurse cooperation for the medication ordering and administration process. *Int J Med Inform.* 2005;74(7-8):629-41.

77. Horsky J, Kaufman DR, Patel VL. When You Come to a Fork in the Road, Take It: strategy selection in order entry. *AMIA Annu Symp Proc.* 2005:350-4.

78. Weir CR et al. A cognitive task analysis of information management strategies in a computerized provider order entry environment. *JAMIA.* 2007;14(1):65-75.

79. Lin CP, Gennari JH. Designing CPOE Systems Using an Ecological Approach. *AMIA Annu Symp Proc.* 2007:1033.

80. Pelayo S et al. Cognitive analysis of physicians' medication ordering activity. *Stud Health Technol Inform.* 2005;116:929-34.

81. Pelayo S et al. Applying a Human Factors Engineering approach to healthcare IT applications: example of a medication CPOE project. *Stud Health Technol Inform.* 2009;143:334-9.

82. Borycki EM, Kushniruk AW. Scenario-based testing of health information systems (HIS) in electronic and hybrid environments. *Stud Health Technol Inform.* 2009;143:284-9.

83. Kushniruk A et al. Integrating technology-centric and user-centric system testing methods: ensuring healthcare system usability and safety. *Stud Health Technol Inform.* 2010;157:181-6.

84. Kushniruk A et al. The relationship of usability to medical error: an evaluation of errors associated with usability problems in the use of a handheld application for prescribing medications. *Stud Health Technol Inform.* 2004;107(Pt 2):1073-6.

85. Kushniruk AW et al. Exploring the relationship between training and usability: a study of the impact of usability testing on improving training and system deployment. *Stud Health Technol Inform.* 2009;143:277-83.

86. Kannry J, Mukani S, Myers K. Using an evidence-based approach for system selection at a large academic medical center: lessons learned in selecting an ambulatory EMR at Mount Sinai Hospital. *J Healthc Inf Manag.* 2006;20(2):84-99.

87. Kushniruk AW et al. Selecting electronic health record systems: development of a framework for testing candidate systems. *Stud Health Technol Inform.* 2009;143:376-9.

88. Beuscart-Zephir MC et al. User-centred, multidimensional assessment method of Clinical Information Systems: a case-study in anaesthesiology. *Int J Med Inform.* 2005;74(2-4):179-89.

89. National Health Service (NHS)-United Kingdom. *NHS Common User Interface.* [cited 2010 Sept. 3]. Available at: www.cui.nhs.uk/Pages/NHSCommonUserInterface.aspx. Last accessed December 2010.

90. National Health Service (NHS)-United Kingdom. *National Reporting and Learning Service | Division of the NPSA - NRLS.* [cited; Available at: www.nrls.npsa.nhs.uk/home/. Last accessed December 2010.

91. CCHIT. *CCHIT Certified 2011 Ambulatory EHR | CCHIT.* [cited 2010 Sept. 3]; Available at: www.cchit.org/certify/2011/cchit-certified-2011-ambulatory-ehr. Last accessed December 2010.

92. Dullabh P, Burke-Bebee S. Emerging Approaches to PHR Design, Development and Use. *AMIA Annu Symp Proc.* 2008:937.

93. Weitzman ER, Kaci L, Mandl KD. Acceptability of a personally controlled health record in a community-based setting: implications for policy and design. *J Med Internet Res.* 2009;11(2):e14.

94. Britto MT et al. Usability testing finds problems for novice users of pediatric portals. *J Am Med Inform Assoc.* 2009;16(5): 660-9.

95. Wang M et al. Personal health information management system and its application in referral management. *IEEE Trans Inf Technol Biomed.* 2004;8(3):287-97.

96. D'Alessandro DM, Dosa NP. Empowering children and families with information technology. *Arch Pediatr Adolesc Med.* 2001;155(10):1131-6.

97. Tjora A, Tran T, Faxvaag A. Privacy vs usability: a qualitative exploration of patients' experiences with secure Internet communication with their general practitioner. *J Med Internet Res.* 2005;7(2):e15.

98. Lee M, Delaney C, Moorhead S. Building a personal health record from nursing perspective. *Stud Health Technol Inform.* 2006;122:25-9.

99. Kim EH et al. Application and evaluation of personal health information management system. *Conf Proc IEEE Eng Med Biol Soc.* 2004;5:3159-62.

100. Bodily NJ, Carlston DA, Rocha RA. Personal Health Records: Key Features Within Existing Applications. *AMIA Annu Symp Proc.* 2007:875.

101. Botts NE, Horan TA. Electronic Personal Health Records and Systems to Improve Care for Vulnerable Populations. *AMIA Annu Symp Proc.* 2007:880.

102. Sox CM et al. Patient-centered design of an information management module for a personally controlled health record. *J Med Internet Res.* 2010;12(3):e36.

103. Cimino JJ et al. *An Evaluation of Patient Access to their Electronic Medical Records Via the World Wide Web.* Proc AMIA Symp. 2000:151-5.

104. Cimino JJ, Patel VL, Kushniruk AW. What do patients do with access to their medical records? *Stud Health Technol Inform.* 2001;84(Pt 2):1440-4.

105. Cimino JJ, Patel VL, Kushniruk AW. The patient clinical information system (PatCIS): technical solutions for and experience with giving patients access to their electronic medical records. *Int J Med Inform.* 2002;68(1-3):113-27.

106. Niazkhani Z et al. Same system, different outcomes: comparing the transitions from two paper-based systems to the same computerized physician order entry system. *Int J Med Inform.* 2009;78(3):170-81.

107. Ash JS, Stavri PZ, Kuperman GJ. A consensus statement on considerations for a successful CPOE implementation. *J Am Med Inform Assoc.* 2003;10(3):229-34.

108. Ash JS, Bates DW. Factors and forces affecting EHR system adoption: report of a 2004 ACMI discussion. *J Am Med Inform Assoc.* 2005;12(1):8-12.

109. Kannry J. *Operationalizing the Science: Integrating Clinical Informatics into the Daily Operations of the Medical Center, in Human, Social, and Organizational Aspects of Health Information Systems.* Kushniruk AW, Borycki E (eds.) 2008, Medical Information Science Reference: Hershey, PA.

CHAPTER 5

State and Regional Health Information Exchange Activities: Current Status and Future Direction

Rachel Block

INTRODUCTION

While much attention has been focused on implementation of electronic health records (EHRs) in specific clinical settings, ensuring that information can flow in standardized and secure ways between those systems is essential to obtain the full value of an EHR or other health IT system. Patients receive services in many different locations within a community and sometimes beyond. EHRs need to capture point-in-time as well as longitudinal information and present information to the clinician or consumer in a useful format (e.g., alerts to schedule regular preventive care services or follow-up lab tests). Some healthcare needs can be met through simple forms of one-to-one exchange of data between EHRs as they are in the paper-based healthcare world, but most of the sophisticated capabilities that are necessary for healthcare improvement (including quality measurement, care management and coordination and population health) will require health information exchange (HIE) across a variety of settings and systems. HIE in turn requires agreement on certain policies and standards in order to achieve interoperability of data and systems.

Coordinated efforts to foster HIE through policy initiatives and technical services have been launched at the state and regional levels across the United States. There are many common elements, but also significant variation, among these efforts, and questions remain as to how they can best be sustained in terms of governance and financing. Federal policies and funding through the American Recovery and Reinvestment Act of 2009 (ARRA)/Health Information Technology for Economic and Clinical Health Act of 2009 (HITECH) and the Patient Protection and Affordable Care Act (PPACA) will encourage further development of health IT adoption and use, as well as HIE, but these policies are not universally applicable. For example, the new meaningful use requirements apply to a limited segment of Medicare and Medicaid participating providers, and participation in the program is voluntary. As a result, state and regional HIE efforts will continue to play an important role in advancing health IT adoption and use while adapting to an evolving policy environment. This chapter will summarize key issues in HIE, provide the current status of state and regional HIE efforts and identify key strategic and operational issues facing HIE programs in the future.

WHAT IS HIE AND WHY IS IT IMPORTANT?

Early policy support for HIE has advanced through a combination of public and private sector efforts. The Institute of Medicine reports on quality and safety in the U.S. healthcare system identified the need for health IT combined with policies and standards to facilitate interoperability and sharing of information within and across disparate healthcare settings. In this context, development of a nationwide health IT infrastructure including HIE was considered an essential building block in support of new systems capabilities, including clinical quality improvement, consumer empowerment and population health surveillance. Widespread use of EHRs and health IT that can collect and transmit data in standardized and useful forms is a necessary precondition for this infrastructure. HIE also supports aggregation of data, which is necessary for quality measures, clinical research, and public health.

The healthcare informatics field has also promoted development and use of data standards to support broader interoperability of electronic health information. Early efforts focused on a variety of voluntary consensus groups that have addressed specific clinical areas (e.g., prescribing and pharmacy data standards) or broader data format and reporting structures (e.g., CCR/CCD). While there has been a great proliferation of these efforts, there has been no regulatory imperative to prioritize or coordinate these efforts, and to enforce the use of standards. As a result, these activities made important contributions to the technical underpinnings of HIE, but this alone was not sufficient to ensure consistent use and therefore ensure broad interoperability across systems.

EARLY MODELS FOR STATE AND REGIONAL HIE

The early state and regional HIE initiatives emerged as a grass roots phenomenon, usually involving clinical leadership, multi-stakeholder collaboration and an incremental approach to building services and value.

Indiana Network for Patient Care (INPC)

INPC was created by the Regenstrief Institute in 1994 with the goal of providing clinical information at the point of care for the treatment of patients in the emergency department (ED). Today, it includes more than 40 geographically separate hospitals, as well as ambulatory practices, public health departments, payers, laboratories and imaging facilities distributed across Indiana, including the Indianapolis metropolitan area and Lafayette and Evansville areas. INPC includes records for more than 10.5 million patients, such as patient registration data for ED visits, inpatient and outpatient hospital encounters, and ambulatory care visits; clinical data, such as laboratory results and immunizations; and free-text notes, including diagnostic studies, procedure results, operative notes, discharge summaries and radiology images. The information in the

INPC follows the patient, not the physician or a specific health system, so physicians can view a patient's previous care information from all participating institutions as a single virtual record. The INPC serves as the backbone for a number of HIE services provided in Indiana by the Indiana Health Information Exchange.

HealthBridge

HealthBridge was launched in the 1990s as an outgrowth of several community-based cost containment initiatives in the Cincinnati area. HealthBridge began with investments from two health plans and five health systems. Each of these five founders provided loans of $250,000 each—a total of $1.75 million—to capitalize the new organization. To ensure there was a return from this investment, each of these five organizations were also given a seat on the board of HealthBridge. In addition to the five founding members, HealthBridge's Board consists of a variety of community stakeholders—employers, physicians, public health, etc.—that have actively contributed to keeping the original vision of using technology and collaboration to improve healthcare quality alive and well for more than 13 years of operation. The governance structure and early investment resulted in HealthBridge becoming one of the best examples of HIE sustainability in the nation. Within five years, HealthBridge was breaking even, and, since 2003, HealthBridge has been a profitable non-profit, earning 5–8 percent over expenses each year.

Today, HealthBridge provides clinical messaging and clinical data Web portal services for more than 90 percent of physicians and acute care hospitals in the community. Remarkably, more than 97 percent of HealthBridge's information exchange is done electronically. Fax and mail accounts for just 3 percent of the information volume sent today through HealthBridge. This level of technology adoption reduces community costs by an estimated $20 million per year.

STATE AND REGIONAL HIE BUILDING BLOCKS

State and regional HIE initiatives are utilizing a common overall policy and technical framework to support health IT interoperability. Several national organizations documented key elements in the framework which includes:

- **Governance:** Most state and regional HIE initiatives operate under a multi-stakeholder governance model, often including some representation from the public sector. Many are non-profit corporations. The operating entity conducts its activities in a transparent and inclusive manner that includes significant community input. Clinicians are integrally involved in governance activities.
- **Policy:** Health information interoperability requires common policies governing data exchange to facilitate "information liquidity." State and regional HIEs have developed and adopted policies to address privacy and security and establish data use protections.
- **Clinical and Administrative Use Cases:** To enhance the value of health IT and HIE, clinical and administrative use cases have been employed as a means to structure data requirements and address workflow considerations in clinical settings, ensuring that HIE can meet real needs in community settings.

- **Technical Architecture and Services:** HIE comprises a combination of "core" and value added services. Core services represent foundational infrastructure required to enable HIE, including identification and authentication of patients and clinicians; security features, such as authorization for use and auditing of disclosures; and mapping of network communication protocols. Value added services address specific administrative or clinical needs (e.g., E-prescribing, lab results delivery, quality reporting).
- **EHR Adoption and Implementation Support:** HIE value is directly correlated to the extent of EHR adoption and use—more EHR adoption translates into more data flowing through an HIE, and more data and users translates into more value for the participants. EHR implementation support covers the full range of activities from facilitating EHR selection, through the implementation process (including planning and executing workflow changes), and finally to the point of demonstrating use of all EHR functions (including decision support).
- **Funding and Sustainability:** HIE funding and sustainability models need to address the full lifecycle of the initiative, from its initial design to a fully operational state. Many initiatives got started with funding from grants, as well as fees from participants; ultimately, all users and beneficiaries should participate in ongoing funding to ensure equity (i.e., eliminate the "free rider" problem, and provide stable, predictable sources and amounts of revenue).

EMERGING TRENDS

In July 2010 the eHealth Initiative published its seventh annual survey of HIE activities across the United States. Nearly 200 organizations responded, including a large number of states and private organizations participating in the State HIE Cooperative Agreement grant program. Highlights from the 2010 survey include the following elements and insights:

- Continued growth in state and regional HIE initiatives, including those that report being "operational" (i.e., beyond planning stage);
- Significant numbers of projects reporting sustainable funding models independent of federal grants;
- A mix of organizational and financial relationships among participants in the HIE;
- Expected benefits have been obtained in a number of initiatives relating to improved administrative efficiencies and reductions in duplicate testing;
- Sustainability remains an ongoing challenge, but meeting government policy mandates is now widely reported as an emerging challenge;
- Functional services delivered have focused on interoperability among EHRs and sharing of patient records;
- Data exchange efforts have focused on medication history, lab results, and ED discharge/summary data;
- Statewide HIEs are focusing on E-prescribing and administrative claims transactions;
- There is a significant increase in patient access to information through HIEs;

- HIEs are addressing privacy and security, including policies and operational processes for patient consent.

CASE STUDY – NEW YORK STATE COMPREHENSIVE HEALTH IT STRATEGY

The New York State Legislature enacted the Health Care Efficiency and Affordability Law for New Yorkers Capital Grant Program (the HEAL NY Program) in 2004 to invest up to an anticipated $1 billion over a four-year period to affect reform and reconfigure New York's healthcare delivery system to achieve improvements in patient care and increase efficiency of operation. The HEAL NY Program is jointly administered by the New York State Department of Health (DOH) and the Dormitory Authority of the State of New York (DASNY). Funding has been made available via state appropriations, beginning with state fiscal year 2006 and pursuant to Section 1680-j of the Public Authorities Law (PAL), DASNY bonding authority in the amount of up to $740 million, as well as through the Federal State Health Reform Partnership (F-SHRP) 1115 waiver which specifically authorizes federal matching funds for this purpose.

The health IT component of the HEAL NY Program is a multi-year, multi-phased program with two primary objectives:

- To identify and support opportunities for development and investment in health IT initiatives on a regional and state level; and
- To identify and support opportunities for restructuring healthcare delivery systems on a regional basis, which includes the use of health IT in a manner that results in improved quality, safety, efficiency and stability of healthcare services.

DOH has supported three prior competitive grant programs (HEAL 1, 5, 10) to advance New York's interoperable health IT infrastructure, and a fourth funding cycle (HEAL 17) was launched in October 2010 (see Table 5-1).

New York's strategy to develop and support this infrastructure comprises three interrelated components—organizational, clinical and technical—which must evolve together to harness the power of health information to support patient care and population health improvements. HEAL 5 marked the beginning of a concerted strategy to lay the foundation for these key organizational, clinical and technical building blocks

Table 5-1: New York State HEAL Grants

Activity	Org	HEAL 1	HEAL 5	HEAL 10	HEAL 17	Total
Community Health IT/HIE Projects	Various	$53M	$95M	$60M	$120M	$328M
Statewide Collaboration Process	NYeC		$5M	$5.3M	$4M	$14.3M
Statewide SHIN-NY Infrastructure	NYeC			$22.8M	$12M	$34.8M
Education and Communication	NYeC			$3.5M		$3.5M
Health IT Adoption Services	NYeC			$3.4M		$3.4M
HIE Accreditation	NYeC				$2M	$2M
Evaluation	HITECH		$5M	$5M	$2M	$12M
Total		$53M	$105M	$100M	$140M	$398M

Source: Statewide Health Information Network for New York

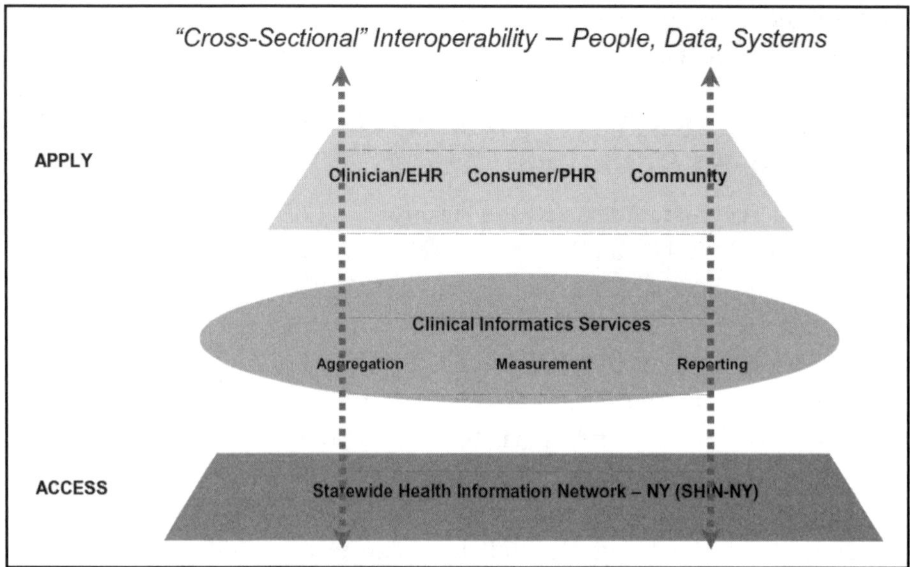

Figure 5-1: Framework for New York's Health IT Strategy

with a particular focus on engaging stakeholders at the community level. This program sought to advance interoperability at all levels of the system as depicted in Figure 5-1.

HEAL 10 is focused on coordination and management of patient care through implementation of the patient centered medical home (PCMH), in conjunction with interoperable EHRs that are linked through the SHIN-NY. HEAL 10 supports the inclusion of all types of healthcare providers, including clinician practices and clinics, hospitals, nursing homes, and other long-term care facilities, as well as home care providers and others. The patient is the center of this coordinated care model, and projects also include health IT for patients to participate in information sharing with all of their caregivers in a safe and secure environment. HEAL 17 intends to build and expand on this foundation of implementation of health IT in support of the PCMH, with particular focus on increasing participation by mental health, long-term care and home health care providers. The PCMH and the care coordination model supported by New York state's health IT infrastructure are depicted in Figure 5-2.

Lastly, New York is at the forefront of clinical excellence and health IT and is well positioned to make effective use of ARRA and other federal funds for health IT, as well as play a significant leadership role and inform the national policy and regulatory framework developed by the United States Department of Health & Human Services (HHS). New York's health IT strategy closely matches the initial key statutory components of the Health Information Technology for Economic and Clinical Health Act that is part of ARRA, including health information exchange infrastructure, which is the SHIN-NY; state designated entities to advance HIE infrastructure, which is the NYeC; and regional extension centers, which are conceptual to New York's Community Health Information Technology Adoption collaborations (CHITAs).

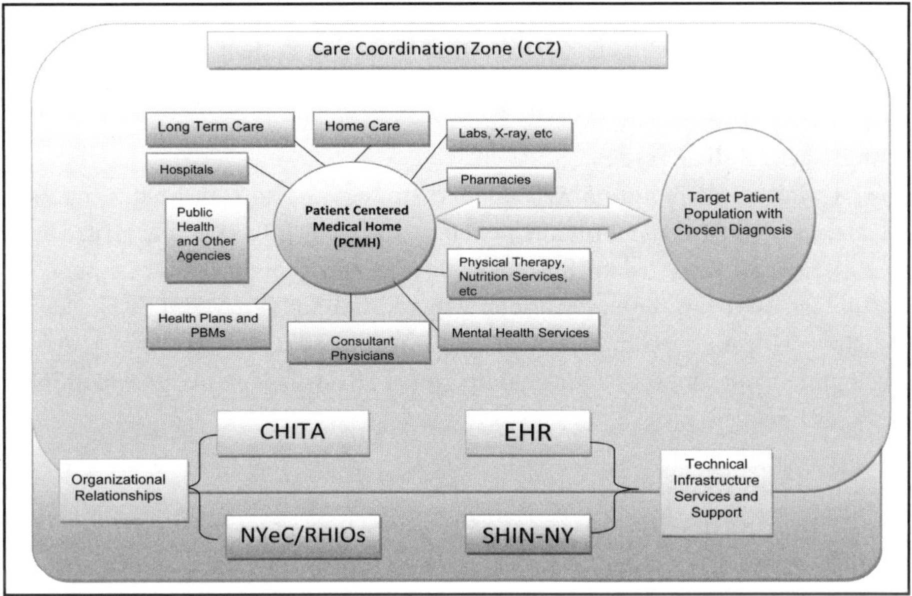

Figure 5-2: PCMH and Care Coordination Model: Care Coordination Zone (CCZ)

FEDERAL POLICIES AND FUNDING

ARRA/HITECH provides an initial framework for federal policies and funding governing HIE in general and state and regional HIE activities specifically. For HIE, the most relevant provisions of ARRA/HITECH are the meaningful use requirements for Medicare and Medicaid payment incentives, and the state HIE Program.

Meaningful Use

The legislative language defining Meaningful Use included three broad characteristics with direct and indirect relevance to HIE:

1. Certified EHR technology (existing certification standards included some HIE functionality);
2. Electronic exchange information; and
3. Collection and reporting of quality data.

The CMS final rule governing Meaningful Use did not prescribe specific HIE models or services as requirements, but many HIEs are exploring ways they can support Meaningful Use so that eligible providers can more readily meet the requirements because they can utilize HIE capabilities.

State HIE Cooperative Agreement Program

ARRA/HITECH authorized funding for the State HIE Program. Administered by the Office of the National Coordinator as a cooperative agreement program, all states are eligible to participate. The original funding announcement identified broad requirements which each state was asked to address relative to its current state of HIE activities reflecting the characteristics of HIE programs outlined earlier (e.g., governance, clinical priorities, etc.). Additional program guidance, issued in July 2010, directed states to focus their efforts on assisting eligible providers to meet Meaningful Use and provide at least one option for three core Meaningful Use functional requirements: E-prescribing, delivery of structured lab results to EHRs and exchange of patient summary records across disparate EHR systems.

Key Strategic and Policy Issues

Successful HIE initiatives require a well-defined strategy, broad stakeholder involvement and support and agreement on key policies to support interoperable HIE. There is enough experience gained to date that emerging state and regional HIEs can incorporate important lessons from the early adopters. In addition to ARRA/HITECH, federal and state health reform efforts may provide additional impetus for HIE efforts. Additional development and support for state and regional HIE will depend on resolution of key strategic and policy issues.

Public Good versus Market Forces

Several early HIEs were developed as a market response to offer more effective and efficient solutions to physicians and others, such as providing a secure and convenient way to obtain lab results. The Nationwide Health Information Network model for secure transport of messages between EHRs is another example of this type of HIE.

However, most state and regional HIEs were established with the broader goals of promoting the development of patient-centered models of care delivery and advancing improvements in population health, both of which require coordination and cooperation among a wide variety of community stakeholders. States are taking on more policy and operational responsibilities for HIE through the Medicaid and public health programs which they administer. The state's role includes:

- Operating or overseeing the state HIE cooperative grant program;
- Providing Medicaid claims data to HIEs and EHRs;
- Establishing Medicaid incentive payments for E-prescribing and patient centered medical homes;
- Modernizing the public health reporting system to support bi-directional data exchange through HIEs and EHRs; and,
- Adopting laws and regulations governing health IT, including HIE.

If HIE is deemed to be a public good, then a host of governance, policy and financing questions move to the forefront, including whether and how services offered in the market place should be regulated or permitted to operate without governance oversight. A public good model for HIE would require that everyone have access to and participate in the same HIE services, that explicit mechanisms would be established to ensure and monitor adherence to common policies among the participants, and that common policies would be established to apportion responsibility for funding the development and operation of HIE services.

Regulation versus Incentives

A separate but related policy debate focuses on the balance between regulation of and incentives for health IT and HIE and how federal and state roles in these areas will be reconciled. For example, the federal government has published regulations that will govern EHR certification, but state HIEs may dictate additional requirements for EHR interoperability above the minimum federal requirements. Mandating provider participation and use of certified EHRs would accelerate the process of health IT adoption and dramatically enhance the value of HIE; however, some providers would face financial hardship to purchase and implement a certified EHR, and it could be argued that more financial incentives should be provided to achieve the goal of expanding health IT adoption and use (including HIE participation). Another option is to blend the two approaches, making participation in HIE a condition to qualify for payment incentives—for example, Vermont enacted legislation requiring hospitals to participate in the statewide HIE if they are participating in the state's Blueprint for Health Initiative, which provides payment incentives for improved management of chronic care.

Consumer Access to HIE

Consumer access to information is another strategic and policy issue facing state and regional HIEs. Consumers generally have legal rights to view their health information from individual providers, and ARRA/HITECH requires physicians to provide consumers with an electronic copy of their information upon request. State laws may vary as to whether and how consumers can access their information—for example, lab results cannot be sent directly to patients but must be provided by the ordering physician. The e-Health Insider 2010 survey documented a clear trend toward HIEs making information more readily available to consumers, but there is little consistency in how this is done. It is expected that consumer engagement measures will increase in the next stages of Meaningful Use requirements. HIE should benefit consumers by making information more readily accessible from a variety of sources; this would alleviate some of the burden on providers as well.

CHAPTER 6

Ambulatory Systems

Curtis L. Cole, MD, and Adam Cheriff, MD

INTRODUCTION

When looked at from the patient's perspective, the ambulatory electronic health record (AEHR) is probably closer to the patient's archetype of "my chart" than its acute care sibling.

Nevertheless, the erstwhile second-class status of the AEHR stems from the socioeconomic history of the EHR. The EHR was born in large, acute care institutions, largely to serve hospital-based providers. Their view, as dictated by reimbursement methods, was encounter-based and focused on procedures and hospital stays. The notion of a single patient flowing through a series of complex encounters across providers over years was absent. So the hospital care delivery flows seemed to take on a disproportionately large role relative to the caretaking place outside it. This view was amusingly captured by Carter in a comparison to inpatient EMR implementations: "Ambulatory care sites tend to be simpler."[1]

The last several years suggest that the perspective on EHRs is changing. In 2005, the HIMSS Ambulatory Care Initiative identified two key trends that point to the centrality of the AEHR (see Figures 6-1 and 6-2).[2]

First is the imbalance in the scale of ambulatory encounters, which are counted in the billions, compared to acute care encounters which are counted in the millions (1.2 billion versus 34 million[3]). Second, ambulatory healthcare expenditures have surpassed acute care expenditures and continue to grow more quickly. The nation spends about 1/10th as much on ambulatory IT as it does on inpatient-based systems.[2] But with the critical importance the Obama administration has placed on the EHR as a tool for reforming healthcare, more physician offices have been incentivized to adopt AEHRs and discouraged from staying with paper.[4,5]

In this chapter, we will explore how the AEHR differs from its inpatient counterpart by focusing on the key functions and workflows it supports. We will examine key executive considerations such as cost, return on investment (ROI) and infrastructure. The chapter closes with a discussion of the status of the industry and where it appears to be headed in the future.

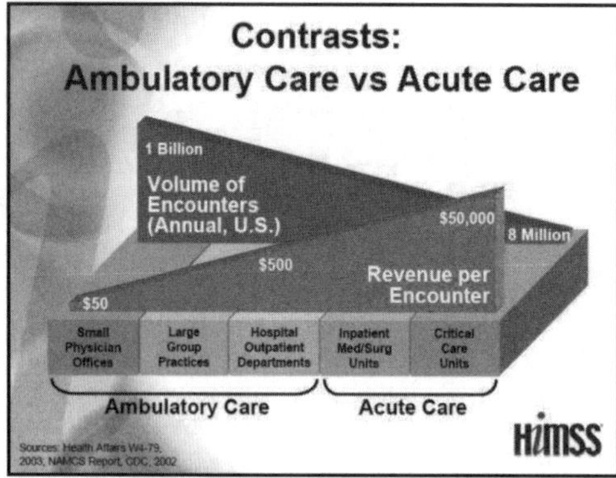

Figure 6-1: Contrasts: Ambulatory Care vs Acute Care

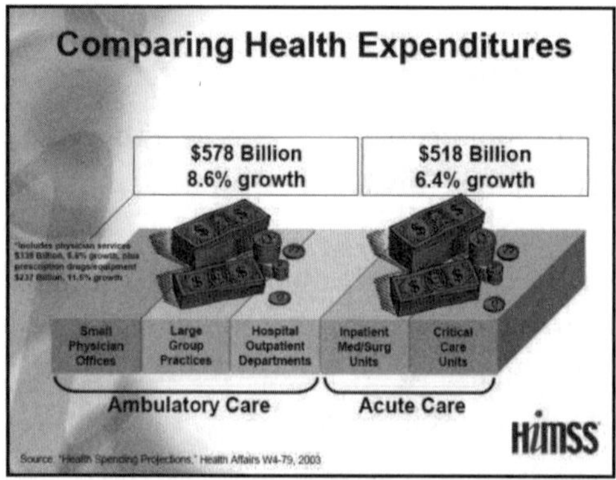

Figure 6-2: Comparing Health Expenditures

HIMSS defines the EHR as follows:

> The Electronic Health Record (EHR) is a secure, real-time, point-of-care, patient centric information resource for clinicians. The EHR aids clinicians' decision making by providing access to the patient health record information where and when they need it and by incorporating evidence-based decision support. The EHR automates and streamlines the clinician's workflow, closing loops in communication and response that result in delays or gaps in care. The EHR also supports the collection of data for uses other than direct clinical care, such as billing, quality management, outcomes reporting, resource planning, and public health disease surveillance and reporting.[6]

While this academic description covers the waterfront, the marketplace boils it down to three categories of systems: practice management systems (PMSs), clinical systems, and biomedical devices. We will examine each category, then briefly consider infrastructure. We will start with practice management system because it is the first system any practice should be implementing (or will need to implement simultaneously with clinical systems). The axiom, "no money, no mission" is certainly applicable in ambulatory medical practices. Clinical systems and biomedical devices are more glamorous and dynamic. Though perhaps the least sexy of all, infrastructure considerations are the foundation for all systems and critical in an ambulatory context.

PRACTICE MANAGEMENT SYSTEM

A practice management system (PMS) focuses on two interrelated concepts: patient flow and the revenue cycle. These are the operational and financial sides of the same coin. They are the outpatient cousins to the inpatient ADT (admit discharge transfer) and patient accounting systems.

Whether you view the PMS through an operations lens or a financial lens, the business begins with patient identification. It is from this starting point the divergence with inpatient systems begins. The concept of "registration" is very different between the inpatient and outpatient world. The conceptual difference is permanence. The ambulatory world treats registration as a persistent beginning to a lifetime record. Patients see their physicians over and over, but they only register once; they reasonably expect their physician to remember them. In the inpatient world, registration is the beginning of a finite stay and is repeated with each admission. Inpatient EMRs may share demographics across stays, but the patient's chart, in many systems, is broken up by hospital admission rather than being a continuous record.

From a systems perspective, the difference is the combination of three related functions: identification, registration and scheduling. Patient identification is increasingly the realm of specialized systems specific to the task known as the electronic master patient index (EMPI). These systems contain a database with a very small amount of identity and demographic data about every patient in their dominion. The job of the EMPI is to make sure that each patient has only one set of data (e.g., first name, last name, birthdate, address, phone number, Social Security number, and insurer), even across multiple systems, specialties, locations and institutions.

Almost all PMSs have some EMPI functionality built in. Large PMSs tend to have more sophisticated functionality. A caveat for executives shopping for a PMS is to make sure this functionality is sophisticated enough to meet your needs or that the system is capable of taking direction from an external EMPI, which is increasingly the preference of large organizations. Too many PMSs are designed with the assumption they are in charge of patient identity, which can lead to significant difficulty when trying to integrate with other systems.

The details of patient identification can be mind numbing, particularly to those who fail to grasp their importance. But ignore them at your peril. The ambulatory world can be deceptively simple in this regard. If you view each practice independently it may be easy to keep a few thousand patients straight without a large number of duplicates. But when you combine practices or try to combine data from patients across practices, you quickly realize that the ambulatory world is very large indeed. The lack of a single identifier makes matching logic more critical. And the well-documented failures and risks of using Social Security numbers make the task ahead look even more challenging.[7,8]

Once the patient is identified, the formal registration can begin. This is the collection of deeper patient demographics, including insurance coverage information, emergency contacts, customer service information such as contact preferences and similar non-clinical information. In the most sophisticated PMSs, insurance eligibility verification may occur at this step in an EDI (electronic data interchange) transaction analogous to a retailer validating a credit card.

Scheduling

In the inpatient world, the process now moves to bed management while in the outpatient world the next job is scheduling. Because patients are admitted to the hospital at a particular time and date, scheduling is inherent in the admission process. For the ambulatory patient, all future encounters will key off the original registration (generally with registration data confirmation and/or necessary updates), and the schedule is the focus of new encounters.

Because the process of scheduling is so tightly linked to registration, it is not surprising that many clinical scheduling systems are integrated with registration systems within the PMS. There are a few key qualities of ambulatory scheduling that differentiate the various systems available on the market. Perhaps the most important is how they differ from non-clinical scheduling systems such as Microsoft Outlook™—which for clarity are referred to here as calendaring systems.

Calendaring systems have been and continue to be used to schedule patient visits/services in the ambulatory context. The main distinction between a scheduling system and a calendaring system is the linkage to the patient record. In a typical business calendaring system, the user cannot quickly locate a whole history of a given patient's appointments, or sort them by type. The appointment is usually free text, whereas in a clinical scheduling system the appointment is with a specific patient already registered in the database.

Clinical schedules are also linked to billing encounters. This is critical from the financial perspective. One of the first interventions in a typical revenue cycle enhancement program is to match charges against the schedule. This is possible manually with a calendaring system but can be made into an automated "missing charge report" in a clinical scheduling product. Another way of looking at this is that the schedule can define the encounter for the billing system.

Clinical scheduling systems typically support complex templates and rules to maximize patient flow and appointment availability. Concepts such as appointment type, bump lists, freeze and thaw, recurring visits, and team care will have variable importance in different practices and specialties. For example, patients on specific chemotherapy protocols or physical therapy routines can be extremely complicated to schedule. Sophisticated clinical scheduling systems can offer appropriate searching algorithms and decision support that can span visits or include resource availability.

Resource linking is particularly critical in procedural areas. For example, in specialties with endoscopes, the availability of the scope itself and the time needed for sterilization must be accounted for by the scheduling system to maximize throughput. Linkage to materials management systems may also be important for inventory and cost controls.

In academic environments, there are complex regulatory rules that must be accounted for to allow compliant billing. For example, the 1969 CMS IL372 supervision regulations require that primary care supervisors oversee no more than four residents at a given time.[9] Without that ratio, the supervisor cannot bill for his or her supervision. Similarly, patients may be part of a clinical trial protocol, and therefore communication regarding a research visit with a clinical trials management system may be important.

Increasingly the most sophisticated practices are providing online access to schedules, with some self-service for patients through Web portals. This is actually not that technically challenging but can interfere with other process controls a practice may have in place. Patients cannot know about complex resource issues, and managed care pre-certifications also can impede delivery of this popular convenience. These barriers can be overcome by enabling patients to request an appointment, which is then managed by scheduling staff or a designated 'health coach.'

The most sophisticated practices use their scheduling systems to track all aspects of clinical workflow. Some systems can parse a variety of wait times, such as time-to-room, time-in-room, time-with-RN and time-with-MD. Some systems use radio-frequency identification (RFID) or other technologies to automate this, though that is hardly mainstream. When used well, these tools provide practice administrators and clinicians the necessary data to optimize patient flow, maximize resource utilization and improve patient satisfaction.

Billing

The core of most PMSs is the financial component. The tools needed to manage billing and accounts receivable are enormously varied due to the wide variety of reimbursement rules and methods throughout the country. The key difference with inpatient systems is the focus on professional fee billing rather than facilities fee billing. One important, and possibly counter-intuitive, feature this may imply is the need for the *ambulatory* PMS to support *inpatient* professional billing. Physicians who see inpatients and do not bill "globally", or through the hospital, send their bills from their office. Therefore, certain types of integration with the inpatient system, such as an ADT interface, may be desirable.

Executives attuned to the current regulatory environment will note the need to synchronize the facility and the professional fee bills in terms of procedure and diagnosis. Given that two staffs, with two different managers, following two sets of rules, using two different systems are responsible for this suggests that it will be fraught with peril. Adding further complexity, multiple specialists may be billing for the same case (e.g., surgery and anesthesia), and different coding systems may be required (e.g., HCPCS and CPT).[10] At this point, few of the systems on the market today are facile at this kind of cross-provider billing reconciliation. If pressure increases toward "global billing" or "bundled payment," hospitals and doctors will be forced to coordinate to unify their bills and determine how to split the fees. This will create new challenges for sites without integrated billing systems.

Today's financial systems put increasing emphasis on capturing data as early in the encounter as possible. The shift from back office to front desk is a major component of revenue cycle enhancement projects. Many systems now automate charge capture at the point of care. There are significant opportunities for both revenue enhancement and cost control by automating this step. Costs fall if you can eliminate charge entry clerks, and revenue rises when the computer helps to appropriately code clean claims.

There is an important architectural decision point here. Should the "encounter form" data (a.k.a. super-bill) be entered into a clinical system or a practice management system? The IT manager who is blind to the actual workflow will generally prefer direct entry into the PMS. Entry into the clinical system will require an interface into the PMS (unless they are the same system).

Understanding the workflow is the key to resolving this question. Most physicians will have little or no need to use the PMS. Therefore, if you want the provider to capture the billing data, it may make more sense to capture it from within the clinical system. Ideally, the billing codes fall out of the documentation, in which case the issue is moot. As discussed next, this remains an ideal more than a reality.

In the past decade, some practices started using PDAs (personal digital assistants) or smartphones to capture charges. These systems may be stand-alone or integrated with a PMS or clinical system. Regardless of the platform, these systems offer another way to eliminate paper encounter forms and capture data more accurately and directly into the billing system.

ROI from these systems stems from the reduction in lost charges and reduced service to posting lag. As such, their value is largely based on the relative inefficiency of whatever paper-based system is in place. Executives need to be cautious when evaluating such systems. Their value is only in capturing revenue that was otherwise never captured or on the time-value of money that was captured late. In some cases, that may be quite large, but it may also be fairly modest where paper systems work well.

In many environments in which part-time clinical employment is the norm, the value may be further mitigated by vendor fees that do not acknowledge the less-than-full-time use of the system. Conversely, in consultation-rich specialties, such systems can be a godsend of convenience to physicians, particularly if they practice in multiple locations. These systems are not needed if the inpatient clinical system can capture the charge and send it to the professional fee billing system. This is usually more convenient for physicians, but hospitals may not have an incentive to build these features if the physician bills separately.

Another nuance executives need to beware of is the definition of the encounter itself. As with registration, terminology here is imprecise and can be confusing. Some prefer to refer to the billable event as the encounter and the face-to-face meeting with the patient as the visit. But the increasing prevalence of phone, Web, and other virtual "visits" makes this topic inherently fluid. Regardless of the term you use to refer to the event, the system must know the rules for the definitions, which are generally determined by the payer and may or may not make sense to the clinician. For example, a nine-month pregnancy may be a single encounter with multiple visits. Similarly, a visit to a physician's office that results in referral to the emergency department may be combined as a single encounter (the "72 hour rule"). A visit to multiple physicians on a single day may be considered a single encounter. The billing system needs to understand these rules. Again, cross-institutional reconciliation may be necessary to ensure complete accuracy in some scenarios.

Managed Care

The most fundamental distinction among practice management systems is support for the various forms of managed care. Practices that take on capitation without a PMS that is fully capable of tracking expenses and supporting risk management are almost certain to fail. Such systems are complex to properly set up and maintain, even when backed by billion dollar insurance companies, which goes a long way toward explaining the falling popularity of this form of reimbursement.

While traditional fee-for-service still exists in some form in most markets, some permutation of managed care is the norm in most areas. While the technology to support managed care exists, it is still very poorly implemented by many PMS vendors. This is, no doubt, in part because few insurance companies support the technology.

The key technologies to support managed care are electronic data interchange (EDI) and robust master file management. The diversity of payer rules, the frequency of changes to the rules, and the frequency with which patients change payers essentially necessitate that providers check eligibility and authorization prior to any service. Despite federal pressure to support EDI, this remains far from ubiquitous.

Many PMS vendors partner with EDI clearinghouse vendors to simplify their own EDI communication. The concept is that providers only need to communicate with one company, which communicates with all the payers on their behalf. Conversely, the payers only need to communicate with a few clearinghouses rather than thousands of providers. The intermediary is therefore more important to the payer than the provider, particularly if your PMS strictly adheres to the transaction protocols.

In theory, Internet standards should allow for direct payer-provider communication. Particularly for large providers, the clearinghouse should not be necessary. Similarly, for small providers who purchase PMS services from a larger entity, such as software as a service (SaaS) or an application service provider (ASP), the clearinghouse should be optional, particularly in the increasing number of markets with very few payers. Payers often mandate the use of a clearinghouse. Further, many vendors charge large transaction fees, which can cut into already slim margins. This practice certainly violates the spirit of laws intended to simplify healthcare communications. Absent stronger regulatory enforcement, inexpensive dis-intermediation will be resisted by the clearinghouses. Executives should pay attention to this issue going forward, as significant efficiencies will be won or lost depending on how the issue of clearinghouses develops.

Claims Editing and Submission

Once the encounter is captured, the next layer of system functionality is charge editing. In many instances, charges may be clean at the point of entry and can quickly flow to the payer. In many other settings, charges must be analyzed for exceptions, discounts, consistency with other claims, the addition of modifiers or other interventions management may want to make before sending the claim. In some systems, these edits can be done in real time and the provider or charge entry staff advised to make changes immediately. In others, the claims are batched and analyzed in bulk. A list of exceptions is created and worked over time.

The goal of editing is to ensure that every claim that is sent to the payer is a clean claim. Sophisticated PMS vendors provide tools that mimic the adjudication rules used by payers and alert the provider to impending rejections before the claim even goes out the door. Clean claims mean no rejections, faster payment, and reduced re-processing costs. Not surprisingly, claim editing is another frequent focus of revenue enhancement efforts. When analyzing the financial return from these efforts, it is important to consider who will be making the charge edits; a highly paid physician or a lower paid biller. This is not to imply that these two efficiencies are necessarily either-or. However, individual workflows need to be well understood before assuming cost reductions. Revenue enhancement may not cut costs and vice versa.

Once through the edit process, a claim is ready to be sent. The ability to print a paper claim remains a requirement of any PMS—if for no other reason than downtime at an intermediary. But most claims today are sent electronically. This may be via a clearinghouse or directly. In either event, logs of the transactions are essential to avoid disputes over lost claims.

The payer now adjudicates the claims, and if a flaw is found the claim is rejected. Here again, there is an opportunity for efficiency if the payer communicates the rejection electronically. Many companies still send rejections via paper. Well-managed practices key these rejections into the PMS with their often obscure rejection codes, so that practice administrators can track the reasons for rejection over time and correct any systematic problems that emerge.

Master File Management

This brings us to the second key technology for supporting managed care: strong master file management. All information systems use a variety of tables and dictionaries to drive the lists and other user interface elements customized to your location or practice. For example, a list of physicians you commonly refer to (or are sent referrals from) is one such provider dictionary. In the world of managed care, keeping track of who is "in plan" and "out of plan" is a major problem. Many providers who have dropped out of plan will tell you that it may take months or even years for their name to disappear from the payer's list, particularly if they are in a shortage specialty.

IT managers are vexed by the need to provide users with accurate data without good sources for the data. Management of referring provider libraries is a good example. This issue is relevant to claims adjudication because of the many nuances of billing that require accurate look-up tables. For example, specialists may need to indicate the license number of a referring physician on the claim or it will be rejected. Therefore the easiest path to clean claims would be a clean dictionary of referring providers.

Many vendors offer portions of these data for sale. But their accuracy may be suspect, and they often lack key information needed to match existing data. States may have good data but often refuse to provide it in a usable form. Assuming one can get usable data, the PMS must be capable of adeptly managing entry adds, changes, and deletes. Updates can be delicate processes (often "all or nothing"), which pose the risk of wreaking havoc on existing record references. The recently adopted NPI (national provider identifier) has helped to some extent, but many problems remain.

Providers, procedures, diagnoses, payers, locations and specialties are all just some of the many master files that need to be managed within clinical and practice management systems. The larger the practice, the more this becomes a critical focus and expense of the team managing these systems. Some can be standardized, but some will always be local, and the ability to customize and control these tables is a key vendor differentiator.

Payment Posting and Contract Management

Of course, most claims are not rejected. The next challenge for the PMS is payment posting. Here again, efficiency would demand electronic payment posting. Reality is far different. The details of payment posting vary considerably. Some providers use bank lockboxes and other services that simplify (or complicate) the process, but the basics are the same.

The payer sends a payment with an EOB (explanation of benefits), typically for many claims at once. The job of payment posting is interpreting the EOB and assigning the correct amount of money to each claim. In large practices with manual payment posting, this may take many full-time employees (FTEs). The procedure is also error prone, making this whole process a ripe target for automation. Barcoding, optical character recognition, and a variety of other technologies have been applied to try to clean up payment posting with varied degrees of success. Rich EDI is probably the most promising solution (short of adopting a single payer insurance plan).

Once posted, there are two more problems the PMS must contend with: overpayment and underpayment. Overpayment most commonly occurs when both the patient and the payer send the provider a payment. This requires a method for refunding which, in many practices, requires a link to a separate accounts payable system.

In today's world of managed care conglomerates, underpayment is the more serious problem. Even within one company, claims may be processed by multiple systems that may not have the current contract and payment policies loaded. Therefore, inappropriate rejections and underpayments are common and often appear to be idiosyncratic. Further, in many states, there is little accountability by regulators. In a study performed at Weill Cornell and Emory, between three and eight percent of all reimbursements from managed care companies were underpaid compared to contract. While this represents tens of millions of dollars to providers, annually payers are only fined a small fraction of this amount by regulators, leaving enforcement of the contract up to the prowess of the provider's management and information technology.[11]

Contract management systems, integrated or added on to the PMS are the provider's defense against these errors. If the PMS knows how much the payer is supposed to reimburse for a given procedure, it can alert the provider to underpayments, individually or systematically. Underpayments of a few dollars are the most insidious, as the cost of reprocessing the claim will exceed the difference collected. This is why tracking underpayments over time is essential, so that underpayments can be addressed in bulk.

Full-featured practice management systems provide many more features and functions. Some provide scanning and document management capabilities. Some manage paper charts in ways analogous to a hospital health information management (HIM) system. Many have sophisticated materials management capabilities, which are particularly important for specialties in which expensive medications or equipment are used.

One final critical feature to any PMS is reporting. The biggest payoff to any information system comes from the ability to extract and manipulate data that have been captured during the routine course of business. Cheaper systems come with preconfigured reports and few tools to manipulate them. More sophisticated systems provide myriad options for extracting data and configuring reports.

CLINICAL SYSTEMS AND BIOMEDICAL DEVICES

The distinction between clinical systems and biomedical devices is becoming both difficult to make and less important. Traditionally, the line between them was apparent. Devices were typically electro-mechanical, diagnostic and procedure oriented. From an IT perspective, they were data sources. Perhaps the most important distinction was that biomedical devices were regulated by the U.S. Food and Drug Administration (FDA). Any changes to their function required recertification. Conversely, information systems were electronic, transaction and documentation oriented, and unregulated in their plasticity.

While some of these distinctions still hold today, their importance is increasingly moot. Clinically, it is completely natural that the systems cardiologists or radiologists use to make a diagnosis should be fully integrated with the systems they use to report their findings. Similarly, from a patient's perspective, the test report is no less part of their medical chart than the note of the physician who ordered the test or procedure.

It is not surprising, therefore, that the marketplaces for these once separate entities are now merging. The leading manufacturers of biomedical devices, such as GE and Siemens, are now also leading vendors of EHRs.

That said, this chapter will not examine further traditional, "know one when I see one," biomedical devices, such as electrocardiography (ECG) and x-ray machines, regardless of how proximal they may have become to clinical systems. One reason for this is that they are still purchased and managed differently in most institutions. But more important, biomedical devices do not fit as cleanly into the major thesis of this section. That is, Clinical Systems are the essential *workflow* managers of ambulatory medicine—or, at least, they should be.

The reason to emphasize workflow is that it is the key to success for executives who need to purchase, implement, and manage these systems. A brief history of clinical systems shows that this was not always the case. In fact, many, if not most, clinical systems on the market today reveal a *modular* orientation that reflects how their development was funded, as much as any well-thought-out technical architecture.

A Very Brief History of the AEHR

The first attempts to build electronic medical records were largely in the outpatient arena. Barnett's landmark work in the 1960s with COSTAR[12] emphasized increasing the availability and organization of medical records. Separate modules for registration, scheduling and the actual clinical encounter form were implemented.

In the 1970s, McDonald at Regenstrief and Stead and Hammond at Duke also developed outpatient medical record systems.[13,14] The Regenstrief system also used encounter form data input similar to COSTAR but pioneered the emphasis on automated reminders. Stead and Hammond's TMR system actually attempted to go paperless, using clerks to enter data.

Throughout the 1970s and 1980s, technology became more affordable and adequate to the task of building medical records. Computers moved from mainframes to mini-computers in the 1970s and from mini-computers to micro-computers in the 1980s. Recall that at this time, most medical centers were organized in a very decentralized manner. Outside the institutions, independent practitioners and small groups were still the norm. Therefore it is not surprising that the medical record systems that developed reflected this departmental and practice-oriented organization. In the 1990s, when graphical programming and database management tools became ubiquitous, these forces of "dis-integration" were even more profound. Commercial systems were specialty focused, procedure oriented, and doctor centric.

Large institutions were installing more centralized systems in hospitals but, even there, the industry was moving toward decentralized client-server designs. The sales teams advocated "best-of-breed"—as much a justification for the way things were as for any nobler architectural reason.

What resulted is the situation most institutions and practices are in right now. Every business unit or clinically distinct entity has (or wants) their own information system that meets their needs. There are significant merits to this approach. Many niche systems do, in fact, meet the workflow requirements of any given specialty far better than general purpose systems that are "customized" for their environment. The needs of a cardiology practice offering echocardiography and cardiac graphics are quite distinct from gastroenterologists offering in-office endoscopy, though both are subspecialties of Internal Medicine. Venture into radiation oncology, physiatry, ophthalmology or almost any other common outpatient medical specialty and you will find radically different functional requirements, workflows and expectations.

This challenge of sub-specialization exemplifies perhaps the most fundamental strategic IT choice facing an executive who manages clinical systems: the choice between an aggregation of interfaced best-of-breed systems versus a monolithic system. If each subspecialty can have a better system for themselves purchased separately, is the total greater or less than the sum of the parts? Does a unified platform offer economies of scale and degrees of interoperability not feasible with multiple interfaced systems?

This struggle is illustrated in the history of results reporting and order entry system discussed in the next section. Fifteen to 25 years ago, many order entry and results reporting systems were separate. Integration now allows "loop closure"; an order is closed when the result comes back. But in ambulatory practices that order from many labs that combine systems, that integration is more complex and costly and might lock you into one laboratory provider.

Order Entry and Results Reporting

The earliest and most basic clinical systems were result reporting systems that allowed viewing of the output of laboratory and other biomedical devices. Lab data are typically numeric and *relatively* easy to categorize and display. Textual results, such as pathology and radiology results, were also fairly analogous to other data routinely managed by early business computers. Graphical results and images arrived later with the more powerful hardware and software required to support these modalities.

Typically absent from simple result reporting systems is any facility for data *entry*. The user interface characteristics required for data entry and data display are radically different, the former being far more challenging. Early monolithic systems had a relatively modest goal of unifying all the entered data into a single repository, while specialized data entry systems were permitted in departmental silos.[15]

More recently, due to the economic power of the physician's pen, many hospitals have focused on order entry systems as the centerpiece of their clinical systems efforts.[16,17] In the ambulatory world, order entry can be a small or insignificant component of the workflow in some specialties. Further, the economic imperatives are very different in the outpatient world (especially with fee-for-service), and the ROI from an order entry system may be harder to realize than at a hospital (with prospective payment). That said, ambulatory order entry is still a big business. Many laboratories will give physicians a results reporting system if they will use their online order entry system. The laboratory gains efficiencies, but they still have to give the physician an incentive to use a potentially less convenient system than paper. In large institutions and practices, order entry systems can be very helpful in controlling the flow of referrals. Order entry systems are all but essential in ambulatory practices under capitation in order to control utilization.

Evidence suggests that ambulatory CPOE can be time neutral to physicians, but not all order entry systems are created equal.[18] The minimal systems, some of which are now free, just write prescriptions. For specialists that prescribe a lot of medications, comprehensive support for refills, including aging and reminders, can be a major timesaver and are frequently the first clinical systems installed. Prescriptions are different from inpatient orders in several respects. The ability to print prescriptions in locally mandated formats is not to be assumed. Inpatient systems also generally have limited formularies, whereas outpatient systems generally need all available drugs. Worse still, in managed care environments, ambulatory systems often have to maintain multiple formularies and distinguish between drugs that are on and off plan. Medicare Part D has made this function almost essential, and yet support within EHRs remains awkward at best.

Inpatient systems tend to be more focused on drips and compound preparations. These exist in the outpatient world as well such as in oncology infusion centers. Such sites need the full medication administration record (MAR) functionality common to inpatient systems. But they are certainly less common and typically less complex than in the inpatient setting. Conversely, ambulatory centers that do dispense drugs often do so without a pharmacist as intermediary. This means that the system must support the functions pharmacists provide. For example, when a sample is given, the system must produce a label with instructions for the patient and log the lot number of the drugs dispensed.

E-prescribing, the transmission of prescriptions electronically, has been rapidly expanding due to recent incentives from the federal government and certain payers. As of this writing, such systems still have a lot of rough edges. The standards were pushed through without fully bi-directional communication, which requires reconciliation of currently incompatible drug vocabularies between pharmacy and physician systems. Therefore acknowledgement, cancellations and some safety features are lacking. Some pharmacies still cannot accept electronic prescriptions, so some systems resort to faxing behind the scenes, which is fraught with security and privacy problems. Still, this is clearly the way most prescriptions will soon be written, and executives would be remiss in not planning for this capability.

Similarly, prescription fill information is becoming available electronically from payers. The availability of this information has the potential to alter physicians' ability to monitor patient compliance. Because ambulatory patients administer their own individual doses and may not submit claims for every prescription filled, the reconciliation of fill data with the original prescription is still imperfect. The potential of this capability to improve care is large, but too little has been done to contemplate the workflow impact these data will have on routine visits. Physicians may object to another uncompensated demand on their time.

For laboratory orders, key features in an ambulatory environment again differ from the inpatient world. Most hospitals send all their lab specimens to one laboratory. In the outpatient world, this may be desirable, but managed care contracts often mandate the use of a particular lab. The ability to control default routing rules based on contracts is a vital revenue control point for sites that maintain their own laboratory.

True integration with multiple laboratories is technically very challenging, but it is also very desirable for many reasons. If the outbound order and the incoming result are linked (loop closure), then there is more potential for sophisticated features, such as alerts and reports. For example, a common cause of malpractice claims is the failure to note an abnormal Pap result. Systems with loop closure can alert a physician both to the arrival of an abnormal result and the *failure* of any result to return after a specified time, thereby diminishing the risk of lost data.

The most difficult aspect of linking to multiple labs is reconciling the coding systems for the orders and the results. As of this writing, there is no satisfactory coding system for either orders or results, and those that do exist are poorly cross-mapped. CPT® is often used when placing orders, but it is too imprecise and incomplete to be used exclusively. Similarly, Logical Observation Identifiers Names and Codes (LOINC®) is emerging as a standard for coding results, but it is also very incomplete and idiosyncratically applied. Certain areas, such as microbiology and transfusion medicine, remain particularly problematic. The National Library of Medicine funded an effort to map CPT and LOINC.[10] While this helped, the fact remains that operations managers faced with multiple laboratories need to commit considerable resources to map procedures and result components. Failure to accurately map the clinical tests can severely compromise the usability of the EHR.

The ability to configure order sets in ambulatory systems is not dissimilar to inpatient order entry systems. Likewise, clinical decision support rules have similar value in both settings. In the outpatient world, there is the additional uncertainty of knowing all medications a patient is taking. This is a topic of considerable conflict in organizations with shared charts. Some specialists object to seeing the full list of medications in their chart, fearing responsibility for drugs they do not prescribe. Of course, this is an issue of legal liability, not medical care. But it can require system managers to jump configuration hurdles before specialists will buy in to a common EHR.

In 2005,[19] The Joint Commission made "medication reconciliation" one of its national patient safety goals. They require that at transitions of care, providers exchange a complete list of the patient's medications. They explicitly include discharge to ambulatory settings. A shared EHR should make this process easier, if not automatic, with the record itself. But the pass-off between EHRs will require a substantial improvement in state of the art interfacing technologies. While technically feasible, today, few systems support this kind of automated reconciliation. The Joint Commission based its recommendation on staffing and process models from the inpatient world,[20] and implementing their ideas outside of hospitals has proven difficult.

Analogous to diagnosis-related group (DRG) reimbursement in inpatient settings, one of the more complex features in ambulatory order entry is "medical necessity" checking. The quotation marks here are to emphasize that the definition of medical necessity is an insurance construct, not a clinical assessment per se. The primary impetus for this requirement comes from Medicare. Through a process called National and Local Coverage Determinations (NCD/LCD – previously called Local Medical Review Policies [LMRP]), Medicare will only reimburse for tests that it deems medically necessary.[21] Since these rules frequently do not meet the needs of individual patients, physicians need to be alerted when they are ordering a test that is not covered. For example, a patient with cancer might need heart tests prior to taking a cardiotoxic drug. It would be clinical malpractice *not* to perform the test, but it may still not be considered "medically necessary" financially.

There are two major reasons to generate NCD/LCD alerts. The first is the intended effect of the regulation: to draw attention to the physician that the test or drug may not be clinically indicated and an alternative should be sought. The second reason is to alert both patient and provider that charges will go unpaid by the carrier. For providers, particularly laboratory and radiology facilities, this can be a key source of uncollected debt. The ordering provider should give the patient an ABN (advance beneficiary notice), which alerts patients how much they are likely to be charged for what the payer may deem unnecessary.

The process for documenting medical necessity is fairly crude. The diagnostic code (typically International Classification of Diseases [ICD-9]) the physician associates with the order (typically coded by CPT®) either matches an approved list designed by the NCD/LCD or it does not. Practices that are very focused on downstream revenue may seek even more sophisticated alerts to question providers who order tests with codes that they may incorrectly be using as "rule outs" rather than using symptom codes. This is presently at the boundary of commercial system functionality.

The last major category of order entry functionality is referrals. These are similar to inpatient consult orders but are a great deal more complex due to third-party reimbursement rules and geographic variation inherent to outpatient care. In many managed care plans, the ordering provider is supposed to solicit an eligibility and pre-approval code before sending a patient to another specialist. Some systems automate this process to some extent, but the rules and documentation requirements are quite variable, making full automation very difficult. If providers find themselves or their staff spending hours soliciting these approvals, executives would be wise to spend as much time renegotiating contracts to simplify and standardize these procedures as they might trying to get the IT staff to automate a chaotic process.

In an ideal patient experience, the referrals can be linked to the scheduling process. This is quite plausible if the order entry system is integrated with the scheduling system and the payer rules allow for such simplification. In reality this kind of service is most likely to be found only in highly integrated care delivery systems, regardless of their IT infrastructure.

DOCUMENTATION

While results reporting and order entry remain the core of many EHRs, the key to the ambulatory medical record is documentation—particularly physician documentation. This is also the most technically difficult challenge for any medical record system for several reasons. The major challenges in medical informatics generally come together in physician documentation. User interface design, workflow management, structured vocabulary, database performance and hardware limitations are all major limiting factors to what we can practically deliver to support the most elemental component of medical care: the doctor-patient interaction.

As with results reporting and order entry efforts already discussed, the first efforts to automate physician documentation were modular. Specific attempts to capture a progress note, a procedure note, a Simple Object Access Protocol (SOAP) note, or a flow sheet have had varying degrees of success. The simplicity of scribbling pen on paper exceeds any EHR, though an EHR can provide legibility, practice standardization, ubiquitous access and clinical decision support.

There is a profound and complex number of nuanced features that need to be added together to build a fully functioning ambulatory documentation system. Not all of these features are needed for every practice or every specialty. Nevertheless, they may be essential to even a single physician in a group, so failure to accommodate the requirement may eliminate the ability to automate that physician in the EHR. This is a key point that is lost on many IT managers and is worth exploring.

There is a difference between essential and non-essential customization. Detailing the many essential and optional functionality offerings in ambulatory systems is beyond the scope of this chapter. More comprehensive lists are readily available elsewhere.[1,6,22,23] Some of the features that illustrate the difference between critical and extraneous customization vary by specialty or setting.

Drawing is a basic element of some physician documentation, such as ophthalmology, that is completely absent in some specialties. Similarly, photography is essential in plastic surgery but optional in most general internal medicine practices. Flow sheets are the primary method of documenting in some specialties, particularly those with repeated visits over a finite period of time, such as obstetrics or in practices focused on a particular disease or procedure, such as diabetes or dialysis. Many "disease management" systems focus on this kind of documentation. Some practices have extensive forms completion requirements, such as general pediatrics or practices with heavy managed care oversight, such as cognitive psychology. Similarly, specialists who perform procedures have very different documentation requirements than those doing evaluation and management. In academia, the ability to extract data generated at the point of care into research databases is critical to the research mission over and above immediate clinical needs. Consultation-heavy practices require robust correspondence support. Any practice with a wide referral base outside the EHR user base will require a scanning system to handle paper brought into the office, while practices that are completely self-contained will have little need for this feature. Practices using physician extenders or supervising residents and students will have complex co-signature requirements.

These kinds of features differentiate systems that can succeed in particular practices and specialties from those that might actually harm productivity by forcing the implementation of a parallel system that works around the oversights. The challenge for the executive is to differentiate these essential business functions from optional features that may slow down implementation and run up costs.

The key to understanding which features provide value and which do not is to examine workflow. This is where systems that deliver functionality in modules reach their limits. All the features in the world can be present in a system, but if they do not hang together for the users in a manner that flows logically within real world use, then the system may cause more harm than good. The National Institute for Standards and Testing (NIST) and CCHIT have published certification requirements that detail the functionality an AEHR should achieve.[24,25] But these requirements say nothing about how the functions work together to achieve a manageable workflow. The Apple Newton introduced amazing new functionality but was practically unusable, so it failed in the marketplace. The unwritten requirement is that all these functions work for the physician without slowing him/her down or compromising his/her sanity.

EHR enthusiasts try to sell these inherently inefficient modular systems by emphasizing the myriad benefits that occur downstream once the initial penalty is paid. These downstream benefits are real and profound. They start with simple legibility, simplified filing and access and the ability to use one data entry point for multiple purposes, such as a progress note and a consultation letter.

These benefits are the essential foundation upon which most present office automation efforts are currently justified. But executives looking for ambulatory solutions today need not stop there. The greatest potential of these systems comes when they can predict where the user will go next and lead the provider through the visit. This is exactly the opposite of a modular system in which the provider may have to disrupt the workflow to search for different functions.

This is beyond the current state of the art in commercial clinical systems. Still, it is where today's executive should be looking when deciding what is needed.[26] Workflow analysis quickly leads to the recognition that system integration is required to make sure data flow in a coordinated manner.

Through the examination of workflow, four additional key functions of clinical systems that go beyond any individual "module" are revealed as essential to the system architecture: messaging, interfaces, decision support and patient data entry.

Messaging

Messaging could, perhaps, be viewed as a module itself. Indeed, if a practice had limited funding, the cheapest and easiest system to implement to increase efficiency would be an instant messaging system. But within a full-featured EHR, clinical messaging can become the central task management tool of a practice. The key difference is the ability to route a message within the context of a patient's chart. This context extends the physician's capacity to utilize support staff, freeing the physician for more productive work. Leading products categorize messages into multiple queues such as new results, orders awaiting co-signature, messages from colleagues and even personal notes about tee times. Messages can go to multiple staff at once to work down a queue and can be rerouted during vacations or for on-call coverage.

Some systems clearly separate messaging from task management. In larger practices, this is probably wise. As the physician workflow progresses along the patient encounter, a variety of tasks queue for the ancillary staff, such as rooming and taking vitals, drawing blood, and processing referrals. How elegantly these processes are integrated with the system will dictate the success of managing the entire practice workflow rather than just isolated pieces of it.

Secure messaging is generally inherent within a given EHR. Communicating between EHRs and over the Internet generally requires different technology, lacking from most existing systems. Communicating with patients through a secure portal is clearly preferred over e-mail and is becoming a standard among top-tier practices.

Interfaces

Interfaces are the glue between modules of non-integrated systems and the mechanism for sharing data across entirely dissimilar systems. The richness and complexity of interfaces is more than enough of a topic for a whole book in itself. The key points executives need to understand about interfaces in ambulatory systems relate to what interfaces can and cannot accomplish and what buzzwords to look out for.

A purely stand-alone system requires no interfaces. Such systems are not uncommon in a small ambulatory setting, though they are quite limited in functionality. We have already reviewed the key administrative interfaces required for practice management. Electronic linkages to insurance companies are mandated by HIPAA (Health Insurance and Portability and Accountability Act of 1996), and federal "meaningful use" guidelines require some interoperability, so the era of stand-alone systems is clearly coming to a close.

Early efforts at interfaces were so-called point-to-point custom interfaces that required coding far too extensive for all but the largest ambulatory providers. In 1979 the American National Standards Institute (ANSI) chartered the Accredited Standards Committee (ASC) X12 "to develop uniform standards for inter-industry electronic interchange of business transactions—electronic data interface (EDI)." In the past 30 years, that body has developed more than 300 business-to-business transaction sets.[27]

In the late 1980s, healthcare joined the EDI standardization process with the creation of HL7 (Health Level 7), a set of semantic standards for exchanging data between healthcare information systems. HL7 was accredited by ANSI in 1994.[28] These standards define many of the key transactions that are necessary to implement clinical and practice management systems. Besides the basic insurance transactions, ambulatory systems generally rely on ADT/Registration and scheduling interfaces, as well as clinical integration with laboratories, radiology systems, transcription providers and pharmacy systems. Other common interfaces include a wide variety of diagnostic devices such as endoscopes, spirometers, EKG systems and similar equipment associated with individual specialties.

Anyone attending to practice workflow quickly realizes that more and better interfaces are critical to physician efficiency.[29] And just as quickly, the deficiencies of current interface standards are revealed. The problems are not dissimilar from those faced in inpatient settings, but the emphasis is typically different.

The first problem is the need for multiple interfaces itself. Interfaces are rarely "plug and play" and even once implemented, they generate error queues and exceptions that require policies, procedures and staff resources to handle. In a large healthcare system, an interface group may be dedicated to these issues. In a small ambulatory practice, this is often impossible and the errors either will go uncorrected or the interface is eliminated.

Ambulatory practices within larger institutions face a related problem of scale. While large IT shops may have the staff to handle implementation and error queues, the priorities of integrating a single obscure medical device may be quite low compared to a new laboratory feed for the whole hospital. But without that device, the single physician or practice cannot do his/her job. For example, it may be easier for a whole hospital to do without an interface to a spirometer than for an allergist or pulmonologist in their private office.

The problem rests in the interfaces themselves. As mentioned earlier, HL7 is primarily a *semantic* standard. It dictates what the message means, not how it is said. There are two problems left unsolved. First, the semantic standards are quite limited. HL7 covers the basics only, and even there enormous flexibility remains such that two vendor systems can both be "compliant" and not be able to understand one another. Second, HL7 does not standardize how messages are sent. This is called *syntax*. HL7 has integrated a widespread syntactic standard called XML into its new standards, which should help ease this problem, though adoption is far from complete.[30]

Presently a debate is raging about the best way to combine semantic and syntactic standards. This has tremendous relevance to executives interested in ambulatory systems. The key argument is between advocates of comprehensive detail versus ubiquitous simplicity. It is not completely unfair to characterize this as a battle between the haves and the have-nots.

Those who have wide-ranging systems with rich feature sets need comprehensive standards to move data between systems. Some of the features laypeople desire or even expect from clinical systems require extremely advanced interfacing techniques. Consider the perfectly reasonable expectation that a patient's laboratory results or medication list should be able to move from physician to physician. To do this without any loss of information would require that we agree to use far more sophisticated semantic standards that include vocabularies for lab tests and medications. As mentioned earlier, vocabularies like LOINC and the RxNorm system are not comprehensive or adaptable enough for use in all settings, so even if they were widely adopted, local customizations would be the norm, adding even more complexity to the interfaces.[31]

Those who have fewer resources, or are just trying to get into the game, are willing to settle for far simpler standards. In 2006 a competing standards-making body proposed a much simpler standard than HL7—ASTM CCR[32] (continuity of care record)—which was embraced by the American Academy of Family Physicians (AAFP). The CCR takes a "snapshot" of patients at transitions of care in an XML document standard. Semantic details are optional, allowing for the basic transmission of information which advocates call "good enough" and critics view as the lowest common denominator. AAFP's first criterion for EHR-related activities is affordability. They are also articulate in advocating plug-and-play compatibility and avoiding "vendor lock."[33] This is largely in reaction to what many perceive as the opposite tendency in HL7. Ironically, while some consider HL7's complexity specifically designed to serve vendor interests, many vendors themselves set up their own advocacy group separate of HL7 in 2004, the HIMSS Electronic Health Record Vendor Association (EHRVA) with promotion of "extensibility to other document types and discrete data" as an explicit goal.[34]

Some reconciliation of these standards has occurred. But the arguments behind this debate are inherent to any standards-making discussion. Standards enable some functions at the expense of flexibility to do other things. Understanding the motives of various vendors who support different standards in different ways is important to determine if they will meet your needs in the long run.

Another HL7 standard, called CCOW (Clinical Context Object Workgroup), shows promise for ambulatory centers in that it can help avoid other costly interfaces altogether. CCOW is a standard for flipping between different applications without requiring a new log on and even carrying the existing patient context. Therefore, a user can move from a laboratory results reporting system to a documentation or order entry system with a few clicks. The actual data stay in each system and cannot flow between them without building specific interfaces. But for sites that lack the resources to deal with all the complexity just described, CCOW may offer enough of the illusion of integration that physicians can still get their work done.

Decision Support

Most modern clinical systems have some form of a rules and alerts engine to improve quality, revenue and compliance. The extent to which data flow across modules dictates the sophistication possible in the delivery of alerts. The simplest systems are passive and post-hoc. They take data already created and analyze them in batch form, generating reports or messages to be responded to after the fact. Such systems remain important today, as we will always want to look backwards or across encounters for diverse reasons, such as drug recalls or auditing.

Modern systems also allow for real-time alerts that can actively modify how care is delivered. A modest amount of research has demonstrated or suggested the efficacy of computerized alerts in improving a variety of quality measures such as vaccination and screening tests,[35,36] reducing over-utilization[37,38] and avoiding adverse events.[39,40] Serious issues remain to be resolved that executives need to understand as this technology is pursued in the future. For example, overwhelming physicians with too many alerts can be counterproductive.[41] Too little research has been done on the relevancy of alerts in subspecialties and in patients with complex comorbidities. The maintenance of the knowledge base that drives complex alerts is costly and potentially dangerous if not done correctly.[42]

Ambulatory systems managers may consider starting with whatever alerts can be purchased in a subscription form, so that the knowledge base is easy to maintain. Drug interactions, medical necessity rules, and formulary lists are some examples of commercially available rule sets. Even some of these will require configuration resources to work optimally. For example, drug-disease interactions will require that problems and lab results are coded in a particular way that the rules engine can detect.

Another area to investigate is pay-for-performance guidelines to which providers are subject in your practice. Another chapter in this book expands on quality issues in greater detail. A few points regarding ambulatory systems are worth reiterating here. First, payers are evaluating performance primarily based on claims data. These data are fraught with peril.

In two samples at our institution, data from the payers were found to be incorrect for more than 90 percent of the patients. Since payers are cutting reimbursements and ranking physicians based on these data, the ability to analyze your actual performance may become critical to maintaining revenue. Such analyses can be quite difficult unless you have highly structured data and excellent documentation compliance from your providers.

Consider the following typical ambulatory quality metrics:

1. Percentage of patients with congestive heart failure currently taking an angiotensin-converting enzyme inhibitor (ACEI) or angiotensin-receptor blocker (ARB).
2. Percentage of diabetic patients with a glycohemoglobin measurement within the past 6 months.
3. Percentage of hypertensive patients with an ophthalmology exam within the past year.
4. Patients older than age 65 years with pneumococcal vaccination.

Performance on all four metrics could be improved with an alert to the provider at the point of care. Further, it is likely that, at some point, a patient could trigger all four alerts, therefore making it easier for the provider to comply than to ignore the alert. This presents the system manager with several technical challenges. First, all the diagnoses need to be coded with sufficient specificity that the correct patients are identified. Second, the laboratory, medication, vaccination and ordering data need to available in a form that includes and excludes the correct patients. Do you want providers to have to slow down and explain to the computer why a particular patient with a particular potassium or renal condition should not get an ARB? If the insurance company is going to make the physician say so, then it is probably worth the effort. If not, it is probably worth coding this out of the alert. Does your system capture enough data from events outside your practice to reliably know if a patient did or did not see the ophthalmologist?

In many instances, payers have access to a broader set of data than the physician caring for the patient. Also payers may be missing data that doctors would like to know is missing—such as the failure to fill the prescription for the ARB or breaking the ophthalmology appointment.

At this time, few systems can respond to all the issues raised by pay-for-performance and quality management initiatives. However, much of the mandated reporting to date has been just to report the performance data, even when they are poor. So, once again, the best the executive can do is learn about the technical issues involved and plan for the optimal combination of solutions for your practice.

Patient Data Entry

The final workflow-optimizing technology to discuss is patient data entry (PDE). Here again, separate modules may exist to give patients questionnaires, allow them to sign consents and authorizations online, or even conduct clinical interviews. Once this technology is integrated into the full EHR, the power to radically alter physician workflow becomes apparent.

If patients can record their complaints; family, social, and past medical history; and review systems online prior to meeting with the physician, several positive consequences will result. Computerized interviews provide more data, allow for asking more sensitive questions, give patients more time; can be adapted for language, hearing impairments, and education level; and when fed into the EHR, they can lower the amount of time physicians spend documenting.[43] Further, by obtaining structured data before the patient is seen, these systems provide clues the computer needs to present physicians with the most appropriate content and structure for their own workflow.

Although these systems are still at the cutting edge of clinical computing today, the very first computer applications for medicine—a half century ago—were patient interviewing tools.[44,45] Clearly the goals of those systems remain compelling today. With the adoption of patient portals rapidly accelerating, these kinds of techniques should become easier. Managers still need to decide individually when the technology will be mature enough to add value ready for their practice.

Infrastructure. The infrastructure issues for ambulatory systems are also similar to inpatient systems but different in emphasis. The scale of ambulatory systems varies from single physician offices to large multi-state groups with thousands of providers. Obviously very different technologies are needed to serve these different constituencies.

Regardless of size, one of the most fundamental questions that needs to be answered early is the degree to which integration is desired in technology and content. Some vendors provide a centralized platform from which huge numbers of users can share a common chart over large geographical distances. Others distribute the systems, often replicating the chart in multiple locations when content needs to be shared. Smart, well-intentioned people can argue the pros and cons of this and a thousand other architectural differences. The key to getting the right solution for your organization is, once again, workflow.

If you know how your organization works (or should work), you can find the right system. If you share a medical record number across disparate sites, chances are you need some kind of centralized system for keeping them in sync. If not, then you do not need to solve this problem, unless you want to share other data. If you have a lot of remote rural sites with variable networking infrastructures, then a system that relies on high bandwidth connectivity is off the table. Conversely, if you are in an urban environment with immense radio interference issues, a system that relies on a crowded wireless network band may not be advisable. If workstation management presents challenges, then a thin-client architecture may be appealing. In settings without the necessary IT staff, this may add complexity rather than reduce it.

Supportability and reliability are other key issues that differ in the ambulatory world. Consider the impact of the loss of a single computer to a busy outpatient center without technical support for 24 or 48 hours. Is that acceptable? Can you afford a shorter time frame? Downtime happens, by accident or design. Does your system provide you with the back-up tools to get by for an hour, a day, a week?

Conversely, diffuse geography may put you at the mercy of an unreliable Internet provider, SaaS, or ASP. In that case your workflow may be forced to accommodate the idiosyncratic infrastructure rather than vice versa.

Interoperability with inpatient records varies in importance by practice and specialty. Security and privacy issues similarly may differ according to the interoperability of the workflow both locally (e.g., nurse and doctor charting on the same patient in the same room) and regionally (e.g., subspecialty referrals across a multi-entity organization).

Earlier, the monolithic versus best-of-breed decision was referenced, as well as repository-based architectures. A related dimension to consider is the segregation of transactional and reporting systems. The system that supports day-to-day operations needs to be oriented toward high speed, single patient transactions. Reporting systems generally look across patients and do not require sub-second response times. Therefore, these jobs are often separated into separate systems.

A detailed discussion of infrastructure is beyond the scope of this chapter. One rule of thumb to keep in mind is that while it may seem expensive, infrastructure is rarely a good place to skimp. Hardware is often the cheapest way to hide the inadequacies of software. But this is only true if you focus on the real bottlenecks as opposed to technical fashion or fads. When selecting infrastructure components, plan for the future but be realistic about the pace of institutional change. Otherwise you risk wasting money on capacity you will not use before it is obsolete.

COSTS AND RETURN ON INVESTMENT AND "MEANINGFUL USE"

Most physician practices now have some form of information technology, but relatively few have a full EHR.[46] Not surprisingly, practice management systems have far greater market penetration than purely clinical systems. As discussed earlier, PMSs provide a direct impact on revenue and cost control. The value of purely clinical ambulatory systems is often more abstract or delayed. Chismar and Thomas have presented an economic model of EHR adoption that illustrates how larger entities, like payers and hospitals, gain more quickly from EHRs than do small providers.[47] Scrutiny of other models that show benefit from EHRs also reveal that the system benefits are greater than those to the individual physician.[48,49] That doesn't mean the value is not present, but given the large start-up costs, physicians are poorly incented to adopt systems that benefit others more than themselves—especially if system adoption costs them more than the prime beneficiaries.

At a very high level, the value of the EHR to society is potentially huge.[50] Enhanced quality, better outcomes, an improved patient experience and lower total costs are all great. But should the individual physician or practice foot the bill? There are plenty of

Barriers	Users n (%)	Imminent n (%)	Non-users n (%)
Financial			
Start up costs	210 (57.8)	82 (73.2)	515 (92.8)
Ongoing costs	205 (55.9)	84 (76.4)	489 (88.3)
Workflow			
Training & Productivity Loss	223 (60.3)	95 (84.8)	475 (85.9)
Loss of efficiency	51 (13.5)	20 (17.5)	127 (22.5)
Technical			
Lack of technical support	220 (58.1)	69 (61.1)	385 (69.8)
Lack of uniform standards	250 (68.1)	81 (74.3)	453 (82.8)
Technical limitation of systems	286 (76.9)	77 (69.4)	436 (80.4)
Privacy or Security Concerns	155 (41.0)	44 (40.0)	309 (55.3)
Personal			
Dissatisfaction with practice situation	285 (74.0)	83 (72.2)	414 (71.1)
Lack of computer skills of physician/staff	207 (54.9)	72 (63.7)	342 (61.2)
Lack of time to acquire knowledge about systems	257 (68.4)	81 (73.0)	446 (79.8)
Physician skepticism	179 (47.6)	57 (51.3)	344 (61.8)

Figure 6-3: Barriers to Health IT Adoption in Ambulatory Practices

Note: This 2009 study by Kaushal et al[51] demonstrated that imminent adopters of EHRs differ from users and non-users, with financial considerations playing a major role.

Adapted from: Kaushal R et al. Imminent adopters of electronic health records in ambulatory care. *Informatics in Primary Care.* 2009;17:7–15.

other barriers to adoption of EHRs including physician resistance to change, concerns about productivity, the complexity of installation and conversion of existing paper medical records (see Figure 6-3).[51-53]

Interest in the adoption and use of EHRs has been greatly enhanced by virtue of recent legislation. As part of the American Recovery and Reinvestment Act of 2009 (ARRA), the Obama administration introduced the Health Information Technology for Economic and Clinical Health Act (HITECH). HITECH designated billions of federal dollars to incentivize the adoption of health IT via grants for education projects that integrated EHR technology into the clinical education of health professionals, funding for strategic health IT projects and bonus payments for providers and hospitals to adopt certified health IT.

In order to promote the adoption of the EHR, the federal government designed a Centers for Medicare & Medicaid Services (CMS) bonus payment program (via Medicare and Medicaid) for both eligible providers and hospitals. The program is designed to make incentives available for five years, with early qualification leading to maximum potential monetary bonus. After 2015, the program will transition to penalties via withholding of escalating percentages of Medicare/Medicaid reimbursement. The EHR incentive program mandates that hospitals and providers use certified EHR technologies in order to qualify for bonuses. EHR certification standards and bodies, described in detail elsewhere in this book, continue to evolve via ongoing national committee work and legislation.

In addition to installing a certified EHR system, providers and hospitals must demonstrate that they are using the technology in a meaningful fashion. The now ubiquitous term "Meaningful Use" refers to this set of important behaviors. Conceptually, the Meaningful Use objectives are those behaviors or functions that promote a core set of health outcome priorities delineated by the federal government. Those key priorities include:

- Improve quality, safety, efficiency and reduce health disparities
- Engage patients and families
- Improve care coordination
- Improve populations and public health
- Ensure adequate privacy and security protections for personal health information

The detailed mechanics of the incentive programs are subject to change and are beyond the scope of this summary. In general terms, the HITECH Act mandated that the Meaningful Use objectives would be defined in stages, with escalating sophistication of objectives and behavioral thresholds. The Stage 1 Meaningful Use criteria assume the capture of clinical information in coded format, use of coded information to track key clinical conditions and coordinate care, implementation of basic clinical decision support tools, and the ability to report clinical quality measures and public health information.

In July 2010, CMS published a final legislative rule that incorporated the comments and feedback of industry experts and stakeholders.[5] This rule defines, in detail, the Stage 1 Meaningful Use requirements. The Stage 1 requirements are nicely summarized by Blumenthal and Tavenner in an editorial published in *The New England Journal of Medicine* that coincided with the publication of the final rule (see summary in Table 6-1).[54] This legislative rule defines fifteen mandatory core objectives and their associated measures. Of the remaining 10 "menu" objectives, a provider or hospital can choose to implement a minimum of five and still achieve Stage 1 Meaningful Use.

Stage 2 and 3 Meaningful Use criteria will be defined in future legislation. It is also likely that the mechanics of the incentive program and the EHR-certification process and standards will continue to evolve. Though the logistics will continue to be refined, the EHR incentive program is likely to have a profound effect on the pace and breadth of national EHR system adoption and feature development.

Money is only one barrier in a properly considered ROI equation. It remains to be seen if the incentives and penalties will be sufficient to overcome other barriers.[55] Physicians also care about quality, time, convenience, regulatory compliance and a host of other issues that must all be taken into account to truly calculate ROI. This is, of course, not feasible and the inadequacy of the literature to date reflects that fact.

For example, some studies show ROI by reducing duplicate orders.[37] Under capitation that is valid but under fee for service, one's revenue might fall. At our center, we recovered millions of dollars of revenue that was going to outside providers that our EHR very gently pointed back inside. The cost was borne by our doctors and the benefit accrued by our hospital. From a business perspective, this is a big win for the medical center, but it will not show up in academic studies of ROI. From society's perspective, this was just a cost shift and not a real reduction in the total cost of healthcare.

Other studies have shown return from up-coding, and the converse is also touted as a benefit by improving regulatory compliance.[56] Other financial benefits include reduced transcription costs, reduced chart pulls, decreased charge-posting costs, pay-for-performance and various other efficiencies.

Table 6-1: Summary of Stage 1 Meaningful Use Requirements

Summary Overview of Meaningful Use Objectives Regulations and filing requirements required to qualify for the EHR Incentive Program are available at the CMS website (www.cms.gov.)	
Core Set Objectives to be achieved by all eligible professionals, hospitals and critical access hospitals in order to qualify for incentive payments	**Measure**
Record demographics: preferred language, gender, race, ethnicity, date of birth, and date and preliminary cause of death in the event of mortality in the eligible hospital or CAH	More than 50% of patients' demographic data recorded as structured data
Record and chart vital signs: height, weight, blood pressure, BMI, growth charts for children 2-20 years	More than 50% of patients age 2 or older have height, weight, and blood pressure recorded as structured data
Provide patients with an electronic copy of their health information (including diagnostic test results, problem list, medication lists, medication allergies, discharge summary, procedures), upon request	More than 50% of requesting patients receive electronic copy of health information within 3 business days
Maintain up-to-date problem list of current and active diagnoses	More than 80% of patients have at least one entry recorded as structured data
Maintain active medication list	More than 80% of patients have at least one entry recorded as structured data
Maintain active medication allergy list	More than 80% of patients have at least one entry recorded as structured data
Record smoking status for patients 13 years old or older	More than 50% of patients 13 years or older have smoking status recorded as structured data
(EPs) Provide clinical summaries for each office visit; (Hospitals) provide electronic copy of hospital discharge instructions upon request	Clinical summaries provided to patients for more than 50% of all office visits within 3 business days; more than 50% of all patients who are discharged from an eligible hospital or CAH who request an electronic copy of discharge instructions are provided it
Implement drug-drug and drug-allergy interaction checks	Functionality is enabled for these checks for the entire reporting period
Implement capability to electronically exchange key clinical information among providers and patient-authorized entities	Perform at least one test of EHR's capacity to electronically exchange information
Implement one clinical decision support rule and ability to track compliance with the rule	One clinical decision support rule implemented
(EPs) Generate and transmit permissible prescriptions electronically	More than 40% are transmitted electronically using certified HER technology
Use computerized practitioner order entry (CPOE) for medication orders	More than 30% of patients with at least one medication in their medication list have at least one medication entered using CPOE
Implement systems to protect privacy and security of patient data in the EHR	Conduct or review a security risk analysis; implement security updates as necessary, and correct identified security deficiencies
Report clinical quality measures to CMS or States	For 2011, provide aggregate numerator, denominator, and exclusions through attestation; For 2012, electronically submit measures
Menu Set Eligible professionals, hospitals and CAHs may select any five choices from the menu list	
Generate lists of patients by specific conditions to use for quality improvement, reduction of disparities, research or outreach	Generate at least one listing of patients with a specific condition
Implement drug formulary checks	The EP/eligible hospital/CAH has enabled this functionality and has access to at least one internal or external drug formulary for the entire EHR reporting period
Incorporate clinical lab-test results into certified EHR technology as structured data	More than 40% of all clinical lab test whose results are positive/negative or numerical format are incorporated in certified EHR technology as structured data
Use certified EHR technology to identify patient-specific education resources and provide those resources to the patient, if appropriate	More than 10% of patients are provided patient-specific education resources
Provide summary of care record for patients referred or transitioned to another provider or setting	Summary of care record is provided for more than 50% of patient referrals or transitions
Submit electronic immunization data to immunization registries or immunization information systems	Perform at least one test of electronic data submission and follow-up submission, for registries that can accept electronic submissions
Submit electronic syndromic surveillance data to public health agencies	Perform at least one test of electronic data submission and follow-up submission, for public health agencies that can accept electronic submissions
Perform medication reconciliation between care settings	Medication reconciliation is performed for more than 50% of patient transitions or referrals
Additional Choices for Hospitals and CAHs	
Record advance directives for patients 65 years and older	More than 50% of patients 65 years or older have an indication of an advance directive status recorded
Submit electronic data on reportable laboratory results to public health agencies	Perform at least one test of electronic data submission and follow-up submission, for public health agencies that can accept electronic submissions
Additional Choices for EPs	
Send reminders to patients (per patient preference) for preventive and follow-up care	More than 20% of patients 65 years or older or 5 years or younger are sent to appropriate reminders
Provide patients with timely electronic access to their health information; this includes lab results, problem list, medication lists, medication allergies)	More than 10% of patients are provided electronic access to information within 4 days of its being updated in the EHR

Adapted from Blumenthal D, Tavenner M. The "Meaningful Use" Regulation for Electronic Health Records. M. *N Engl J Med.* Available at: www.nejm.org. (10.1056/NEJMp1006114). *Perspective.*

Critics of these studies abound.[57] Costs of implementation are difficult to accurately account for. Once live, there are hidden costs rarely accounted for in any analysis. Dealing with temporary employees is far more complex in an automated environment in which training is more complex and less intuitive than in the paper world. Conversely, benefits such as integrated access to reference materials or sophisticated reporting capabilities are extremely difficult to assign value to in a finite period of time. Even the cost of the software itself is hard to standardize and is almost always overemphasized as a cost relative to the much higher intangible costs such as disruption, morale effects and functional losses from system deficiencies.

For our faculty practice at Weill Cornell, we attempted to address some of these issues by looking at bottom line measures of productivity. We implemented a commercial EHR between 2001 and 2007. We compared monthly visit volume, charges and work relative value units (wRVUs) before and after each provider's EHR implementation go-live date. We also compared these data to a group of physicians who did not implement, though they had too many confounding variables to be considered formal controls. Our data matched the anecdotal impression in the industry showing that those practitioners who adopted the EHR had a statistically significant increase in average monthly patient visit volume (9 visits per provider per month), while the non-adopter cohort's visit volume was statistically unchanged. Likewise, while both groups had significant increases in average monthly charges, only the adopters showed a statistically significant increase of this in wRVUs (12 per provider per month).[58]

While these and other data suggest that EHRs do not harm productivity and probably help it, we believe the value of the EHR ultimately needs to be judged in the same way as an elevator in a skyscraper. It has become an essential tool of the trade.[59] Too few ROI analyses ask what the ROI is of the analysis itself. Like the word processor and the typewriter, e-mail and the fax machine, or cars and the horse, the EHR will come and will transform ambulatory care. Today's executives need to manage the change, not attempt to justify it.

That said, predicting the future direction of the ambulatory EHR industry is relevant. Vendors still rapidly come and go. The technology is evolving rapidly. What you buy today will be obsolete soon. Expect it and plan accordingly. Assume your vendor will change and protect your data and your investment in the knowledge it took to automate your practice. As a rule of thumb, only 20 percent of implementation costs are vendor fees. Not all of the remaining 80 percent is lost if you need to change vendors. Wise process redesign will deliver value now and in the future, independent of the specific technical platform. The delayed returns from automation will also translate from one system to the next, as they come from the EHR technology itself, not from any given brand.

The current round of vendor consolidation is marketed as a chance to increase interoperability, particularly with the biomedical devices made by the large conglomerates buying EHR vendors. But we may also see dramatic reductions in serviceability if these vendors oversimplify and cut the wrong costs. Will their size and oligopoly power destroy innovation? Consider the conflicting incentives facing just one vendor with multiple product lines and seemingly competing interests. Will a vendor that sells MRIs and EHRs support an EHR to help reduce the overutilization of expensive MRIs—a business with far more profit potential than software? Large health IT software vendors are also employers who need to control medical insurance costs. Interoperability with competitors would reduce healthcare expenditures but might cause loss of market share. How large health IT vendors balance their own internal conflicts could have as much an impact on the future of the industry as technology itself.

The technology is also hard to predict. The big problems facing informatics for the past 35 years have not fundamentally changed. The nature of the human-machine interface, the physical limits of hardware and the complexity of medical vocabulary are still problems today. The expansion of the EHR outside academia only adds new problems of scale, configurability, flexibility, complexity, control, and ever-lower fault tolerance.

The next generation EHR, evolving today, is focused on integration, standards, ubiquity, mobility, reliability, quality, outcomes and, of course, workflow. Dangers to look out for include oversimplification, information overload, alert fatigue, overdependence and depersonalization. The next generation of ambulatory care is also emerging today full of potential opportunities and dangers. And as a key part of that future, the ambulatory electronic health record is surely both an opportunity and a danger.

FREQUENTLY ASKED QUESTIONS

Q: My consultants and vendor advise me to "keep it vanilla" to stay on time and under budget, but my physicians all demand customizations that sound clinically reasonable. How do I balance these conflicting demands?

A: Customization is often the most difficult management challenge of an implementation. If you want a single EHR to span diverse specialties, then you will have to customize to some extent, unless you are comfortable with ophthalmologists and cardiologists being reduced to a lowest common denominator, which is unlikely to result in high-quality care. Conversely, yielding completely to subspecialty customization can defeat the purpose of unifying the patient record and indulge wasteful, often dangerous intra-specialty variation that high-quality institutions are trying to reduce. There is no easy answer, and the answer will change as both computer technology and medical expertise advance.

Q: We can't afford to build custom templates for every subspecialty workflow. The physicians currently dictate, but some of the ROI for the EHR is supposed to come from eliminating transcription costs. Can we use voice recognition instead?

A: Voice Recognition (VR) is perpetually three years away. Consider how the following sentence written silently might sound to a patient if it were spoken to VR instead: "The unkempt, malodorous, obese patient, appearing older than her stated age complained of an old liver." Do you want to say this in front of her? Didn't she really complain of a cold shiver?

Even if accuracy was improved, voice recognition is still expensive and time consuming to set up, slow to navigate and requires time for proofreading. In terms of long-term ROI, it produces text, not structured documentation, so the value of the data are lower, particularly in systems that otherwise offer advanced features like alerts, coding assistance, and complex reporting. Still, many physicians are accustomed to dictating their notes; for physicians who cannot type, this can be a tempting intermediate step toward a more complete EHR. Physicians who are not facile with computers will struggle just as much with voice recognition as they would a conventional EHR—so the applications are still limited. For users with upper extremity disabilities, this technology may be essential.

ADDITIONAL READING

Markle Foundation. *Connecting for Health.* Working Group on Accurately Linking Information for Health Care Quality and Safety. Linking Health Care Information: Proposed Methods For Improving Care and Protecting Privacy. February 2005. Available at: www.connectingforhealth.org/assets/reports/linking_report_2_2005.pdf.

Woodcock E. *Mastering Patient Flow: More Ideas to Increase Efficiency and Earnings.* Medical Group Management Association (MGMA); October 2003.

REFERENCES

1. Carter JH (ed). *Electronic Health Records: A guide for clinicians and administrators.* 2001 Philadelphia: American College of Physicians –American Society of Internal Medicine.
2. Leavitt M. Ambulatory Care: *IT's Emerging and Growing Fast.* HIMSS Annual Conference; Feb 14, 2005. Dallas, TX. http://www.himss.org/content/files/2005proceedings/sessions/edu007.pdf. Accessed March 19, 2006
3. U.S. Census Bureau. *The 2010 Statistical Abstract: National Data Book. Tables 160 and 162.* Available at: http://www.census.gov/compendia/statab/cats/health_nutrition/health_care_utilization.html. Last accessed July 2010.
4. American Recovery and Reinvestment Act of 2009. PUBLIC LAW 111–5—Feb. 17, 2009.
5. Medicare and Medicaid Programs. *Electronic Health Record Incentive Program.* Department of Health & Human Services/Centers for Medicare & Medicaid Services 42 CFR Parts 412, 413, 422, and 495 CMS-0033-F, RIN 0938-AP78.
6. *HIMSS Electronic Health Record Definitional Model,* Version 1.1. HIMSS Electonic Health Record Committee. Available at: http://www.himss.org/content/files/EHRAttributes.pdf. Last accessed March 2006.
7. Carpenter PC, Chute CG. *The Universal Patient Identifier: a discussion and proposal.* Proceedings: The Annual Symposium on Computer Applications in Medical Care; 1993:49-53.
8. *Social Security Numbers.* Electronic Privacy Information Center. September 2004. Available at: www.epic.org/privacy/ssn. Last accessed March 2006.
9. *Physicians at Teaching Hospitals Audits.* Available at: www.aamc.org /advocacy/library/ teachingphys/phys0040.htm. Last accessed March 2006.
10. Available at: http://www.nlm.nih.gov/research/umls/mapping_projects/loinc_to_cpt_map.html. Last accessed December 2010.
11. Zall RJ. The truth about managed care: the silent provider discount. *Managed Care Quarterly.* 2004;12(1):11-5.
12. Grossman JH, Barnett GO, Koespell TD. An automated medical record system. *JAMA.* 1973;263: 1114-20.
13. McDonald CJ, Overhage JM, Tierney WM et al. The Regenstrief Medical Record System: a quarter century experience. *Int J Med Inf.* 1999;54:225-253.

14. Stead WW, Brame RG, Hammond WE et al. A computerized obstetric medical record. *Obstet Gynecol.* 1977;49(4):502-9.

15. Clayton PD, Sideli RV, Sengupta S. Open Architecture and integrated information at Columbia-Presbyterian Medical Center. *MD Computing.* 1992;9(5): 297-303.

16. Ash JS, Gorman PN, Seshardri V et al. Computerized physician order entry in US hospitals: results of a 2002 survey. *JAMIA.* 2004;11:95-99.

17. Cutler DM, Feldman NE, Horwitz JR. US adoption of computerized physician order entry systems. *Health Affairs.* 2005;24(6):1654-63.

18. Overhage M, Perkins S, Tierney WM et al. Controlled trial of direct physician order entry: Effects on physicians' time utilization in ambulatory primary care internal medicine practices. *JAMIA.* 2001;8(4):361-71.

19. Available at: http://www.jointcommission.org/PatientSafety/NationalPatientSafetyGoals. Last accessed May 2006.

20. Rozich JD. Standardization as a mechanism to improve safety in health care. *Joint Commission Journal on Quality and Safety.* 2004;30(1):5-14.

21. Available at: http://www.cms.hhs.gov/center/coverage.asp. Last accessed March 2006.

22. U.S. Department of Health & Human Services Health Resources and Services. Administration Bureau of Primary Health Care. *Functional Requirements for Electronic Medical Records and Disease Management Systems.* Available at: http://bphc.hrsa.gov/chc/emrspecs.htm. Last accessed March 2006.

23. Drury B. Ambulatory EHR Functionality: A Comparison of Functionality Lists. *JHIM.* 2006; 20(1):61-70.

24. Test Method for Health Information Technology. Available at: http://healthcare.nist.gov/use_testing/index.html. Last accessed August 2010.

25. CCHIT Certified 2011 Ambulatory EHR Certification Criteria April 7, 2010. http://www.cchit.org/certify/2011/cchit-certified-2011-ambulatory-ehr. Last accessed July 2010.

26. East TD. The EHR paradox. *Frontiers of Health Series Management.* 2005; 22(2):33-5.

27. Schrotter FE. ASC X12 25th Birthday Celebration: 25 Years of Business to Business Accomplishments. Keynote Address. June 7, 2004 Chicago, Il. Available at: http://public.ansi.org/ANSIOnline/Documents/News%20and%20Publications/Speeches/. Last accessed March 2006.

28. Available at: www.HL7.org. Last accessed December 2010.

29. Walker J, Pan E, Johnston D et al. *The Value of Health Care Information Exchange and Interoperability.* Health Affairs Web Exclusive. January 19, 2005. http://content.healthaffairs.org/cgi/content/abstract/hlthaff.w5.10. Last accessed March 2006.

30. Mead CN. Data Interchange Standards in Healthcare IT –Computable Semantic Interoperability: Now Possible but Still Difficult. Do We Really Need a Better Mousetrap. *Journal of Healthcare Information Management.* Winter 2006: 20(1). 71-78.

31. Available at: http://www.nlm.nih.gov/research/umls/rxnorm_main.html. Last accessed March 2006.

32. ASTM Committee E31 on Healthcare Informatics.Available at: http://www.astm.org/cgi-bin/SoftCart.exe/COMMIT/COMMITTEE/E31.htm?L+mystore+kprv3048. Last accessed March 2006.

33. Available at: http://www.centerforhit.org/x174.xml. Last accessed March 2006.

34. Available at: http://www.himssehrva.org/ASP/statements.asp. Last accessed March 2006.

35. McDonald CJ, Hui SL, Tierney WM. Effects of computer reminders for influenza vaccination on morbidity during influenza epidemics. *MD Computing.* 1992;9:304-12.

36. S Shea, W DuMouchel, Bahamonde L. A meta-analysis of 16 randomized controlled trials to evaluate computer-based clinical reminder systems for preventive care in the ambulatory setting. *J Am Med Inform Assoc.* 1996;3(6):399-409.

37. Bates DW, Kuperman GJ, Rittenberg E et al. A randomized trial of a computer-based intervention to reduce utilization of redundant laboratory tests. *Am J Med.* 1999;106:144-50.

38. Harpole LH, Khorasani R, Fiskio J et al. Automated evidence-based critiquing of orders for abdominal radiographs: impact on utilization and appropriateness. *JAMIA.* 1997;4:511-21.

39. Gandhi TK et al. Adverse drug events in ambulatory care. *New Engl J Med.* 2003;348:1556-64.

40. Gurwitz JH et al. Incidence and preventability of adverse drug events among older persons in the ambulatory setting. *JAMA.* 2003;289:1107-16.

41. Weingart SN et al. Physicians' decisions to override computerized drug alerts in primary care. *Archives of Internal Medicine.* 2003;163:2625-31.

42. Koppel R, Metlay JP, Cohen A et al. Role of Computerized Physician Order Entry Systems in Facilitating Medication Errors. *JAMA.* 2005;293:1197-1203.

43. Bachman JW. The patient-computer interview: a neglected tool that can aid the clinician. *Mayo Clin Proc.* 2003;78(1):67-78.

44. Brodman K, van Woerkom AK, Erdmann AJ et al. Interpretation of symptoms with a data-processing machine. A.M.A. *Archives of Internal Medicine.* 1959;103:776-82.

45. Brodman K, Erdmann AJ Jr, Lorge I et al. The Cornell Medical Index; an adjunct to medical interview. *JAMA.* 1949;140:530-34.

46. DesRoches CM, et al. Electronic health records in ambulatory care—a national survey of physicians. *N Engl J Med.* 2008;3;359(1):50-60. Epub.

47. Chismar WG, Thomas SM. The economics of integrated electronic medical record systems. *Medinfo.* 2004;11(Pt 1):592-6.

48. Wang SJ, Middleton B, Prosser LA et al. A cost-benefit analysis of electronic medical records in primary care. *Am J Med.* 2003;114:397-403.

49. Miller RH, West C, Brown TM et al. The value of electronic health records in solo or small group practices. *Health Affairs.* 2005;24(5):1127-37.

50. Hillestad R et al. Can electronic medical record systems transform health care? Potential health benefits, savings, and costs. *Health Affairs.* 2005;24(5):1103-17.

51. Kaushal R et al. Imminent adopters of electronic health records in ambulatory care. *Informatics in Primary Care.* 2009;17:7–15.

52. Gans D, Kralewski J, Hammons T et al. Medical groups' adoption of electronic health records and information systems. *Health Affairs.* 2005;24(5):1323-33.

53. Miller RH, Sim I. Physicians' use of electronic medical records: barriers and solutions. *Health Affairs.* 2004,23(2):116-26.

54. Blumenthal D, Tavenner M. The "Meaningful Use" Regulation for Electronic Health Records. *N Engl J Med.* Available at: www.nejm.org. Last accessed July 2010 (10.1056/NEJMp1006114). *Perspective.*

55. Rosenfeld S, Bernasek C, Medelson D. Medicare's next voyage: encouraging physicians to adopt information technology. *Health Affairs.* 2005;29(4):1138-46.

56. Barlow S, Johnson J, Steck J. The economic effect of implementing an EMR in an outpatient clinical setting. *JHIM.* 2004;18(1):5-8.

57. Walker JM. Electronic Medical Records and Health Care Transformation: EMR supported health care transformation is too immature for credible estimates of its costs or benefits. *Health Affairs.* 2005;24(5):1118-20.

58. Cheriff AD et al. Physician productivity and the ambulatory EHR in a large academic multi-specialty physician group. *International Journal of Medical Informatics.* 2010;79: 492–500.

59. Goodman C. Savings in Electronic Medical Record Systems? Do It For the Quality. *Health Affairs.* 2005;24(5):1124-26.

CHAPTER 7

The Personal Health Record

Glenn Martin, MD

> The personal health record (PHR) is an electronic, universally available, lifelong resource of health information needed by individuals to make health decisions. Individuals own and manage the information in the PHR, which comes from healthcare providers and the individual. The PHR is maintained in a secure and private environment, with the individual determining rights of access. The PHR is separate from and does not replace the legal record of any provider.[1]

INTRODUCTION

This definition of a personal health record (PHR) from the American Health Information Management Association (AHIMA) can be criticized for being prejudiced as it is limited to electronic formats. It can be dismissed as grandiose, for it calls for universal access. It can even be called too optimistic as it suggests that a PHR can meet all of these goals and yet be secure and private. However, this definition is a good place to start as it highlights how the focus and expectations of PHRs have changed over the years. Initially, the PHR was a collection of paper, either completed by or maintained by the patient or a family member. As PHRs evolved to include digital forms, they were primarily seen as a patient-controlled space for which the individual could collect and collate information and ultimately decide to share all or parts of the information. It has become clearer that in terms of functionality, the value of the PHR lies in its interactions and management functions.[2] In this sense, it becomes less of a "repository" and a personally maintained health record and more a set of information and integrated tools that allow the patient to interact with providers through secure messaging, appointment scheduling, and medication refill requests, and to provide a platform within which health monitoring, incorporation of at-home medical monitoring device data, and decision support and education can occur.

While there are abundant variations on the definition, they are frequently silent on many of the key defining characteristics of the PHR. What will be the content and from where exactly will that information come? How current and accurate can the information be? How will the information enter the PHR? What will be the structure of the information, and what will hold or transmit the PHR? In fact, all of these issues are still evolving. Those discussions about the PHR should at least take place in the context of three overarching concepts:

- The players and the environment
- Trust
- Truth

THE PLAYERS AND THE ENVIRONMENT

PHRs do not exist in a vacuum. They are held, managed or controlled by patients, used by physicians and other healthcare providers, and operate in an increasingly electronic and interoperable healthcare environment. While arguably simplistic, the way these three interact with a PHR can be characterized by the following:

Patients Are Not Medical Historians

Humans constantly demonstrate that they will not always do the right thing, even when the benefits are apparent. This is especially true when they are asked to do something that will only be used infrequently and only when something bad is happening. A good example is drawing up a will or completing a healthcare proxy. In the usual situation neither is hard to do, nor are they lengthy or expensive to generate. The need for healthcare proxies is communicated to the public regularly and is a focus of patient education through the nation's hospitals. Both documents can be of great benefit, yet many people do not complete them. The same can be said of the records organizers found in most personal financial software.

A patient's ability to understand, collect and organize medical information is usually limited. The average individual cannot be expected to recognize the importance of the individual items of his/her medical history. Nor can they be expected to actively collect that information from a variety of providers and sources—some electronic, some paper-based—and keep it regularly maintained. Even if the PHR is easy to use, collecting the data from a variety of sources—many of which will still maintain or transmit the information on paper—can be tedious and ultimately incomplete.

There is at least one examination of the layperson's efforts to populate an electronic record from paper sources.[3] The authors demonstrated that accuracy of the data transfer was dependent on the type of data entry. Guided and limited fields (e.g., pull-down selections) were more accurate than data that allowed for free text entry. Not surprisingly, data entries that required more knowledge and sophistication (e.g., the medical indication for a medication being prescribed) proved to be problematic. Similarly, the layman demonstrated problems in entering lab data when units (e.g., mg/mL) were needed or the normal range for the results had to be entered in order for the test to be interpretable.

Providers Have Limited Resources, Financial and Temporal

Most providers will not invest money in systems that are neither proven nor have a readily apparent return. Money is not the only limiting factor, as providers operating in the current managed environment frequently find that their scarcest resource is time. Integration into the office workflow is a key success principle.

A study conducted in 2007 of practicing physicians in Nebraska and South Dakota is informative.[4] Of physicians who were using EHRs, 18 percent reported some of their patients were using electronic PHRs. However, only 7 percent of those same physicians reported that they used the information the patients had entered into their own PHRs. This percentage was even lower for physicians without EHRs.

Any successful PHR that requires physician input has to be inexpensive from the physician's perspective and cannot take an appreciable amount of time from a provider or staff. Ideally, it would be integrated into an existing electronic medical records system, assuming the physician or hospital already has one. This does not define the current state but does represent the government's financially incentivized future.

The American Recovery and Reinvestment Act of 2009 (ARRA) provides significant funding, approximately $34 billion, to eligible providers and hospitals to promote the adoption of health IT. To be eligible for funding, the health IT must meet certain "Meaningful Use" criteria, many of which are specifically chosen to improve care coordination and better engage patients and families in their healthcare. Among the many criteria in Stage I of the program, certain directly impact PHRs: Provide patients with an electronic copy of their health information (including diagnostics test results, problem list, medication lists, medication allergies) upon request (may be through a PHR or patient portal).

- Provide clinical summaries for patients for each office visit (may be through a PHR or patient portal).
- Enable the capability to exchange key clinical information (for example, problem list, medication list, allergies, and diagnostic test results) among providers of care and patient authorized entities electronically.
- Provide patients with timely electronic access to their health information (including lab results, problem list, medication lists, and allergies) within three business days of the information being available to the provider (may be through a PHR or patient portal).

While the criteria for Stages 2 and 3 of the program are not specified in the final rule published July 28, 2010, the rule makes clear that subsequent stages will be "focusing on decision support for national high priority conditions, patient access to self management tools, access to comprehensive patient data through robust, patient-centered health information exchange and improving population health."[5]

Thus it likely that the trend of having the provider's electronic system, or the linked HIE, do the information collection and collating, and from there, through a patient portal or direct physician to patient transfer, allow the patient access to his/her personal health information, will accelerate.

Murphy Looks Over Information Systems

Information systems are complex operations with many failure points. Inaccurate information can enter the system, the software can malfunction and the hardware can crash. Murphy's Law dictates that this will happen at the worst possible time. We will limit this discussion, however, to those times a PHR must be created, updated or accessed.

As such, a good PHR must be able to cope with system failures; in fact, it should help overcome them. A PHR accessible only on the Internet cannot work if the network is down or cannot be reached or if the server hosting the record is down. Recent events in the United States, such as Hurricane Katrina and the 2003 Northeast blackout, amply demonstrate the vulnerability of computer networks and records. A PHR that has at least some of the most pertinent information offline (e.g., on a secure flash-drive or smart card) can work without a network. In fact, it can even help repopulate a medical record if there is truly a catastrophic failure.

TRUST

An effective PHR can only work well in an environment in which trust is established, or at the very least, issues of trust are well thought out and managed. A patient will only maintain a PHR if he/she believes that the information will be securely stored and only used for his/her benefit in circumstances with his/her approval. In the current environment, patients are bombarded by reports of massive loss of private and sensitive data. Losses have occurred in the financial and service sectors by healthcare organizations and governmental agencies (see Table 7-1).

Losses have occurred via the Internet, corporate networks, and lost backup tapes and computers. The increasing use of flash drives has made it easier to download and transport stolen data. While it has made it easier to transport data for legitimate purposes, it also makes it more likely that those data will be lost or stolen. Robust encryption technology exists and is even available as open source freeware (e.g., Truecrypt). However, it frequently is not used or paired with utterly inadequate passwords.

A provider can only use the information on a PHR when he is convinced it actually pertains to the patient in front of him. The use of photo identification and incorporating biometric IDs will surely help achieve this confirmation. However, the complications of making identity matches from online data are well known and still an area of active concern. Furthermore, the provider must be assured that the information is reasonably complete and accurate and that its limitations are readily apparent (e.g., date of last update, sources of information, whether sensitive information such as HIV or substance abuse is even initially incorporated or can subsequently be masked). While it is true that these issues exist in the standard paper environment, they are amplified by the use of electronic media.

Neither the patient nor the provider will readily accept a PHR unless access control and the uses of the information are established and enforced. Recent history has taught us a clear lesson: owners of prescribing information (large pharmacy chains and pharmacy benefit managers) have sold this information to the pharmaceutical industry. While the information has been stripped of patient identifiers, the prescribing habits of individual physicians is routinely examined and used to make marketing decisions including visits and calls by the sales force. This practice, while legal, has enraged many physicians, prompted action by multiple state and national medical societies, and even prompted legislative remedies to be introduced at the state level.[8]

The Patient Privacy Rights Foundation published its first report card of PHRs.[9] By reviewing the privacy policies published on their websites, the foundation did its "best to decode PHR privacy policies and spell out what control you have over your infor-

Table 7-1: Reported Data Incidents[6]

2005
- 152 incidents and 57,700,000 records
  - 11% (17) healthcare facilities/companies

2006:
- 315 incidents and nearly 20 million records
  - 13% (41) healthcare facilities/companies

2007
- 446 incidents and 127,725,343 records
  - 14.6% (65) healthcare facilities/companies; 3.1% records 4,005,233

2008
- 656 incidents and 35,691,255 records
  - 14.8% (97) healthcare facilities/companies; 20.5% records 7,311,833

2009
- 498 incidents and 222,477,043 records
  - 13.7% (68) healthcare facilities/companies; 5.1% records 11,311,818

As of 8/4/2010
- 400 incidents and 13.144.029 records
  - 29.8% (119) healthcare/medical; 12.4% 1,636,400 records
- Home Supportive Services program

UCLA:
- June 2004 incident involved 145,000 blood donors via unencrypted laptop

MSMC:
- July 2005 incident involved more than 10,000 research patients with more than 6,000 SSN exposed
- Stolen desktop with password protected unencrypted
- Recovered and not accessed

Providence Home Services:
- January 2006 incident involved 365,000 patients via unencrypted back-up tapes

University of Pittsburgh Medical Center:
- January 2006 incident involved the demographic information of 700 patients on one of six stolen computers; medical conditions not in the file

State of Washington Health Care Authority:
- In January 2006, 6,000 health screening reminder postcards were sent to 6,000 public employees with their Social Security numbers printed on them

PricewaterhouseCoopers/University of Texas M.D. Anderson Cancer Center
- In November of 2005, the private health information and Social Security numbers of nearly 4,000 patients were compromised after a laptop containing their insurance claims was stolen from the consultants

YMCA:
- May 2006 incident involved more than 65,000 YMCA members from Rhode Island and Seekonk, Massachusetts
- Information lost on a stolen laptop included credit card and debit card numbers, checking account information and Social Security numbers
- Also lost were the names and addresses of children in YMCA daycare programs and medical information about the children, such as allergies and medicine taken

Department of Veterans Affairs:
- As many as 26.5 million veterans were placed at risk of identity theft after an intruder stole an electronic data file containing their names, birth dates and Social Security numbers from the home of a Department of Veterans Affairs employee in May 2006 (*The Washington Post*, May 23, 2006)

Table 7-1: *(Continued)*

Healthnet

- A hard drive with seven years of personal and medical information on about 1.5 million Healthnet customers was lost in March 2009 and reported in November 2009.
- Information included claims data and physician information. In July 2010 Healthnet agreed to pay the state of Connecticut at least $250,000 and implement stronger consumer protections after being sued by the state over the loss of data of more than 440,000 Connecticut members. (*New Haven Register*, July 7, 2010)

University of Texas at Arlington

- A file server at the University of Texas at Arlington was compromised four times from February 2009 through February 2010 leaving health data on 27,000 students, faculty and staff potentially exposed. The data included records of students, faculty and staff that received or filled a prescription through the Student Health Center from 2000 on. Names, addresses, prescription names, amounts spent and diagnostic codes were potentially vulnerable. (*Dallas Business Journal*; Author: Jeff Bounds; Date Published: 7/23/2010[7])

Adapted from www.IDTheftcenter.org

mation." Only one product received a grade of A, and "PHRs Offered by Employers and Insurers" received a grade of F. While the accuracy of the report is hampered by methodologic issues and reflects the clear advocacy agenda of the foundation, it does underscore the perceived unresolved issues of trust that color the PHR environment.

Patient concerns about the use of private information that affects insurability and employability have already had an impact on HIV testing and genetic testing for susceptibility to diseases (e.g., cancer, Alzheimer's dementia). Without clear protections and adequate technologic safeguards, it is likely patients will not consent to assembling a PHR—or if they do, they may edit it extensively to remove pertinent and possibly life-saving information. For example, there are potentially life-threatening medication interactions that can occur with drugs used in the treatment of HIV infection and severe mental illness. To not include these medications or mention the diagnoses in the record can actually increase the possibility of medical errors if the healthcare provider relies on the PHR when performing an interaction check before prescribing or dispensing.

There have been recent changes to the HIPAA regulations that impact PHRs.[10,11] If the PHR is maintained by a healthcare entity, then it is covered by HIPAA, with all of its associated security requirements, breach notification responsibilities and financial and criminal penalties. If the PHR is maintained on behalf of the covered healthcare entity by another party (i.e., a business associate), then the PHR is also covered by HIPAA and the business associate is directly responsible for being compliant with HIPAA security rules and is liable for civil and criminal penalties. Health information exchange (HIE) organizations that provide transmission services to covered entities are now considered business partners. This new inclusion is particularly germane as the evolution of the PHR is increasingly toward tight integration with, or data provision by HIEs. PHRs that are maintained by other businesses are not covered by HIPAA and include, for example, Microsoft HealthVault and Google Health.[12]

TRUTH

The benefits of the widespread use of PHRs to promote patient safety and speedy, accurate and cost-effective medical care are dependent on the quality of the information provided in the record. If the information is not considered reliable, it cannot be used. If it is not considered current and appropriately comprehensive, its usefulness is seriously constrained.

Is It Accurate, and What Does That Mean?

Any physician who treats a patient with multiple medical records from multiple providers knows that the information is rarely consistent. There are gaps and contradictions in the record. Patients may recall something one day to one provider and recall it a bit differently at a later date or in different circumstances. Significant family and early developmental history given to a psychiatrist is likely to be different than that given to a cardiologist evaluating chest pain. One entry of a side effect entered by a provider or a patient may very well be documented by someone else as an allergy. Not infrequently, a patient will report something to a physician who will subsequently conclude that it is not accurate. The amount of daily exercise or alcohol consumption being reported may not reflect reality. In the record maintained by the physician, this discrepancy may be noted and explained. How these entries are to be reconciled in a comprehensive record is not always clear, especially when it is the patient who has ownership and control of the PHR.

These issues of data reconciliation have been explicitly addressed by collaborations among stakeholders in the state of Illinois. One outcome has been the concept of the "Community System of Record" that would be the maintained "source of truth." Envisioned as a link between provider-maintained EHRs and PHRs, one of the functions would be "Closed-loop clinical messaging to permit the patient, providers and institutions to identify inconsistencies, lack of completeness, and potential safety issues…Each one is tracked until mutual resolution."[13]

Corrections

Occasionally mistakes will enter a record; entries can be placed in the wrong chart, information can be misread or mistyped. Other times, interpretations of findings can change. Initial readings of radiology procedures, pathology reports, and other tests can be changed in the normal course of medical care when they are reviewed by a more experienced practitioner or more information becomes available. The ability to update and correct a record but not erase the "electronic audit trail" is needed. In addition, HIPAA gives patients the right to ask for corrections and edits of their information. If the provider does not wish to amend the record, the patient has the right to have a statement of disagreement incorporated into the record. Solutions to track and incorporate these changes into shared information that populates a PHR are not obvious.

Is It Complete? Who Decides, and How Do You Let Others Know?

In a perfect world, patients would feel comfortable with all necessary information being available in their PHR, and all doctors would be comfortable feeding their information to it. This does not reflect reality. Some patients will only want to share some information because of privacy concerns, modesty, or fear of stigmatization. A patient might decide to block his/her HIV status but not know that allowing for a complete medication list—essential for maximizing patient safety by reducing medication interaction problems—actually reveals the diagnoses to a medical professional and others. How should this be recorded? Should all records be blocked from having certain information, or should a notation be made that some of the record is being voluntarily withheld? Obviously, these different scenarios have different interpretations, as a clinician might conclude that a non-answer is meaningful. Some doctors would not want to have the full diagnoses or pathology results available to all patients, as occasionally good judgment and patient preference compel less than full disclosure. Even if the information will be fully disclosed to the patient, it is likely that having it appear first in a patient portal or PHR without a face-to-face discussion would be ill-advised.

Even if the record is complete, it is reasonable for a patient to withhold certain information from certain providers. Few would challenge the reasonableness of a decision not to share a history of sexually transmitted diseases with a podiatrist being consulted for a bunion. Accepting this and implementing it are two different things, however, especially if the user interface does not allow for easy access control at such a detailed level. Not giving access at all is one thing; selecting portions of a PHR to share is a much greater technical challenge.

HOW TO STORE A PHR

Paper Records

While paper records may not fall within the definition of a PHR in an electronic age, they represent a valid alternative for many individuals (see Table 7-2). Paper has the advantage of being familiar and portable. In fact, the forms many patients are given at the beginning of an office visit to record basic health information is a rudimentary PHR. Completing a form can be done by the most unsophisticated members of the population and can be updated with minimal cost and time by anyone given access.

Paper forms have many limitations, though. Updating them is not automatic and may require a dedicated and organized family archivist. They are relatively bulky and are not likely to be carried by a patient in all circumstances where a PHR would be of value. Without access to a photocopier or scanner, there is inadequate back-up of the records, making loss or destruction very disruptive. If misplaced, the documents are easily read by the finder without need of a password or security software. Forms are generally completed with handwritten notations that may not be legible. With time, paper and ink can become difficult to read and are susceptible to environmental damage.

Paper forms are also less than ideal for integrating information from multiple sources and assembling it in an organized fashion with each update. One has only to contemplate a multi-year medication history—with repetitive scratch outs, misspelled

Table 7-2: Characteristics of Paper PHRs

• Portable and controllable (until lost)	• Too much or too little
• Not easy to collate and summarize	• Handwriting
• Never around when you need them	• Source and timeliness of information

names and illegible dosing instructions and dates—to see the limitations. Even if a record is well maintained, there is also the risk of providing too much information. Data overload at the point of care can make the information almost useless as the busy clinician cannot take the time to wade through a comprehensive notebook of information.

Computer-based Records

Clearly the equivalent of a paper history form can be placed on an individual's computer (see Table 7-3). For years, financial software has included a vital records section where one could organize the contents and locations of documents, accounts and contacts. The records remain on the individual computer but can be printed out for remote use or prepared as an electronic file for e-mail transmission. Templates for use on local computers are readily available.[14]

Table 7-3: Characteristics of Computer-based PHRs

- Need a computer and the desire to use one
- Interface has to be easy, obvious and friendly
- Still have to print it out to use it, though it could be e-mailed
- Hope the computer maven is not the incapacitated patient

Unlike paper, there are no issues with handwritten entries and illegibility. Well designed, it will allow for adequate space to enter all information in correct fields and promote ready access to both a current snapshot and a historic overview of the patient's health. Backups can be done efficiently and, at least in theory, automatically. Updates could be prompted at regular intervals, either by the software or via e-mailed reminders by healthcare providers. Security can be built into the software being used, or the files can be encrypted by readily available products.

The limitations of data entry remain paramount. The patient or family member has to have access to a computer and want to use it. The patient will have to take the time to assemble the necessary information and enter it. This will frequently require entering technical information in a jargon that is unfamiliar. Even if the jargon is not a problem, the provider who will eventually use the information must be wary of simple typos, transposition of numbers, and other transcription errors. A chronically ill patient with multiple specialists has the daunting task of frequent update.

As with paper, it will still require the patient to have a copy of his PHR with him when he visits the doctor or hospital. This requires planning, and in an emergency situation this may not be possible. If it is the computer user who is ill, remaining family members may not have ready access to the PHR and password, or have the know-how to access and print it. It is possible to e-mail the file to a physician, but unless a secure form of transmission is readily available, there are significant security risks associated with an open transmission.

Table 7-4: Characteristics of Web-based PHRs

• Same issues of data entry, unless tightly integrated with data sources • Can it import information from other systems or the individual's computer files? • Who controls it, and can you trust them? • Will they stay in business? • Need a computer and a functioning network to enter and retrieve, especially during disasters!

The Web

Many of the limitations of a PHR stored on a patient's personal computer can be mitigated by storing the information online using a Web-based service (see Table 7-4). If properly designed, data entry can be facilitated, and storing and presenting the information in a variety of sensible formats is quite feasible. The patient does not need to remember to take his/her PHR with him, as it would be available from any Internet-attached device throughout the world. Linguistic challenges can be addressed by multiple versions of the forms. For example, the patient in New York completes the form in English. If he should take ill abroad, the French-speaking physician on the Ivory Coast could call up the patient's PHR using the French template. The answers would be in English, but the French online version would at least have the questions and field names in French.

Storing the information remotely does raise a host of security concerns, as the patient is no longer the sole holder of the record. Patients are rightly concerned about the possible loss of online records. Even if not stolen, there is precedent in the online information storage business of commercial enterprises going out of business with such rapidity that records were lost before they could be retrieved by their owners.

Security for any PHR stored online or on electronic media is a balance between competing compelling concerns. The information must be secure and unusable without permission of the patient. Yet, the information has to be readily available to healthcare workers in an emergency situation in which the patient's medical condition prevents him from providing a personal identification number (PIN). Ideally, the online service provides a form of "break the glass" security in which an authenticated provider can access the record without the patient's PIN, and an audit log records the emergency retrieval.

In addition, an online storage solution is only useful if the online location is accessible at all times. This requires the practitioner to have a functioning Internet hook-up and for the storage site to be up and running. Even scheduled maintenance is a challenge; unlike financial sites that can safely do maintenance in the early hours of a weekend morning, a PHR may be needed 24/7. Finally, there are many situations for which an accessible PHR could be life-saving, but Internet access is not guaranteed (e.g., ambulances in poor wireless data service areas, disaster response and blackouts).

Devices

Over the past several years, portable storage has become both physically smaller and quantitatively larger. Increasingly flash drives and miniature hard drives are used in the business and consumer environment. Smart cards, though not as popular in the United

Table 7-5: Devices for the PHR

• Form Factors	• Considerations
– USB sticks, key chains, etc.	– Need to carry them
– CDs	– Need to update them
– Smart cards	– Need to be able to read them
– Smartphones, iPods, MP3 players	– Need to secure them from loss

States as the rest of the world and with more limited data capacity, also have their place in information storage and identity authentication. PHRs can be stored on any of these media, even if that was not their original intent. For example, most MP3 players and cell phones will also allow for a data file to be stored. Smartphones, because of their integrated functionality, will be discussed in the next section.

The advantage that this group brings to the PHR is their easy portability and large capacity (see Table 7-5). The data entry issues outlined in the previous groups remains as does the password control conundrum. To be most useful, the device has to be readable on a computer without special preinstalled software and should operate on a multitude of operating systems. Portability is a two-edged sword. By carrying the device, the patient avoids the perceived risk of online storage and can be in greater control of access to the PHR. However, the patient has to remember to carry the device and avoid its loss. In addition, the updating process is another risk point in the system, since the data will most likely have to be entered via a computer connection.

Form factor is important when considering an appropriate device. It has to encourage someone to carry the device, yet, as importantly, at the same time protect it from environmental damage. Flashdrives, while small, are not tiny. Incorporating them into key rings is a popular approach. More recently, a drive and USB interface contained within a silicon bracelet has been promoted as an alternative.

Compact disks have been distributed to patients with excerpts of their medical record. They have the advantage of holding a great deal of information and they are inexpensive; however, they generally do not allow for patient updates. To be useful in a portable format that a patient is likely to carry at all times, the smaller "business card" size CD version has to be used. Durability in a wallet remains a concern.

Smart cards represent another form that has proven user acceptance. They are the size of a standard credit card and the incorporated integrated chip's size, location and interface are governed by accepted international standards. Data storage is limited. Typical chips hold 64k, but larger chips are now available. The chips are designed to be tamper resistant and usually incorporate some form of data encryption. The chips also contain microprocessor components that allow their use as SIM cards in phones and as debit cards and identity cards. In fact, multiple uses with one card are allowed.

Hybrids. Different storage locations can be combined for increased functionality, availability and durability. A device can be used to download and store either a complete copy or an excerpt of a PHR that is primarily stored online or on a desktop computer. The device can serve as a backup, as well as a means of transporting the information to a provider here or abroad when a patient is not comfortable with electronic transmission or the physician does not have access to effective electronic information exchange. For PHRs primarily stored online, a smart card or USB device may be used as the authentication token to allow access, while at the same time storing information for those times when network access is not available.

Smartphones represent a new opportunity for PHR hosting. They provide a mechanism for local storage, as well as online access to Web-based PHRs. In addition, the information can be viewed directly on the screen, a clear advantage when pressed for time over CDs USB drives, etc. And finally, anecdotally many emergency department physicians will say that smartphones are always available. Joggers, for instance, may not be carrying their wallets when a medical emergency strikes, but they will have their phones!

There is a comprehensive assemblage of available options.[14] Information includes links to the vendors and online sites with information on pricing, etc.

Connectivity.[15,16] Stand-alone systems are characterized by a lack of direct connectivity to data sources. Data entry is generally manual and unless scanned images are uploaded, or certain medical devices are connected (blood pressure, blood sugar, peak flow, etc.), keyboard re-entry of information by the patient populates the PHR.

Other PHRs are considered tethered, usually to an individual provider or health system, or to an insurer. Access is Web-based generally through a patient portal. The source of information is typically uni-directional from the host toward the patient, though added functionality such as messaging, appointment scheduling, claim inquiry, etc., may be provided. Information from the patient is either not accepted or, if it is, it is generally segregated from the rest of the record. Data are frequently not coded or structured in a way to readily support exchange even if it is downloadable by the patient. The extent of the information is limited to the information held by the host. Insurers provide claim information, but claims information is very limited. Physicians frequently do not code for all diagnoses, and problems addressed at a given visit and "rule-out" diagnoses that are eventually discounted can make way their way into the claims record. Provider records are likely to be more complete, but unless they are robustly linked to laboratory, imaging, and prescribing data, they are also very limited.

Integrated or interoperable PHRs, while less common at the moment, hopefully represent the future state. Information will be available from a multitude of sources—providers' EHRs, laboratories, pharmacies, insurers, medical devices and the patient themselves. Data will be structured so they can be integrated within the PHR. As a result, data sources complement each other and do not needlessly overlap and obscure the information the patient needs. Ideally a patient can track and trend a laboratory value, e.g., cholesterol level, overtime no matter which physician ordered the test and which lab performed it, whether it is part of a lipid panel, a general metabolic panel, or a stand-alone test. The hosts of these PHRs are likely to be multiple. Health information exchanges are by their very nature designed to integrate and share data among providers. They are well positioned to make the information available to patients through portals and expand their data sources to include patients. Third parties, such as Microsoft HealthVault and Google Health, are also providing spaces for data to be stored and shared among insurers, medical device vendors, pharmacies, healthcare organizations and patients. For all, though, the need for interoperability standards and sustainable business models remain the challenge.

In the Field

In addition to polling users, efforts have been made to examine deployed PHRs, their characteristics and actual use. The Medical Library Association/National Library of Medicine (NLM) Joint Electronic PHR taskforce conducted an evaluation that initially located 117 unique PHRs.[17] After eliminating 26 as either defunct, not as of yet operational, or not meeting the pre-established definition of the PHR, 91 products were evaluated; 54 percent were found to be stand-alone products, while 26 percent were tethered to some form of electronic health information record maintained by an insurer or provider. Forty-three percent of the products were on some form of mobile device, but they were unable to locate products specifically catering to smartphones. Presumably some of the tethered products would be available through the smartphone browsers, even if specific applications were not developed as of yet. In general, the PHRs were free to the patient, though many were limited to plan members, care recipients, etc. PHRs that involved devices or portable media typically involved a fee. Not surprisingly, PHR vendors did charge a fee to the employers, health providers or insurance plans that then made the service available for free to their users. The librarians noted that approximately half of the PHRs evaluated offered consumer health information to their users from a wide variety of sources, with the NLM's MedlinePlus being the most frequently linked resource.

Revolution Health, founded in 2005 by AOL co-founder Steve Case, notified users of its online PHR product at the end of January 2010 that they were shutting down the product. Users were given until the end of February to logon, prepare PDFs of their records, and print them for their files. After that date, the files would be removed. The PHR model required patients to enter and maintain their record, and the fact that the information had to be converted to PDF and printed underscored the lack of interoperability. Company management cited underutilization as the reason to discontinue. The tedious manual data entry process, lack of interconnectivity with data sources, and poor usability of the product were seen as contributing to the product's demise.[18]

CONTENT AND STANDARDS

For a PHR to yield the greatest benefit, it has to have sufficient information to be useful, enough organization to allow easy access and viewing, and ideally have been built in such a way as to allow for interoperability with existing electronic medical records (EMRs). In the past few years, there have been several efforts underway to guide the development of PHRs in this direction.

The American Health Information Management Association (AHIMA)[19] advocates that individuals establish their own PHR using freely provided paper forms and various electronic formats. The suggested content for a PHR is found in Table 7-6. In addition to content recommendations, there are links to a variety of products that can help assemble, organize and hold a PHR. However, standards to promote interoperability are not provided.

ASTM Continuity of Care Record (Standard E2369-05)

The Continuity of Care Record is a standard specification that has been developed jointly by ASTM International, the Massachusetts Medical Society, the Healthcare Informa-

Table 7-6: PHR Content (adapted from AHIMA)

- Personal identification, including name, birth date and Social Security number
- People to contact in case of emergency
- Names, addresses, and phone numbers of your physician, dentist and other specialists
- Health insurance information
- Living wills and advance directives
- Organ donor authorization
- A list and dates of significant illnesses and surgeries
- Current medications and dosages
- Immunizations and their dates
- Allergies
- Important events, dates and hereditary conditions in your family history
- A recent physical examination
- Opinions of specialists
- Important tests results
- Eye and dental records
- Correspondence between you and your provider(s)
- Permission forms for release of information, operations and other medical procedures
- Any information you want to include about your health—such as your exercise regimen, any herbal medications you take and any counseling you may receive.

tion and Management Systems Society, the American Academy of Family Physicians, the American Academy of Pediatrics and the American Medical Association. As stated in the scope of the standard, "The Continuity of Care Record (CCR) is a core data set of the most relevant and timely facts about a patient's healthcare.[20] It is to be prepared by a practitioner at the conclusion of a healthcare encounter in order to enable the next practitioner to readily access such information. It includes a summary of the patient's health status (e.g., problems, medications, allergies) and basic information about insurance, advance directives, care documentation and care plan recommendations. It also includes identifying information and the purpose of the CCR. It is intended to foster and improve continuity of patient care, reduce medical errors, improve patients' roles in managing their health and assure at least a minimum standard of secure health information transportability."[21]

This standards effort addresses both the content of information in the record as well as the format of the CCR. Specifically, the content is designed to be machine- and human-readable. The content is envisioned as being entered by the provider with the idea that the information would be used and updated by other providers when they render care at the time of a transfer or consultation. Additionally, the information would be available to the patient as a record of recent care.

The CCR core data set consists of three parts:

- **The header:** It contains basic information about the source and use of the information. It includes a unique CCR identifier from the provider, the date/time the record is written, the name of the patient, from and to fields, and the purpose of the record (e.g., transfer, discharge, patient record). The identifiers

Table 7-7: Continuing Care Record Core Data Set

• Insurance	• Medical Equipment
• Advance Directives	• Immunizations
• Support	• Vital Signs
• Functional Status	• Result
• Problems	• Procedures
• Family History	• Encounters
• Social History	• Plan of Care
• Alerts	• Healthcare Providers
• Medications	

are nether universal patient or provider identifiers, though nothing in the standard precludes their use should they be established and accepted.

- **The body:** It contains patient administrative/demographic and clinical sections. Highlights of the content are found in Table 7-7. The content is comprehensive, yet generic. Clinical extensions are planned to allow for more specificity in different clinical situations. HIV and Ob/Gyn extensions are currently being developed.
- **The footer:** It contains detailed information about the "actors," that is, essentially any person or organization mentioned in the record. Details about any external sources referenced in the CCR will also be included here (e.g., the location of a healthcare proxy). Free text comments that do not fit into the defined content field in the body can be entered here. Finally, there is a location for all needed digital signatures.

Interoperability

When the CCR is presented on paper, the only mandated structure is the inclusion of the core data elements. When used in an electronic format, strict adherence to a W3C XML schema and the associated Implementation Guide is required. The syntax is not specific to healthcare. There is a prohibition of the use of XML tag attributes to contain data. All data in the CCR must be tagged. Both of these decisions were made to make the CCR consistent with the general computer industry and Internet practice. All of the XML and tags within the CCR are human-readable as well as machine-readable, and the CCR stores human-readable text as text strings or structured data.

By building the CCR as a collection of discrete data elements, the information can be viewed, sorted, filtered and otherwise organized without changing the content or the integrity of the data. By using the appropriate XML syntax, the CCR can be read in a Web browser, an XML-aware cell phone or an XML-enabled word processing document. It also allows the data elements to be reused by others as it facilitates incorporation into other medical records (even those otherwise incompatible with the source EMR) and data exchange repositories.

Harmonization

Like ASTM, Health Level Seven, Inc. (HL7)[22] is another standards developing organization (SDO) accredited by the American National Standards Institute (ANSI). As part of its mission to "create standards for the exchange, management and integration of electronic healthcare information," HL7 has approved Clinical Document Architecture (CDA), Release 2.0. The CDA is a document architecture standard designed to represent medical legal healthcare encounter documents in a standardized format using XML. As such, it is a standard looking at a large variety of healthcare documents—and not just the CCR. To facilitate wide acceptance and promote industry-wide functionality and interoperability, HL7 and ASTM have a memorandum of understanding (MOU) in place to coordinate efforts to harmonize the CDA and CCR. Out of these efforts should evolve the ability for the seamless transformation of CDA XML syntax to CCR syntax with no data loss.

Additional efforts are underway to coordinate security standards for these portable XML formats. Both ASTM and HL7 are working with a third ANSI SDO National Council for Prescription Drug Programs to harmonize the needed standards for E-prescribing (SCRIPT).

However, even with these efforts at harmonization, the entire issue of controlled medical vocabularies remains a continuing source of frustration to achieving full interoperability. This is well laid out in the following excerpt from the Center for Healthcare Information Technology:

> To reach true data interoperability, vocabularies and semantic interoperability need to be defined and *tightly* controlled. The CDA (Version 3, under development) and the CCR are designed to support detailed semantic interoperability. There is a lack of definition, agreement and constraint, however, on existing healthcare vocabularies within the healthcare industry, which prevents CDA (Version 3, under development) and the CCR from providing constrained (interoperable) semantics. ASTM, HL7, NCPDP and X12 are all coordinating efforts with SNOMED (Systemized Nomenclature of Medicine) and other entities to define interoperable vocabularies and semantics. Note that this involves constraining and controlling the unfettered use of vocabularies and the explosion of terms within vocabularies as much as defining vocabularies. The lack of vocabulary standardization, and even more importantly, constraints, is a critical barrier to overall healthcare standard harmonization and true interoperability.[17]

USERS' AND POTENTIAL USERS' VIEWS, USAGE PATTERNS AND OUTCOMES

Over the past several years, online surveys have been conducted to assess the current use of PHRs and the American public's likelihood of adopting them. One of the first studies was conducted in spring 2003 by the Foundation for Accountability on behalf of the Connecting for Health Initiative of the Markle Foundation.[23]

The survey solicited more than 1,200 online households. Key results are as follows:

- Only 1.5 percent had a PHR on their computer, and an additional 0.5 percent had a PHR online.

- People with chronic illness were more likely to say they would use a PHR than other respondents (65 vs. 58 percent, respectively).
- More than 60 percent of respondents would use one or more of the following features: e-mail communication with their physicians, tracking immunizations, check for errors in their records, transfer information to a new physician, and getting and tracking test results.
- More than 60 percent of the respondents felt that a PHR could achieve one or more of the following aims: better understanding of physicians' instructions, preventing errors, getting more control of their care, helping patients ask better questions, and changing how patients take care of themselves.
- More than 90 percent of respondents answered that they were very concerned about security of their PHR, though only 25 percent said they do not use a PHR because of these concerns. More than 40 percent of healthy respondents would not want lab results online because of security concerns.
- More than 90 percent of respondents felt that their medical providers and hospitals should be able to access their PHR, but only 65 percent felt the same about their insurance companies. Interestingly, 58 percent of respondents were comfortable with their physician hosting the online PHP, but only 15 percent felt that way about their insurance plan and even fewer (12 percent) wanted the government as the host.

Another poll conducted in the fall of 2005 revealed similar results. Approximately 60 percent supported the creation of an online PHR and would use it for the purposes outlined earlier. Approximately 20 percent would not use such a service.[24]

More recently, an online poll was conducted of 2,000 general consumers by Health Industry Insights, an IDC company.[25] The poll took place November/December 2005 and had a 55 percent response rate. The poll shows how few people are actually using PHRs and some of the obstacles to widespread acceptance:

- Only 17 percent have used a paper or electronic PHR.
- 52 percent have not even heard of a PHR.
- Of those without a PHR, more than 80 percent are uncertain when they would start using one.
- Of those with some form of PHR, 60 percent are on paper, 28 percent on their computer, and only 5 percent are Internet-based.
- If a health plan offered a PHR with data sharing with providers, more than 57 percent of respondents would prefer to "opt-in" to data sharing, while 26 percent would be comfortable with an "opt-out" design.
- 62 percent were comfortable with having a "complete" PHR, with others expressing a reluctance to include sensitive lab results or mental health and substance abuse records.

The California HealthCare Foundation commissioned Lake Research Partners to conduct an online national consumer study on health IT from December 18, 2009, through January 15, 2010.[26] A total of 1,849 adults nationwide took part and findings pertinent to PHRs were:

- 44 percent of respondents or their family members maintain some records of the medical history, treatments, medicines or other health information.

    - 4 percent are solely computer based
    - 14 percent are a mix of paper and computer files.
- 7 percent have used a website to get, keep or update their health information.
    - 26 percent used a site sponsored by the healthcare provider
    - 51 percent used a health insurance plan sponsored site
    - 13 percent were unsure
    - 4 percent were employer sponsored
- In a shift from the 2003 survey results, a little over one-third of respondents would be interested in a site sponsored by a non-profit or a "government group like Medicare," only 25 percent were interested in a site sponsored by a "company like Google or Microsoft or their employer", and 58 percent were interested in sites sponsored by their physicians and 50 percent from their insurers.
- 41 percent of non-PHR users were somewhat or very interested in using such a website for themselves, while 48 percent of caregivers were interested for the person the help provider cared for, yet 61 percent of non-users agreed that they "don't need this (a PHR) to handle my health needs."
- More than 70 percent of non-PHR users endorsed that they "would be worried about the privacy of their health information if it were online," and even 40 percent of website PHR users were very/somewhat worried about the privacy and confidentiality of their information.
- Online PHR users did feel there were healthcare benefits:
    - 56 percent of PHR users say they now know more about their own health
    - 40 percent say they were compelled to ask a question they would not otherwise have asked.
    - 38 percent feel more connected to their physicians.
    - 32 percent did something to improve their health.

The study by Zhou et al. on the health benefits of the secure e-mail feature of the robust suite of online services found at Kaiser Permanente's tethered online patient portal[27] provides some evidence to collaborate the healthcare benefits users reported in the previous survey. Conducting a retrospective examination of e-mail use and Healthcare Effectiveness Data and Information Set (HEDIS) criteria for diabetes, hypertension, or both, they found that two years after implementation approximately 25 percent of all members in the region with access to the portal had registered for its use, and 7.2 percent had used secure physician-patient e-mail. They evaluated 35,000 patients versus matched controls. The authors concluded, "For patients with diabetes and hypertension, the use of secure patient-physician e-mail was associated with an increased likelihood that patients would meet each of the nine HEDIS measures. In addition, when compared to matched controls, the use of e-mail was associated with a 2.0–6.5 percentage-point improvement in HEDIS performance." It must be noted that this real-world study is limited by its inability to completely control for self-selection biases, nor could it control for other features of the portal including reminders, access to lab results and patient instructions. In other words, perhaps the "better" more adherent patient is more likely to use the portal and e-mail in the first place. Or, it was not the e-mail per se, but the whole package of features that was associated with the better outcome. In either case, there is support that the use a robust portal/tethered PHR helps the engaged user improve health outcomes.

Cleveland Clinic's experience with use of their eCleveland Clinic MyChart is also informative.[28] At the time of their study, 63,295 people had registered for the free tethered PHR. Of those, 12,101 (19 percent) had never logged onto the system after registration. Registered users were more likely to be Caucasian and married than registered never-users. The researchers concluded that other factors, e.g., physician or family encouragement, computer skills, etc. which were not examined in this study are probably more important to explain the decision to first use the system. However, the study did find a robust correlation between the number of diagnoses listed in the problem list, as well as the number of clinical encounters with the number of total logins and the frequency of use. Not surprising, the sicker patients were more likely to use the system more frequently. This bears out some of the survey data and common sense: healthy people are less likely to see the need for using a PHR and will use it less frequently.

While it appears that a majority of Americans see the utility of a PHR, at least in theory, few have actually established one in any form. This number has increased over the years but it has clearly lagged behind the general acceptance of online living, be it e-mail, social networking, commerce or banking. The vast preponderance of people continue to have security and trust concerns. This leads many to limit (1) where they would allow their records to be stored—there is clear preference for Web-based PHRs to be sponsored by providers, followed by insurers; (2) what they would want in those records—approximately 15 percent of adults say they would hide something from their physician if they knew the information would be shared, even without identifiers, and another 33 percent say they would consider withholding information; (3) and who they would allow to access their PHR—only 31 percent would feel comfortable sharing information without identifiers with health insurance plans, researchers, companies, and others.[26] Some of these decisions would limit the usefulness of the PHR, and/or the business model to support them, and underscore the need to address these concerns head-on if this tool for patient safety and better medical outcomes is to be widely adopted.

A CASE STUDY: SMART CARDS AT THE QUEENS HOSPITAL NETWORK

History and Design

The Queens Health Network (QHN) consists of the two public hospitals and multiple affiliated clinics in the borough of Queens, New York City. The borough has a population of nearly two million people and is widely considered to be the most ethnically diverse county in the United States. By the nature of their public mission, the city hospitals have an obligation to treat all comers regardless of their ability to pay. As a result, the city hospitals treat a disproportionate number of undocumented residents and transients with questionable "official" documents who historically have shown a certain fluidity of identity based on immigration, criminal and insurance pressures. In addition, there are immigrants from more than 100 countries speaking more than 150 languages and dialects in Queens County—more tongues than are spoken at the United Nations. No matter how extensive the translation services available on-site at the hospitals or readily accessible by phone are, the production of a clear comprehensible medical summary at the time of care, especially emergency care, is a particular challenge in this environment.

The administration at QHN recognized that high-quality safe patient care required a stable longitudinal identity, more so than an officially sanctioned one. From a patient care perspective, in other words, it is arguably less important to know if someone is really John Smith and more important to know his/her records are stored as John Smith and that he is the same John Smith from visit-to-visit. As such, the decision was made to use photographic ID. With that identity check in place, attention was paid to the other administrative savings that could be accrued by using this new card. In addition to embossing the patient's name and ID number, a bar code was added to the front of the card and a magnetic stripe was added to the back. The embossed information allowed for the card to be used in those paper-based activities found in some hospital areas, as well as a back-up in the event of a computer systems failure. The magnetic stripe contained the same information but was designed to allow for rapid front-desk registration while eliminating transcription errors. The bar code was included as implementing technologies for faster laboratory and pharmacy services was contemplated.

The network also realized that because of the mobility of the population and the relatively close proximity of other hospitals in the borough, there was a good chance that patients received care in multiple settings. This would be especially true in the emergency department (ED) setting, an area that tended to be heavily used as the population often looked to the ED as the gateway for nonurgent primary care. To verify our impression that there were a substantial number of "mobile patients," we reviewed the billing records for one of our participating Medicaid managed care plans (see Table 7-8). The review showed that more than 20 percent of all ED visits of patients that had chosen our network as their primary healthcare provider had occurred outside of the city hospital system. Since managed care patients should be more likely to return to the home facility, the network took this number as a lower-end estimate for the care-seeking mobility of the patient population.

Within the Queens Health Network, the two hospitals had access to the complete electronic record at either facility, but this access was not available to the other emergency departments in the borough. The city hospitals tend to treat patients that are sicker than average, primarily because of the health burden of poverty and an inability to consistently receive coordinated primary and chronic disease care. As a result, many patients are on multiple medications for multiple conditions. Given the complexity of patients' medical care, coupled with the high percentage of those who do not use English as their primary language, the network concluded that our patients were at a higher risk of a medical miscue from adverse medication interactions, therapeutic duplications, and delayed diagnoses caused by incomplete histories and information at the point of care outside our network.

For all of the reasons summarized in Table 7-9, the decision was made in spring 2003 to incorporate a smart chip into the card. A standard 64k chip was selected, as it was the largest readily available and seemed to be large enough to record a comprehensive medical summary with room left for an ECG. The technical details of the chips and supporting hardware and software are found in Table 7-10. The key design points

Table 7-8: QHN Out-of-Network ED Visits

In 2002, 1,847 of 8,786 (21%) ED visits were out-of-network (non-HHC).

2002 Enrollees of a Selected Health Plan	
Vendor	**ED Visits**
Jamaica Hospital	348
Saint Vincent Catholic Medical Centers	317
Catholic Medical Center Physician Services, PC	244
NY Flushing Emergency Practice Plan	175
Mount Sinai Medical Center	139
NYH Medical Center of Queens	103
Wyckoff Heights Medical Center	90
Long Island Jewish Radiology	50
The Brooklyn Hospital/Caledonian	28
Brookdale Emergency Physician Associates	26
North Shore University Hospital	25
New York Presbyterian Hospital	20

Table 7-9: What Are the Issues We Try to Confront?

- More timely information = better care
- Multi-ethnic population with more languages than the UN
- Identity confusion
  - Common names
  - Deliberate errors
- Multiple problems with multiple medications
- Out-of-network ED visits

Table 7-10: Technical Issues

- 64k open platform smart card compliant with the following standards:
  - Java Card 2.1.1
  - Open Platform 2.0.1
  - ISO 7816
- Application also utilizes the following:
  - PC/SC compliant smart card reader
  - Private key algorithms (3-DES)
  - Standard Windows applications
  - TCP/IP communications
  - Software was written using Java and C++

are that the system was smart-card–standard compliant and that we used off-the-shelf products. The credit card sized Health Connection itself is seen in Figure 7-1.

Having decided to create a card capable of storing health information, it became necessary to determine both the information to be recorded and the format. The format selected was a simple text file. It required no particular viewing software, no on-site support, and it reflected the lack of clear accepted standards for such a record. Since that time, the CCR standard has evolved. It has become more accepted, reflecting a significant advance in allowing for the merging of information from different sources and for more sophisticated viewing options but still within standard browser software.

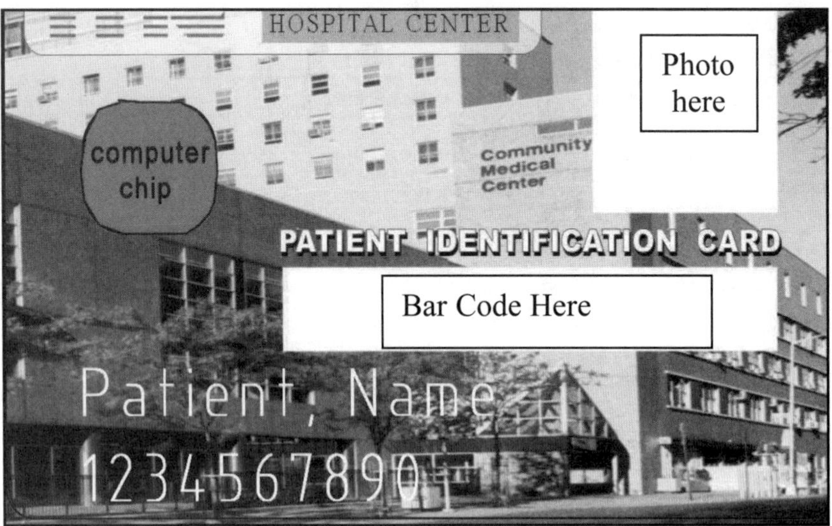

Figure 7-1: The Health Connection Smart Card

Content

Content decisions were made by polling emergency physicians within the network to determine the minimal data set that would be of use in an emergency. From those discussions, the following content was agreed to:

- Demographic information
- Emergency contacts
- Problem list and allergies
- Active medications
- Complete, relevant lab results

Problems were generally consistent with CPT/ICD-9 nomenclature, though free text problems were allowed. The date of the problem's activation was included, a move that was quite necessary, as the network physicians do a good job adding problems but a poor job of marking them resolved. Allergies included the type of allergen and the symptom. Active medications came from the network's EMR and included all medications prescribed at discharge, active outpatient medications or those prescribed within the last 60 days. It did not include medications from other sources. Laboratory results included standard metabolic and hematologic results, therapeutic blood levels, coagulation studies and culture and sensitivity results. The microbial culture and sensitivity results were not written to the card if more than 30 days old. For other laboratory results, the last version of any test available on the EMR was written to the card with the date on which it was performed.

While ED physicians were clear in their desire to have an image of an ECG on the card, this was not accomplished during the pilot. It was possible to condense the image to an appropriate size, but we were stymied by our inability to smoothly integrate the writing of the ECG information into the update workflow.

Privacy and HIPAA Considerations

A decision was made not to include financial or insurance identifiers on the card. During its initial rollout, it was felt that the risk of economic data theft would adversely affect the acceptance of the cards. The plan was to include the information once the cards were accepted and the security issues had been re-analyzed, post rollout. Since the information written on the card was a simple text report written from the EMR, such changes were fast and easy to accomplish. Likewise, HIV status was not included on the cards. Medications used almost exclusively in the treatment of HIV conditions were included if prescribed, as the clinicians felt the safety gains of having them included were worth the security risks.

Patient confidentiality and HIPAA concerns were addressed in the design of the program. No patient was forced to accept a Health Connection card. An informational brochure and video were developed in several languages. Before the patient sat for his/her picture, consent was obtained. Patients were asked to acknowledge the following statement:

> I accept the Elmhurst Health Connection Card (the "Card") and I acknowledge that it is my decision whether to disclose the information contained on the Card to another facility. I also understand that I am responsible for securing this card. In the event I become incapacitated and I am unable to communicate with my treating healthcare provider, I hereby grant consent to Elmhurst Hospital Center and participating facilities to: (1) access all of the information contained on the Card to assist in my treatment; and (2) to contact the emergency contact person contained thereon.

Nonemergent use of the card is completely controlled by the patient, as he chooses with whom to give the card to access the information. Emergency care, when the subject is unable to give consent, is covered by the statement the patient signed when accepting the card. Information on the chip was encrypted with private key algorithms (3-DES). To read the card, specific software is needed that generates the unlocking PIN from an algorithm that uses the medical record number as the sourcc. That software was only distributed to local PCs in observed areas within the network, and eventually in two or three PCs in participating emergency rooms.

The Pilot

The goals for the pilot were to answer the following questions:

- Could a photo ID Health Connection card with a smart card chip be issued within the workflow of an outpatient clinic?
- Could the card be reliably updated with information from the EMR and within the workflow of the hospital?
- Would patients treated at a city hospital with a wide range of ethnic and socio-economic origins accept and use the card?
- Could other hospitals in the borough be convinced to install Health Connection card readers and software in the emergency departments?

The Health Connection smart cards were issued in the medical primary care clinic at Elmhurst hospital. Updating was to occur at any clinic visit throughout the hospital or at the time of an inpatient discharge. For a variety of reasons, the ED was not a designated update location at the start of the pilot. The ED was not using the general EMR, so discharge medications would not be available at the time of update. Many lab results are still pending at time of discharge from the ED. Finally, given the nature of the ED, it was felt that a negative effect on patient flow due to burdens associated with updating was not advisable.

Process Results

- Cards were issued beginning in August 2003. In the first two years, approximately 10,000 cards were issued. Using two cameras and two card embosser/initializers, approximately 270 cards were issued weekly at peak periods.
- Card retention by patients has proven to be excellent. During a single two-day period, all patients registering in the clinic were reviewed. Of the 228 patients who had previously been issued a card, only 2 did not have their card with them at this subsequent hospital visit. In over 2 years, with more than 14,000 cards issued, fewer than 50 have had to be replaced due to loss.
- Card updating has been more of a challenge. When examined, 78 percent of cards were updated at a clinic visit. No data are available for updates at time of discharge from inpatient service. This number reflects an assessment done outside a period of staff education or reminders about the importance of updating cards. We were pleased to see that the update process itself was easily performed by nonclinical personnel at the time of patient checkout. The process takes less than a minute and requires a minimum of keystrokes. The update software checks to make sure the information being written to the card is from the appropriate medical record before allowing the write to proceed.

Patient Acceptance

As shown in Table 7-11, subjects were given an anonymous questionnaire to demonstrate both their knowledge of the card and their acceptance. Only subjects with the card were polled. The results support the notion that patients were comfortable carrying a photo ID with health information stored in a chip. Their knowledge of what was actually on the card was imprecise with errors in both directions. In fact, the card held no insurance information, but it did carry basic demographic information and medical information. Subjects were in overwhelming agreement that having a card of this sort was important and agreed to use it. This is despite a significant, but clear, minority of subjects who were "very concerned" about having medical information on the card. An unexpected finding was how comfortable patients were with the photo ID despite the fact that many were in the country with less than complete legal authorization. When asked follow-up questions, subjects indicated that the ID was often helpful to them when establishing their identity in nonhospital settings. At the time of the survey, most subjects did not know which hospitals could read the card. This was not surprising as deployment of the readers was still ongoing, and there was no educational attempt made by the institution to educate card-carrying patients during the transaction period.

Table 7-11: Patient Survey

	% English (N=32)	% Spanish (N=51)	% Total (N=83)
What information do you think is on the card?			
• Address and telephone number			
– Yes	69%	78%	75%
– No	22%	14%	17%
– Not Answered	9%	8%	8%
• Medical Information			
– Yes	72%	57%	63%
– No	9%	18%	14%
– Not Answered	19%	25%	23%
• Insurance Information			
– Yes	50%	57%	54%
– No	22%	24%	23%
– Not Answered	28%	20%	23%
Do you carry the card with you at all times?			
• Yes	75%	88%	83%
• No	16%	4%	8%
• Not Answered	9%	8%	8%
			0%
Do you have concerns about having your medical information on the card?			
• None	50%	80%	69%
• Slight	22%	12%	16%
• Very Concerned	25%	2%	11%
• Not Answered	3%	6%	5%
Would you give it to a doctor or nurse in an Emergency Room?			
• Yes	91%	94%	93%
• No	6%	2%	4%
• Not Answered	3%	4%	4%
If you would not give it to a doctor or nurse in an Emergency Room, why not?			
• I don't want physician or nurse to see all the information about me.	9%	0%	4%
• I'm not sure what is on it.	16%	8%	11%
• Other Reason	6%	8%	7%
• Not Answered	31%	51%	43%

Table 7-11: *(Continued)*

	% English (N=32)	% Spanish (N=51)	% Total (N=83)
Would you be willing to spend additional time at the hospital to make sure your card is updated?			
• Yes	94%	82%	87%
• No	3%	0%	1%
• Not Answered	3%	18%	12%
• 5 minutes	31%	22%	25%
• 10 minutes	13%	14%	13%
• 15 minutes	6%	20%	14%
• 20 minutes	16%	14%	14%
• 30 minutes	22%	14%	17%
• No, I would not be willing to wait extra time to update my card	3%	14%	10%
• Not Answered	0%	2%	1%
Is having a photo ID important to you?			
• Yes	91%	100%	96%
• No	9%	0%	4%
Is having a card with your medical information on it important to you?			
• Yes	91%	92%	92%
• No	9%	4%	6%
• Not Answered	0%	4%	2%
Do you know which hospitals can read the card?			
• Yes	50%	31%	39%
• No	50%	67%	60%
• Not Answered	0%	2%	1%

Health Systems Acceptance

Issuing cards that cannot be read by emergency departments in other hospitals does not advance the cause of health data exchange, nor does it promote the patient safety gains of having point-of-care information access. Initially, readers were installed in the emergency departments of the nine other municipal hospitals throughout New York City. Outreach to the other hospitals in the borough of Queens was then attempted. Interestingly, the demonstration to the emergency department followed a pattern—after one minute of demonstration, the clinical utility was apparent to the clinicians and the conversation shifted to the practicalities of installing readers and discussing ways for the other institutions to issue their own cards. No institution turned down a request to install the readers. Installation involved installing the read-only software on two or three PCs (usually at triage or admitting, the nursing station, and a doctor's office) and connecting the smart reader, a plastic device with an USB interface costing less than $20.

As a result of the success of the pilot, the hospitals that participated in the pilot agreed to participate in a regional health data exchange with smart cards as an important backbone for data exchange and identity verification. Two of the local hospital systems planned to issue their own interoperable cards as part of this project. This project had been selected for New York state matching funding as part of the HEAL NY initiative.

Because of the momentum generated by the acceptance of the card by multiple institutions in Queens, it has been possible to partner with QHN's academic affiliate, Mount Sinai School of Medicine, and our commercial partner, Siemens, to develop "the Patient Health Card" with increased functionality. Specifically, the new card system allows multiple hospitals to update the card and to have the information—including an ECG—stored in a CCR-compatible format. Delivery and wide deployment of the new card and software was delayed after Siemens withdrew from the project as their worldwide interest in smart cards waned secondary to events overseas. Despite this setback to the project, Mount Sinai, with other vendors, continues to develop the card and works to integrate it into the clinical workflow and strategic IT vision of the medical system.

The Future

By its very design, the pilot was not equipped to demonstrate the actual clinical and economic utility of the card. Information at the point of care should reduce medical errors, the need for excess tests and help avoid unnecessary admissions. All of these outcomes have the effect of reducing medical costs. Most of the benefits of data exchange at the time of the service—even if restricted to a limited data set—are outlined in Table 7-12.

Table 7-12: Patient Safety/Cost Savings

- Avoid unnecessary testing, either by having a test result available or by better selected testing, as the information available makes the list of differential diagnoses that are much shorter and precise.
- Avoid drug-drug interactions from the inadvertent use of a drug that interacts with a substance the patient is already taking at the time of treatment.
- Avoid allergic reactions, as even food allergies can sometimes predict allergic reactions to medications (e.g., egg allergy and inoculations, seafood allergies and dyes used in radiology).
- Avoid misidentification and increase the speed of registration and treatment for all those with cards.
- Avoid unnecessary admissions from medical misadventures, as well as more complete information at the time of evaluation.

Future Functionality

As the new smart card is being developed, the ability to capitalize on the added functionality of this advanced PHR will allow for the outcomes detailed previously and at the same time provide multi-application support. While still maintaining the PHR and providing point-of-care information to providers in multiple settings such as nursing homes, private offices, disaster scenes and ambulances, the card may also facilitate integration with the following:

- Secure electronic prescriptions
- Disease and case management programs
- Insurance verification and authorization
- Security/identity component for health information exchanges
- Security/identity component for in-hospital kiosk use to provide patient entered registration and health history information

REFERENCES

1. AHIMA e-HIM Personal Health Record Work Group. The role of the personal health record in the EHR. *Journal of AHIMA*. 2005;76(7):64A-D. Available at: http://library.ahima.org/xpedio/groups/public/documents/ahima/bok1_027539.hcsp?dDocName=bok1_027539. Last accessed August 2010.
2. Johnston D, Kaelber D, Pan EC et al. A Framework and Approach for Assessing the Value of Personal Health Records (PHRs). *AMIA 2007 Symposium Proceedings* 374-378.
3. Kim MI, Johnson KB. Patient entry of information: evaluation of user interfaces. *J Med Internet Res.* 2004;6:e13.
4. Fuji KT, Galt KA, Serocca AB. Personal Health Record Use by Patients as Perceived by Ambulatory Care Physicians in Nebraska and South Dakota: A Cross-Sectional Study. *Perspectives in Health Information Management*. 2008;5;15.
5. Medicare and Medicaid Programs. Electronic Health Record Incentive Program; Final Rule 42CFR Parts 412,413,422 et al. Available at: http://edocket.access.gpo.gov/2010/pdf/2010-17207.pdf. Last accessed December 2010.
6. Available at: http://www.IDTheftcenter.org. Last accessed December 2010.
7. Available at: http://www.bizjournals.com/dallas/stories/2010/07/19/daily42.html. Last accessed December 2010.
8. Zoutman DE, Ford BD, Bassili AR. A call for the regulation of prescription data mining. *CMAJ.* 2000;163(9):1146-8.
9. Available at: http://patient privacy rights.org/personal-health-records/. Last accessed August 2010.
10. Available at: http://www.ihs.gov/NonMedicalPrograms/BusinessOffice/documents/2010pres/FIOAhandoutI.pdf. Last accessed August 2010.
11. Available at: http://www.hhs.gov/ocr/privacy/hipaa/understanding/special/healthit/phrs.pdf. Last accessed August 2010.
12. Available at: http://www.google.com/intl/en-US/health/hipaa.html. Last accessed August 2010.
13. Pringle S, Lippit A. Interoperability for electronic records and personal health records. *JHIM.* 2009;23:(3)31-37.
14. Available at: http://www.myphr.com/index.php/start_a_phr/choose_a_phr. Last accessed December 2010.
15. Detmer D, Bloomrosen M, Raymond B et al. *Integrated Personal Health Records: Transformative Tools for Consumer-Centric Care.* BMC Medical Informatics and Decision Making. 2008,8:45.
16. Vincent A, Kaelber D, Pan E, Shah S et al. A Patient Centric Taxonomy for Personal Health Records. *AMIA 2008 Symposium Proceedings* 763-7.
17. Jones DA, Simpson JP, Plaut DA et al. Characteristics of personal health records: findings of the Medical Library Association/National Library of Medicine Joint Electronic Personal Health Record Task force. *J Med Libr Assoc.* 2010;98(3): 243-9.

18. Available at: www.fiercehealthit.com/story/revolution-health-kills-its-phr/2010-02-01. Last accessed August 2010.

19. Available at: www.myPHR.com. Last accessed December 2010.

20. ASTM E2369-05. *Continuity of care record (CCR); the concept paper of the CCR.* Available at: http://www.astm.org/COMMIT/E31_ConceptPaper.doc. Last accessed August 2010.

21. *Essential Similarities and Differences Between the HL7 CDA/CDS and ASTM CCR.* Available at: www.centerforhit.org/PreBuilt/chit_ccrhl7.pdf. Last accessed August 2010.

22. Available at: www.hl7.org. Last accessed December 2010.

23. Markle Foundation. Connecting for Health: the Personal Health Working Group, final report. Available at: www.markle.org/downloadable_assets/final_phwg_report1.pdf. Last accessed August 2010.

24. Markle Foundation. Attitudes of Americans Regarding Personal Health Records and Nationwide Electronic Health Information Exchange. Available at: www.markle.org/downloadable_assets/research_release_101105.pdf. Last accessed August 2010.

25. *Health Industry Insights. Health industry Insights Consumer Survey.* Available at: www.idc.com/downloads/HIIConsumersurveyePHRs_Q&A.pdf. Last accessed August 2010.

26. *Consumers and Health Information Technology:* A National Survey Source. Available at: www.chcf.org/publications/2010/04/consumers-and-health-information-technology-a-national-survey. Last accessed December 2010.

27. Zhou YY, Kartner MH, Wang JJ et al. Improved Quality at Kaiser Permanente Through E-Mail Between Physicians and Patients. *Health Affairs.* 2010;29:(7):1370-75.

28. Miller H, Vandenbosch B, Ivanaov D et al. Determinants of Personal Health Record Use. *JHIM.* 2007;(21):3,44-8.

ADDITIONAL READINGS AND RESOURCES

American Health Information Management Association (AHIMA). *My PHR Website.* Available at: www.myphr.com/.

Northern Illinois Physicians for Connectivity and the Chicago Patient Safety Forum, Series of Essays on Personal Health Records titled *A Community View on How Personal Health Records Can Improve Patient Care and Outcomes in Many Healthcare Settings.* Available at: www.niu.edu/rdi/pdf/personal_health_records_and_patient_care_2009.pdf.

U.S. Department of Health & Human Services, Medicare's Personal Health Record (PHR) Programs. www.medicare.gov/navigation/manage-your-health/personal-health-records/personal-health-records-overview.aspx?AspxAutoDetectCookieSupport=1.

U.S. Department of Veterans Affairs. *My HealtheVet Website.* Available at: www.myhealth.va.gov/mhv-portal-web/anonymous.portal?_nfpb=true&_nfto=false&_pageLabel=mhvHome#.

CHAPTER 8

Health Information Exchange

Jason S. Shapiro, MD, and Gilad Kuperman, MD, PhD

INTRODUCTION

Health information exchange (HIE) refers to the movement of health information across a network of otherwise unaffiliated healthcare stakeholders. These stakeholders may include hospitals, ambulatory practices and clinics, skilled nursing facilities, home care agencies, payers, commercial laboratory and radiology facilities, public health agencies and patients. HIE allows patients' information to follow them as they migrate about the healthcare system. Regional health information organizations (RHIOs) typically refer to the organizations that create HIEs or other forms of interoperability among various stakeholders within a given region. The RHIO provides the governance structure and management to create and operate an HIE network. Various efforts are underway to bring regional HIE networks and other data sources together into a cohesive national network of healthcare stakeholders, sometimes referred to as the Nationwide Health Information Network (NHIN). The federal government has funded several rounds of NHIN demonstration projects involving RHIOs and health IT vendors.

HIE holds the promise of reducing resource utilization (e.g., duplicate diagnostic tests, potentially avoidable hospital admissions), improving safety and quality (clinical decision support that operates on a region-wide data set), and, through both of these, improving efficiency and lowering overall healthcare costs.[1-6] Much evaluation work is needed in order to prove these promises will come to fruition once the investment to build these networks is made.

HIE is necessary because patients often move among multiple providers, payers and other stakeholders.[7,8] This "crossover" or migration of patients leads to fragmentation of their health records across multiple locations that are historically not interconnected or interoperable.[9] The fragmentation leads to gaps in information for the clinician at the bedside,[10,11] and because clinicians have difficulty obtaining data from outside of their own organization,[12] this may in turn lead to problems with safety, quality and efficiency.[13]

The clinical use case for HIE generally refers to bringing relevant health information to the clinician at the bedside. This has typically been achieved through a "portal," a stand-alone results review application, but the portal may impose some significant workflow integration issues because it requires the clinician to perform a separate task that is not part of his or her normal routine. Increasingly, attempts are being made to import the HIE data directly into various EHRs, allowing clinicians to view the data in their own native application in a more seamless way.

In order for the clinical use case to have any real benefit for a given patient, there are two fundamental prerequisites: (1) the patient must have been to more than one site in the exchange, and (2) the patient must have a condition that is sensitive to the addition of external data through HIE. The first point is rather obvious; if a patient has not been to another site prior to the current visit, there will be no information for the clinician to look up through HIE. As for the second point, if a patient comes to the emergency department (ED) with an ankle sprain, any information available from another site is probably not relevant; the clinician will examine and possibly x-ray the patient's ankle with no need for outside historic information from another site. There are also a number of secondary use cases in which health data are used for purposes outside of direct clinical care[14] that leverage the data already being aggregated through the HIE in support of the clinical use case for other "secondary" purposes. These will be discussed in more detail next.

To assure that RHIOs are able to interact with each other and not just create silos of data at a higher level, the federal government has supported various initiatives intended to promote the development of a nationwide health information network.[15] The first project, known as the NHIN Prototype Architecture project, funded four projects from 2005 to 2007, each of which demonstrated architectures to interconnect three communities. The main findings of the NHIN Prototype Architecture project was that nationwide interoperability was possible without a large central technical infrastructure, without a single nationwide patient identifier and without a large central administrative structure. The project outlined the data and security protocols that RHIOs would need to adhere to in order to participate in a nationwide health information network.

The subsequent project in the Nationwide Health Information Network program was the NHIN Trial Implementation, which took place from 2007 to 2008. In this project, 20 operational RHIOs interoperated to support the exchange of summary patient data as well as the support of the eight specific interoperability use cases that had been identified by the American Health Information Committee. The use cases included transmission of laboratory data into an EHR, access by a clinician at an emergency department to a patient's summary record, transmission of quality data, support of biosurveillance, transmission of medication data to support medication reconciliation and transmission of a patient's data into his or her PHR. The NHIN Trial Implementation project successfully demonstrated the exchange of summary data and the use cases; however, mock data had to be used because the data use agreements needed to support exchange of live data among all the participants had not yet been developed.

The HITECH Act, passed in 2009, contains incentive funding for the meaningful use of certified EHRs. The stage 1 Meaningful Use criteria were finalized in mid-2010 and contain several objectives that depend on interoperability. The Meaningful Use criteria provide flexibility for exactly how interoperability may be achieved. One approach to achieving interoperability would be to implement the protocols that were developed under the NHIN Trial Implementation; however, one criticism of NHIN Trial Implementation is that the data exchange protocols were overly complex. To address this criticism, the Office of the National Coordinator for Health IT has initiated the NHIN Direct project. The goal of NHIN Direct is to develop interoperability specifications to support stage 1 meaningful use that are simple and can be integrated directly into EHRs. The vision for NHIN Direct is that one authorized provider would be able to send data to another authorized provider. This would be much like an e-mail interaction, although with robust security and authorization mechanisms. As of this writing, several issues with NHIN Direct remain to be addressed, such as how an "address book" would be created and maintained and how security policies would be developed and implemented.

Although NHIN Direct appears to be a promising approach for the stage 1 meaningful use criteria, there are many aspects of interoperability that it does not address. Most notably, NHIN Direct is a "push" of data from one provider to another; it does not allow all of the patient's data to be retrieved. Aggregation of a patient's data is something that likely will be required by later stages of meaningful use, and different approaches to interoperability will be required.

OVERVIEW OF HEALTH INFORMATION EXCHANGE ARCHITECTURE

Health information exchange may be enabled under a number of different technical models, including a centralized model, a hybrid peer-to-peer model and a standards-based document sharing model.

In smaller markets with one dominant provider organization (i.e., one large academic medical center) and/or one dominant commercial payer, a centralized data model may predominate. In this model, the dominant stakeholder creates a centralized server that hosts its own data and a master patient index (MPI) that allows patients to be identified across stakeholder organizations based on a demographic look-up using elements such as last name, first name, date of birth and last known address. In a centralized model, the affiliated stakeholders (ambulatory practices, smaller community hospitals, commercial labs, etc.) allow their data to be stored on the centralized server and are given access to the same server in order to view data. This is a fairly simple technical architecture compared to the others and, in markets in which this has been possible, may decrease overall installation and operating costs.

Commonly, in larger markets for which there is no predominant provider or payer, HIE employs a federated peer-to-peer model using "edge" servers that are either real or virtualized (see Figure 8-1). These edge servers sit behind the firewall at the "edge" of each healthcare stakeholder's IT infrastructure. All the edge servers in a given exchange use a common data model and are securely connected using encryption or encrypted virtual private networking (VPN) tunnels, allowing them to function collectively as a distributed data repository. All clinical data are stored on the edge servers, and each healthcare stakeholder maintains stewardship of their institutional data. At the hub of the system, there are typically a few centralized services: (1) an MPI that performs look-ups of patients based on demographic data and maintains a table that links a patient's visits at the various sites, (2) a record locator service that creates pointers to the various data for a given patient on multiple edge servers and allows these data to be served up

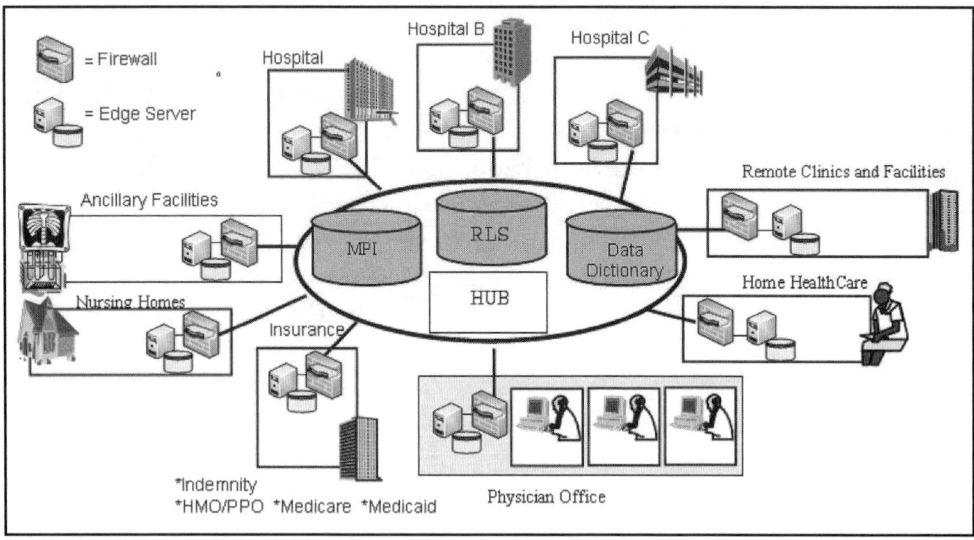

Figure 8-1: Health Information Exchange Architecture

and presented to the clinical user on a Web page, (3) a data dictionary to support terminology services, look up functions using translation tables, mapping to standards and data normalization, and 4) various security, auditing, and reporting functions.

Increasingly there is also a model using XML document standards for sending and receiving data. This model may function similarly to the hybrid peer-to-peer model described earlier insofar as there is a centralized hub with an MPI to identify individual patients and determine where they have been, but in this case there are no edge servers. Instead, each healthcare stakeholder organization is able to produce an XML document abstract of the patient's data from their native systems, often an EHR. This document standard allows the patient's data to be sent between systems in a common format that can then either be displayed for viewing or imported into the requesting stakeholder's native system. Common standards being developed for this purpose include the Continuity of Care Record (CCR), which is an XML instantiation of a standard specification developed jointly by the American Society for Testing and Materials (ASTM), the Healthcare Information and Management Systems Society (HIMSS) and various other professional associations and vendor organizations. The CCR contains various sections, including patient demographic information, insurance, problem lists, medication lists, test results and care plans. Other commonly discussed standards include the Continuity of Care Document (CCD), which is an HL7 CDA implementation of the CCR. In some instances, these XML document interoperability standards are used to create simple data-sharing networks to support more narrow use cases such as closed loop referral networks, secure provider-to-provider communication systems, and results delivery services.

NYCLIX: A CASE STUDY IN HIE

Origin

The New York Clinical Information Exchange (NYCLIX) is a large RHIO in the New York City metropolitan area that has implemented an HIE capability.[16] NYCLIX began in 2004 out of the Health Information Technology Working Group of the Greater New York Hospital Association, a trade association in New York that represents nearly 250 hospitals.[17] NYCLIX members currently contributing data to the exchange include 11 academic medical centers and home care and ambulatory organizations. NYCLIX employs a hybrid peer-to-peer architecture and, as of August 2010, contains records for more than 3 million unique patients, of whom nearly 250,000 have been to more than one NYCLIX site.

Clinical Use Case

The original mission of NYCLIX was to:

1. Build an extensible infrastructure to enable the sharing of clinical data among healthcare provider and public health organizations in the New York region in a way that improves the quality, efficiency, and safety of patient care and assures they are consistent with emerging federal frameworks for such systems, and in a manner that preserves patient confidentiality and privacy.
2. Use the infrastructure to implement an application that allows healthcare providers in emergency and ambulatory settings to access the clinical data at the point of care in a way that improves the healthcare of the people in the community.
3. Use the infrastructure to standardize and increase the efficiency of disease surveillance and public health reporting.
4. Evaluate the impact of the data exchange capability on the cost, quality, and safety of patient care, as well as patient and provider satisfaction.
5. Identify the technical, legal, governance, advisory, and business issues that would allow the initiative to be extended to other healthcare settings and also to be financially sustainable.

This original set of aims laid the framework for the clinical use case, some secondary use cases, and also anticipated many of the challenges that RHIOs face as they implement HIE.

The exchange currently has demographic data, diagnoses, and next-of-kin information from all sites and laboratory results and radiology reports from all hospital participants. There is also a heterogeneous mix of additional data elements from some sites, including hospital discharge summaries, medications, cardiology reports and EKG reports.

Adding data elements and sites to NYCLIX is a priority; however, the main focus over the past year has been to improve workflow integration and promote adoption and usage. Some of the keys to achieving these goals are to find ways to notify the treating clinician that there is NYCLIX data available on a given patient *before* he or she begins the encounter, either through a flag that pops up in an electronic record or tracking board or through the use of automatically printed patient summaries in instances in which most of the workflow is still on paper. Such notification is very important, because once the clinician has started to interview and examine the patient and formulate a differential diagnosis and treatment plan, the benefits of HIE will likely begin to diminish. Additionally, finding ways to integrate the NYCLIX portal into the workflow is a near-term priority. One solution under development is to create a secure pass-through or "deep link" that allows users to automatically authenticate and launch the

NYCLIX portal from an EHR directly into a particular patient's NYCLIX record with one mouse click. If the clinician only has to hit one button to access NYCLIX data from within their regular workflow application, adoption and usage should increase.

Funding and Sustainability

NYCLIX was initially funded by the National Library of Medicine under an Integrated Advanced Information Management Systems (IAIMS) planning grant and then under the New York State Health Care Efficiency and Affordability Law for New Yorkers (HEAL NY) as an awardee of a HEAL-1 contract.[18] Using these initial funding mechanisms, NYCLIX planned, developed and implemented a hybrid peer-to-peer network, initially to enable an emergency medicine use case, and subsequently rolled out the capability to multiple other specialties. NYCLIX has maintained an operating budget based mainly on dues from the participating members and has continued to develop new capabilities beyond the clinical use case through new funding opportunities as they arise. Some of these capabilities will be discussed next under secondary uses of HIE data. Developing a sustainable business model that supports ongoing operations and research and development for expansion of the exchange continues to be a challenge for NYCLIX and many RHIOs around the country.[19,20]

Governance

The governance structure of an RHIO permits it to function across otherwise non-affiliated stakeholders who, in many markets, may be in direct competition with one another. The NYCLIX governance structure, shown in Figure 8-2, was created in spring 2005 and has evolved over time. NYCLIX applied for and became a 501(c)(3) not-for-profit organization incorporated in New York state. NYCLIX established a board of directors comprising representatives from each member organization and a chair, vice-chair, and secretary who are elected annually, each for a one-year term. The board then adopted a set of bylaws to establish rules and standard operating procedures by which NYCLIX and the board may function.

The board also established an Executive Committee, comprising the board chair and four additional board members who rotate through the Executive Committee and serve one-year terms. The Executive Committee is charged with decision-making authority between regularly scheduled board meetings and advises the board on matters of strategic significance to the organization.

NYCLIX also has a number of committees that serve operational functions and act in an advisory capacity by bringing policy recommendations to the board within their various areas of expertise. Working groups are also often convened to address new issues and challenges that arise as NYCLIX embarks on new projects and breaks new ground.

Clinical Advisory Committee. The Clinical Advisory Committee was initially comprised of clinical representatives from the EDs of all member sites. It has since expanded to other clinical domain experts. This group has provided clinical insight for strategic initiatives, working groups to help with requirements analysis for the clinical use case, design and testing of the graphical user interface, and ongoing input on platform functionality. The Clinical Advisory Committee has also served as a point of

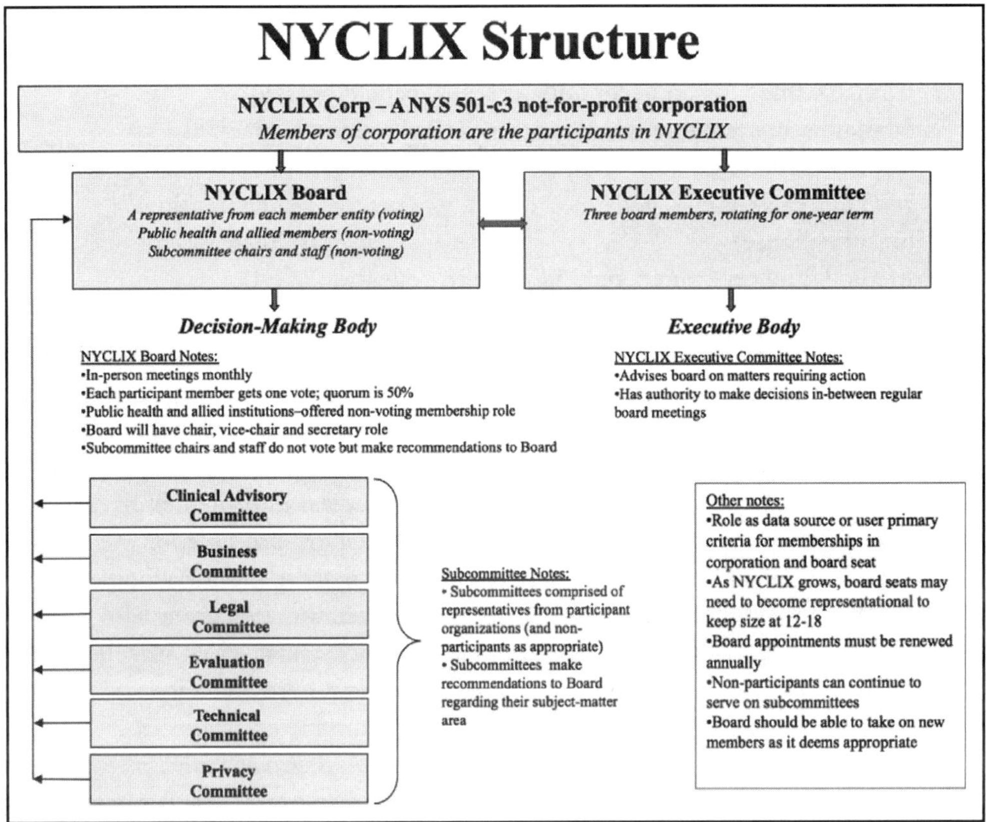

Figure 8-2: Governance

contact for evaluation work conducted using surveys and semi-structured interviews of future and current users, and its members have served as clinical champions advocating for HIE capability within their organizations.

Business Committee. The Business Committee has been charged primarily with seeking new strategic contracts and forming new alliances. This work has included meetings with pharmaceutical companies, payers and others to discuss potential partnerships and ways to help fund ongoing HIE-based projects.

Legal Committee. Initially, the Legal Committee was comprised of legal counsels from member organizations, but NYCLIX has since retained professional counsel to perform many of its legal tasks. Prior to becoming a funded operation with an annual operating budget, the Legal Committee was invaluable in helping guide the organization. Originally convened to help draft the organization's bylaws, participant agreement and various business associate agreements, the Legal Committee went on to help advise the organization on many matters, including compliance with state and federal law, and much of the work that the Privacy Committee has since carried forward.

Evaluation Committee. The Evaluation Committee was convened shortly after NYCLIX began and has been actively researching all aspects of HIE, including measuring resource utilization before and after NYCLIX implementation with the hypothesis that HIE will decrease duplicate diagnostic testing and potentially avoidable hospital admissions. Other evaluation goals include:

- Clinician information needs and perceived benefit of HIE
- Workflow analysis and optimization of HIE adoption frameworks
- Impact of consent on opt-in rates and data availability
- Secondary use of HIE-generated data (e.g., research, public health/ biosurveillance)
- Methods and experimental design for the evaluation of HIE
- Overall and condition-specific crossover rates

The NYCLIX Evaluation Committee has published on many of these topics[12,21-29] and has many ongoing evaluation projects working with survey data and large datasets derived from NYCLIX and other sources.

Technical Committee. The Technical Committee is comprised of IT experts from each site, including chief information officers, chief medical information officers and other IT leaders. The Technical Committee was primarily responsible for the vendor selection process, including an initial Request for Information and a grading exercise to help choose the organization's primary technology vendor. This group also proved instrumental during vendor contract negotiations since many of its members had industry experience. The Technical Committee continues to provide ongoing strategic advice whenever technical decisions are made or problems are encountered.

Privacy Committee. The Privacy Committee comprises privacy officers from each NYCLIX member organization. The committee created the NYCLIX Privacy Policy which was voted on and adopted by the NYCLIX Board. Meetings of the Privacy Committee are held bi-monthly during which time federal and state regulatory issues are discussed and policies affecting privacy issues are held to a vote. The Privacy Committee then makes recommendations to the board, which makes final policy decisions.

NYCLIX has a commitment to protecting the privacy rights of participants in the exchange. An opt-in consent model was adopted as required by the New York State Department of Health (NYS DOH), which mandates that patients are given an informed consent to participate in HIE and to have their data accessed at the point of care through the RHIO. Most NYCLIX member organizations have now adopted the NYS DOH-recommended consent form, which includes translations into 14 languages.[30,31]

SECONDARY USE OF HIE DATA

Through secondary use, sometimes referred to as "re-use," HIE may enable data already collected as part of the clinical use case to be "re-used" for another, secondary use case. These use cases may be broken down into four distinct categories: Research, Industry, Quality Reporting, and Public Health.

Research

Using HIE-generated data for research can support two major functions. The first is in cohort identification. Suppose a researcher wants to look at a particular age range of patients who have a specific medical condition and take a particular class of medication. Before applying for funding to embark on a prospective randomized control trial, the researcher could potentially use the database generated by HIE as a retrospective tool and create a query to see how many patients might be available for a multi-center study that spans the stakeholder organizations within the RHIO. This data may be used for preliminary analyses and power calculations in planning for the prospective study.

The second research use is in the performance of retrospective analyses. In this case the researcher is not just using the data generated by HIE as a preliminary tool but is using the data to test hypotheses and answer specific research questions.

Industry

The pharmaceutical industry is very interested in leveraging HIE-generated data for secondary use in two particular ways. The first is for clinical trials enrollment, which could also be considered a *research* use, but in this case, the research is funded and/or performed by the pharmaceutical company. They could use a decision engine within the RHIO that automatically alerts a clinician when a particular patient meets the inclusion and exclusion criteria for a drug trial. Clinicians could then use automated tools to help their patients enroll in the trial if desired.

Another use is in pharmacovigilance or stage 4 drug trials. Drug manufacturers are required to conduct stage 3 trials, enrolling tens or even hundreds of thousands of patients in order to make sure a drug is safe before it is released on the market. Following the drug's release, the company is required to conduct a stage 4 trial, which is essentially surveillance for additional adverse events once the drug is being used by millions or tens of millions of patients. This has been a difficult requirement for the drug companies to comply with, since traditionally there have not been any good data sources for this kind of wide-based surveillance. In this instance, the HIE could be used to look for patients on the drug who experience various adverse events based on lab values, new diagnoses or other measures.

Quality Reporting

Quality reporting can be broken into four distinct categories. The first is *patient-level quality reporting*. This refers to disease management of individual patients by individual providers or larger organizations (i.e., the patient's health plan). For instance, if a primary care physician is taking care of a panel of patients, including several hundred diabetic patients, the RHIO could use the HIE data to generate a report for the treating physician that aggregates each patient's relevant clinical data from multiple organizations, such as lab data from multiple sources, an ophthalmology consultation and a podiatric consultation, and structure the report in such a way that the clinician can quickly assess how well the patient's disease is being managed and if there is any trend over time.

The second is *provider-level quality reporting*, or pay-for-performance. In this instance, quality measures are implemented and run against all of the data in the exchange. An individual physician's compliance with and performance on these quality measures are used as a direct metric for reimbursement from various insurance plans. An example would be the percentile rank of a physician as compared with his or her peers regionally. Compliance with the guideline that his or her diabetes patients have a certain level of glucose control as evidenced by their hemoglobin A1C, or that a certain number of his or her patients receive screening for colon cancer via colonoscopy after age 50 is assessed. There have been some successful pilots that have implemented this model and are showing promising results.[32]

Next is *organizational-level quality reporting*, which refers to reporting requirements of providers and other organizations that might participate in HIE. Examples of this might be use of the HIE-generated data for present-on-admission requirements. For hospitals to be reimbursed, they must prove that certain conditions, such as bed sores, were present on admission and not caused as a result of the patient's hospital stay. Another example, which is also part of *public health* secondary use (discussed next) is compliance with mandated public health reporting of reportable diseases. Every state has a list of diseases that, once diagnosed clinically or by laboratory tests, must be reported to the appropriate public health agency. In many instances, reporting rates are far below 100 percent. The RHIO could be used to automatically report these conditions and to monitor organizational compliance with the reporting requirement.

Finally is *population-level quality reporting*. This falls under secondary use cases for both *quality reporting* and *public health*. Many public health agencies use campaigns to improve various aspects of the public health. Examples of this are smoking cessation, diabetes management, and decreasing the spread of HIV. A public health agency can use HIE-generated data to produce a population health-reporting data warehouse and use this as a tool to measure the effectiveness of its public health interventions.

Public Health

There are a number of secondary use cases for HIE-generated data in public health. Several such uses have been mentioned earlier, including mandated laboratory and clinical reporting of reportable diseases and population health quality reporting. Other examples include biosurveillance for bioterrorist attacks and pandemic diseases, such as novel flu, patient look-up functions to let family members know if a loved one was seen in a hospital following a mass-casualty event, data access for providers caring for patients displaced following a natural disaster, or uses of HIE-generated data to monitor the spread of antibiotic-resistant organisms to slow their spread.

De-identification of HIE-generated Data for Secondary Use

In some instances, such as in research, there may be a requirement for the HIE-generated data to be de-identified for secondary use. In such cases, typically all data elements considered personal health information (PHI) under the HIPAA Privacy Rule must be removed from the research database by an "honest broker" prior to its delivery to the research team.[33] The honest broker is a person who regularly has access to the database for operational purposes but is not part of the research team. It is also possible to create a de-identified research data warehouse from the data that could serve as a more self-service tool for researchers by applying a tool on the front end that allows researchers to generate their own queries against the data.

SUMMARY AND CONCLUSIONS

Health information exchange is a method by which health data are made interoperable between otherwise separate healthcare stakeholders and their health information technology implementations. HIE allows patient data to be accessed across institutional boundaries and has the potential to improve efficiency by decreasing duplicative services and safety and quality by bringing information to the bedside that could prevent potentially harmful medical errors.

Many challenges continue to exist before a nationwide health information network becomes fully operational, with interoperable electronic health records pushed out to every nook and cranny of the healthcare system. Consistent privacy and consent policies need to be developed that will allow RHIOs to interoperate amongst themselves and across state lines. Sustainability and funding issues must be addressed, since the financial benefits have yet to be proven in a meaningful way. Until we can show clearly to whom the financial savings will accrue (i.e., providers, payers, patients, employers or the government), it will be difficult to determine how these projects should be funded. Although the federal government recently allocated billions of dollars to health IT and HIE, it is still only a fraction of the estimated costs.[34,35] Finally, the issue of standards is ever present in health IT. Standards are necessary to make the implementation of these networks simpler and the services that they can provide more powerful. Although much progress has been made in recent years, there is still much work to be done.

Health information exchange use cases, such as the ones described here, are often fairly narrow in breadth, targeting only a small region or at most a state, and often narrow in scope. However, successful RHIOs have focused on expanded use cases. It is likely that these HIE use cases will prove to be temporary measures in hindsight, once the necessary technology, infrastructure, and sustainable funding is in place and the full vision of a truly wired healthcare system can be attained.

REFERENCES

1. Stewart BA, Fernandes S, Rodriguez-Huertas E et al. A preliminary look at duplicate testing associated with lack of electronic health record interoperability for transferred patients. *JAMIA.* 2010;1;17(3):341-4.
2. Overhage JM, Dexter PR, Perkins SM et al. A randomized, controlled trial of clinical information shared from another institution. *Ann Emerg Med.* 2002;39(1):14-23.
3. Stair TO. Reduction of redundant laboratory orders by access to computerized patient records. *J Emerg Med.* 1998;16(6):895-7.
4. Campbell J. Inappropriate admissions: thoughts of patients and referring doctors. *J R Soc Med.* 2001;94(12):628-31.
5. Eriksen BO, Kristiansen IS, Nord E et al. The cost of inappropriate admissions: a study of health benefits and resource utilization in a department of internal medicine. *J Intern Med.* 1999;246(4):379-87.
6. Siu AL, Sonnenberg FA, Manning WG et al. Inappropriate use of hospitals in a randomized trial of health insurance plans. *N Engl J Med.* 1986;13;315(20):1259-66.
7. Greater New York Hospital Association. [newsletter on the Internet]. New York: *GNYHA Members Initiate Clinical Data Exchange Project.* 2005 Jul [cited 2005 Nov 9].
8. Finnell JT, Overhage JM, Dexter PR et al. Community clinical data exchange for emergency medicine patients. *AMIA Annu Symp Proc.* 2003;235-8.
9. Institute of Medicine. Committee on Quality of Health Care in America. *Crossing the Quality Chasm: A New Health System for the 21st Century.* Washington, DC: The National Academies Press; 2001.
10. Stiell A, Forster AJ, Stiell IG et al. Prevalence of information gaps in the emergency department and the effect on patient outcomes. *CMAJ.* 2003;169(10):1023-8.

11. Smith PC, Raya-Guerra R, Bublitz C et al. Missing clinical information during primary care visits. *JAMA*. 2005;293(5):565-71.

12. Shapiro JS, Kannry J, Kushniruk AW et al. Emergency physicians' perceptions of health information exchange. *JAMIA*. 2007 Nov;14(6):700-5.

13. Institute of Medicine. Committee on Quality of Health Care in America. *To Err Is Human: Building a Safer Health System*. Washington, DC: The National Academies Press; 2000.

14. Safran C, Bloomrosen M, Hammond WE et al. Toward a National Framework for the Secondary Use of Health Data: an American Medical Informatics Association White Paper. *JAMIA*. 2007;14(1):1-9.

15. Nationwide Health Information Network: Overview 2010 Aug 20 [cited 2010 Aug 30] Available at: http://healthit.hhs.gov/portal/server.pt/community/healthit_hhs_gov__nationwide_health_information_network/1142. Last acccessed December 2010.

16. The New York Clinical Information Exchange (NYCLIX) 2010 [cited 2010 Jun 29] Available at: www.nyclix.org. Last accessed December 2010.

17. Greater New York Hospital Association 2010 [cited 2010 Jun 29] Available at: http://www.gnyha.org/.

18. Health Information Technology (HIT) Grants - HEAL NY Phase 1 2006 May [cited 2010 Jun 29] Available at: http://www.health.state.ny.us/technology/awards/. Last accessed December 2010.

19. Adler-Milstein J, McAfee AP, Bates DW et al. The state of regional health information organizations: current activities and financing. *Health Aff.*(Millwood.) 2008;27(1):w60-9.

20. Migrating Toward Meaningful Use: The State of Health Information Exchange—A Report Based on the Results of the eHealth Initiative's 2009 Sixth Annual Survey of Health Information Exchange 2009 [cited 2009 Sep 11]. Available at: http://www.ehealthinitiative.org/ehealth-initiative-releases-results-2009-survey-health-information-exchange.html-0. Last accessed December 2010.

21. Friedmann BE, Shapiro JS, Kannry J et al. Analyzing Workflow in Emergency Departments to Prepare for Health Information Exchange. *AMIA Annu Symp Proc*. 2006;926.

22. Shapiro JS, Vaidya SR, Kuperman GJ. Preparing for the Evaluation of Health Information Exchange. *AMIA Annu Symp Proc*. 2008;1128.

23. Shapiro JS, Vaidya S, Lovett P et al. The Presence of Two Sets of Troponin Cardiac Biomarkers Within 24 Hours of Emergency Department Registration Is Highly Sensitive and Specific for Initial Identification of Rule-Out Acute Coronary Syndrome Patient Cohorts in Clinical Research. *Acad Emerg Med.* (Abstract) 2009;16[4, Suppl 1], S85. [Abstract].

24. Vaidya S, Shapiro JS, Lovett P et al. Acute coronary syndrome cohort definition: troponin versus ICD-9-CM codes. Future Cardiology Forthcoming.

25. Genes N, Shapiro JS. Two Troponins: Defining and characterizing a resource-intensive ED cohort using a clinical datamart. *American College of Emergency Physicians*. 2009. [Abstract]

26. Shapiro JS, Bartley J, Kuperman G. Initial Experience with Opt-in Consent at the New York Clinical Information Exchange (NYCLIX). *AMIA Annu Symp Proc*. 2009. [Abstract]

27. Shapiro JS, Genes N, Kuperman G et al. Health information exchange, biosurveillance efforts, and emergency department crowding during the spring 2009 H1N1 outbreak in New York City. *Ann Emerg Med.* 2010;55(3):274-9.

28. Shapiro JS, Kannry J, Lipton M et al. Approaches to patient health information exchange and their impact on emergency medicine. *Ann Emerg Med.* 2006;48(4):426-32.

29. Shapiro JS. Evaluating public health uses of health information exchange. *J Biomed Inform.* 2007;40(6 Suppl):S46-9.

30. New York Statewide Collaboration Process (SCP). New York Health Information Security and Privacy Collaboration (HISPC). *Recommendations for Standardized Consumer Consent Policies and Proce-*

dures for RHIOs in New York to Advance Interoperable Health Information Exchange to Improve Care. 2008 Nov [cited 2010 Jun 29] Available at: http://www.nyehealth.org/files/File_Repository16/pdf/Consent_White_Paper_20081125.pdf. Last accessed December 2010.

31. New York eHealth Collaborative SCP. *Privacy and Security Policies and Procedures for RHIOs and their Participants in New York State.* Version 2.0 2009 Nov 13 [cited 2010 Jun 29] Available at: http://www.nyehealth.org/files/File_Repository16/heal5/PrivSec_PPs_V2.pdf. Last accessed December 2010.

32. *Quality Health First.* 2008 [cited 2010 Jun 30] Available at: www.qualityhealthfirst.org. Last accessed December 2010.

33. *De-identifying Protected Health Information Under the Privacy Rule.* 2007 Feb 2 [cited 2010 Jun 30] Available at: http://privacyruleandresearch.nih.gov/pr_08.asp. Last accessed December 2010.

34. Walker J, Pan E, Johnston D et al. The value of health care information exchange and interoperability. *Health Aff.* (Millwood) 2005;Suppl Web Exclusives:W5.

35. Kaushal R, Blumenthal D, Poon EG et al. The costs of a national health information network. *Ann Int Med.* 2005;2,143(3):165-73.

Chapter 9

Identity Management

Jonathan Leviss, MD

IDENTITY MANAGEMENT STORIES

The issue illustrated by Case #5 was first presented by Dr. David Brailer, National Coordinator for the Office of Health Information Technology during his keynote address to the American Medical Informatics Association's Spring Congress (2005, Boston, Mass.). None of the other cases in this chapter were based specifically on individual occurrences, although all were influenced by true scenarios.

Case #1

A new physician at a hospital performs rounds on patients admitted by her practice. Although she has admitting privileges at the hospital, she has not yet received her access to the clinical information system. In order to review patients' lab results and order medications in the hospital information systems, she uses the username and password of another physician in her group.

Case #2

A leading health system initiates a project to evaluate emergency medicine physicians for management of community-acquired pneumonia. Since all medication orders are entered by physicians, using a computerized practitioner order entry system (CPOE), the CPOE records are used to compare antibiotic selection and timing of orders with recommended guidelines. Antibiotic order reports assign 90 percent of all medications to one physician per shift, although three to five physicians staff each shift.

Case #3

A clothing store sales clerk who takes medications for post-traumatic stress disorder falls from a ladder and is taken by ambulance to the local emergency department for treatment of a compound fracture. On day #2 of hospitalization, the patient deteriorates, requiring medical sedation and transfer to the ICU. Although the patient's medical record is accessible through the health system's EHR, his psychiatric record is restricted, and the clinical care team is unaware that he is withdrawing from clonazepam.

Case #4

A southeastern state website used by pharmacists to track prescription drug abuse was illegally accessed; the violators demanded $10 million in exchange for returning the records of 8 million patients. U.S. federal and state authorities began a criminal investigation.

Case #5

Two hospitals that serve the same community have implemented a data exchange capability to share information about patients. At one hospital, the physicians are required to use fingerprint biometric scanners in order to sign on to the clinical information system; at the other, physicians use passwords. A particular patient's data can be accessed by caregivers at both institutions despite the different authentication requirements at the individual hospitals.

Case #6

A large Florida health system notifies 12,500 patients treated in a gastroenterology clinic that a laptop containing their medical information, including Social Security numbers was stolen.

Questions to Consider

- Which of these identity management cases are important to clinical care?
- Which of these cases are governed by regulations about patient confidentiality and the security of patient data?
- Which are important to your patients' desire for privacy of health data?
- Which of these identity management cases would provoke public concern and loss of confidence in your health system's ability to serve a community?
- What is *identity management*?

INTRODUCTION

As a society of consumers and providers of healthcare, we struggle with the balance between adequately safeguarding PHI and providing appropriate access to the same information so that people stay healthy and receive quality healthcare. Developing and maintaining policies, procedures, expertise and technologies to address this conflict is a complicated, yet increasingly important task.

In 2008, the Office of the National Coordinator for Health Information Technology (ONC) stated:

> If individuals and other participants in a network lack trust in electronic exchange of information due to perceived or actual risks to individually identifiable health information or the accuracy and completeness of such information, it may affect their willingness to disclose necessary health information and could have life-threatening consequences.[1]

Similarly, in 1993, the American Medical Association stated:

> While the legal and ethical principles may not change, the risks to confidentiality and security of patient records appear to differ between paper-

> and computer-based records. Breaches of system security, the potential for faulty performance that may result in inaccessibility or loss of records, the increased technical ability to collect, store, and retrieve large quantities of data, and the ability to access records from multiple and (sometimes) remote locations are among the risk factors unique to computer-based record systems. Managing these risks will require a combination of reliable technological measures, appropriate institutional policies and governmental regulations, and adequate penalties to serve as a dependable deterrent against the infringement of these precepts.[2]

Over a 15-year span, our regard for the importance of healthcare identity management has not diminished, yet most health systems struggle with safeguarding patient information from inappropriate use. The public awareness of healthcare privacy issues, spurred in part by the HIV/AIDS epidemic and the passage of HIPAA, combined with the rapid growth of the electronic exchange of personal information, irreversibly elevated the importance of identity management in healthcare for regulators, privacy advocates and the lay public. Continued international, national, and local news reports about identity theft have further enhanced the focus on this issue. The passage of the HITECH Act by the United States Federal Government in 2009, which began a $32 billion investment by the federal government in health IT, furthered the mandate for managers of healthcare data to protect them closely. The following chapter will serve to introduce and explain the core concepts of identity management in healthcare, review best practices and solutions to address them, and highlight areas of remaining uncertainty.

Identity Management requires:

- **Security**—Prevent unauthorized individuals from accessing patient data.[3]
- **Privacy**—Prevent individuals authorized to access patient data from using or releasing that patient data inappropriately.[3]
- **Efficiency**—Enable authorized individuals to appropriately access and use patient data quickly and easily, both individually and in groups.

While *security* and *privacy* (illustrated in Figure 9-1) are healthcare identity management requirements by law (as regulated primarily by HIPAA), *efficiency* is a healthcare identity management requirement for busy physicians, nurses, and other providers to care for patients in fast-paced and high-stress health systems. In general, HIPAA and other privacy and confidentiality regulations require vigorous supervision of *who* is authorized to do *what* with *which* patient information and raised public awareness of the ability for patient information to be exposed. In July 2010, after 15 years of debate about HIPAA's value and effectiveness, ONC reinforced HIPAA's authority on the regulation of privacy and security of PHI. ONC published its Final Rule interpretations for the Medicare and Medicaid Electronic Health Incentive Program funded under the HITECH Act (commonly known as the "Meaningful Use" guidelines). In the Final Rule, ONC asserted that certified EHRs must be able to "protect electronic health information"[4] as required by HIPAA; certified EHRs are required for use by providers and hospitals in order to receive the HITECH Medicare and Medicaid funding for health IT.

Additionally, contemporary quality improvement efforts in healthcare require that clinicians and patients have faster, less expensive, and more complete access to patient

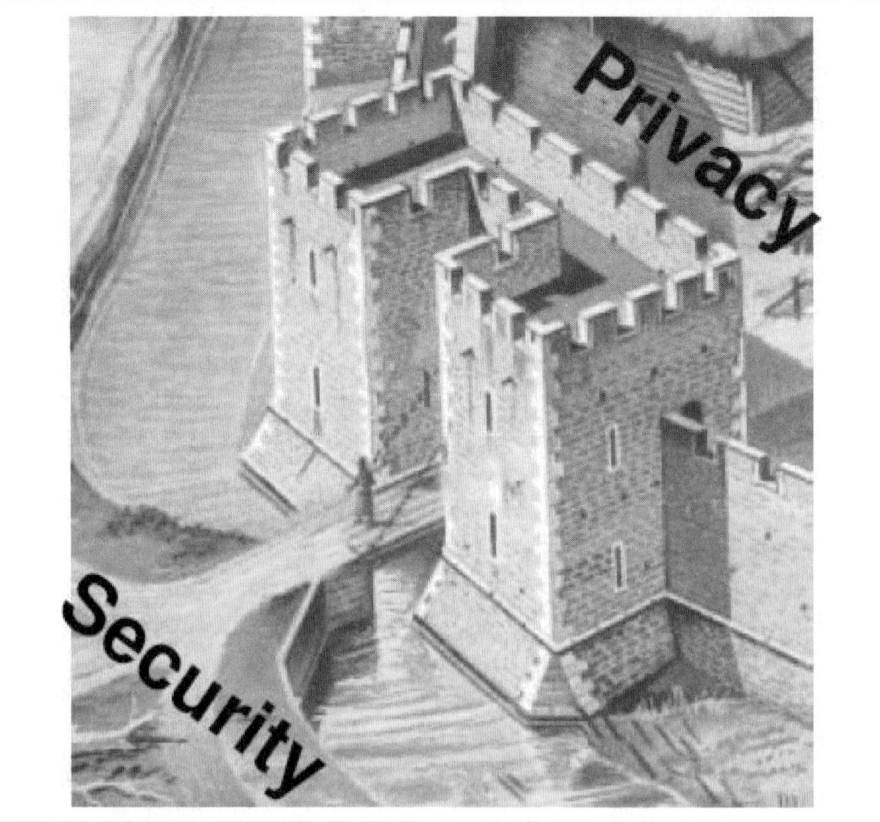

Figure 9-1: Security and Privacy[1]

information, whether captured in paper or electronic format. Many of these quality improvement efforts require that a health system identify which treatments a patient received, at what point in the care process and by whom, so that care processes can be measured, analyzed and improved. The alignment of quality drivers plus security drivers has increased the need for effective healthcare identity management solutions.

Identity Management means:

- Knowing how to identify people, places, and things
- Knowing that an individual is who he or she claims to be
- Knowing what they are allowed to do
- Knowing to whom they are related
- Knowing what staff are allowed to do in a manner related to the roles of others
- Knowing how to create identities
- Knowing how to maintain identities when circumstances change

Recognizing that the critical issue in delivering healthcare is treating the patient, addressing privacy and security effectively and efficiently can be daunting tasks.

IDENTITY MANAGEMENT LIFECYCLES

The components of identity management exist together in a continually revolving lifecycle (Figure 9-2).

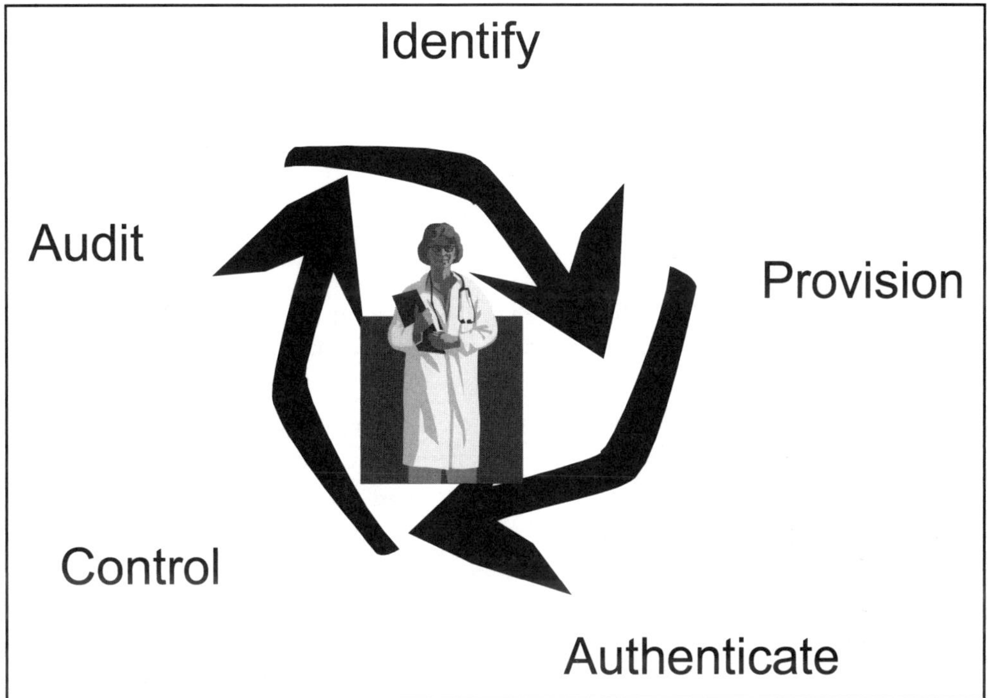

Figure 9-2: Components of Identity Management

Identify

- Dr. Gomez arrives at the Medical Staff Office with two photo IDs. The staff person retrieves her completed credentialing file, photocopies the ID cards and hands Dr. Gomez a letter to bring to the Security Office for a hospital ID to be issued.
- Mr. Marks presents to the Ambulatory Surgery Admitting Office on the day of an elective procedure. He shows the registration clerk a letter from his surgeon, his health insurance card and a driver's license, after which he is registered as a patient.
- Nurse Chang administers an intravenous antibiotic to an inpatient and then returns to her mobile laptop. Her RFID (radio frequency identification)-enabled hospital ID badge identifies her to a mobile computer, and she logs the medication administration in the clinical information system.

Identification is the first step for any person or thing to enter into an identity management system. Health systems use many methods today to identify new individuals, whether the individuals are newly hired employees, newly credentialed physicians, patients to be admitted for care, or visitors of patients. Most often, paper documentation is presented to a "trusted" individual at an appropriate access point. The trusted individual reviews the relevant identification information or documents and then records that the individual is who he or she claims to be. An identification card with a photo, such as a state-issued driver's license, is commonly used to identify an individual. Other documentation might include a birth certificate, a passport, or another government-issued document. A newborn infant upon delivery from the mother will often receive a hospital-issued bracelet or anklet even before leaving the delivery room; direct observation is used to determine that the infant is the same as the person named in the hospital's medical record. For a known individual within a health system, technology such as an RFID card or badge might facilitate how an individual is identified to an information system in order to provide an efficient workflow.

Provision

- The Department of Medicine sends a request to the IT Office for Dr. Gomez to establish accounts in the hospital e-mail, the clinical information system and the quality reporting system, with privileges appropriate for an attending physician.
- The Clinical Information Systems Office creates a physician account for Dr. Gomez in the requested information systems; a hospital-issued smart phone is configured for Dr. Gomez to securely download patient information from the hospital's electronic patient record.
- A recent HIPAA security audit by an outside firm reports that more than 27,000 user accounts exist in a hospital's clinical information systems. The same audit reports that clinical, nonclinical, employed, and affiliated staff only amount to 15,000 individuals. The Information Systems Office is not able to account for the difference.

Once a health system identifies an individual, the health system must assign to that individual a role and access privileges for information systems (in addition to other processes and assets necessary for the role). Provisioning is the act of assigning a role and granting user privileges, such as a case manager with access to patients' problem lists and care plans. One way that hospitals provision staff is by creating and managing individual accounts in the hospital information systems. Roles and accounts may be provided for:

- Access to paper or electronic medical records (e.g., all physicians receive access to medical and general psychiatric records, but only substance abuse treatment providers might have access to records from an alcoholism treatment program)
- Distribution of equipment (e.g., all respiratory therapists receive mobile phones, but in the pharmacy department only managers receive them).
- Applications (e.g., physician accounts in a CPOE system allow ordering and documentation of administration of medications, while nurse accounts only allow documentation of the administration of medications)
- Relationships between individuals (e.g., a physician admits a prominent member of the local clergy to the hospital, and his entire physician coverage group receives access to the patient's medical record, while other physicians who are not part of the coverage group do not receive such access)
- Preferences (e.g., a patient prefers for a primary care physician to order prescription medications from a pharmacy near the train station used to commute to work, while another prefers to use the health system pharmacy)

Through effective provisioning policies, procedures and technologies, a health system manages the roles and/or privileges of an individual, even as the roles and privileges evolve through the course of the individual's interaction with the health system.

Patients are transferred from one provider to another or one inpatient unit to another; nurses and other employees change departments, responsibilities, and roles, or might be supplied by a staffing agency for a limited amount of time; and physicians gain privileges to perform new procedures, or even retire or leave the health system. Each step requires re-provisioning of an individual's role and account(s) within a health system; additionally, a process must occur to de-provision user accounts when an individual leaves a health system, either temporarily or permanently. Many departments are involved in the decisions and processes to provision and de-provision roles and privileges for individuals at a health system, such as human resources, a credentialing or medical staff office, a clinical department, a security office, and IT. A person's assigned department might have the responsibility of notifying another department of a change in role or a termination of employment; that department might process the change and then relay the new status to IT or a security office. An analyst in this final office might perform the actual modification of the individual's accounts and roles in the health system information systems.

Authenticate

- Nurse Kelly types his username and password to sign on to the computer so that he may record the medications he administers to patients on the Cardiology Unit.
- In the ICU, Respiratory Therapist Staples approaches a bedside computer. The RFID-enabled ID card on her coat enables the computer to display her name on the sign-on screen; she places her thumb on a biometric fingerprint reader and is signed on to the ICU information system.
- A finance clerk has forgotten his password to the hospital billing system. On an intranet site, he answers questions about his dog's name, the color of his car, and his favorite ice cream to reset his password and regain access to his accounts.
- A nurse looks on the bottom of a keyboard to find a user name and password that colleagues share to access the hospital's PACS in order to review a patient's chest x-ray.

An identified and provisioned user must still authenticate, or prove that "you are who you say you are" to be able to exercise the privileges associated with a role. Depending on the role and the associated privileges, the authentication process might be simple or complex. The presentation of an ID bracelet attached to a patient's wrist, a typed username and password, RFID cards and readers, biometric fingerprint scanners and smart cards that must be swiped through a card reader are all examples of different technologies and procedures for authentication. These examples illustrate how an individual can be required to authenticate using the formula: something *you have*, something *you know*, or even something *that is part of you and unique to you*. The important principal is that only one identified individual is able to authenticate as that individual. Different technologies offer advantages and disadvantages, depending on the need for security and privacy for a particular level of access, combined with a specialized workflow's need for efficiency. If a back room office staff is restricted so that only ICU staff are allowed to enter, a list of patients and bed numbers may be considered secure even if posted continuously on an open monitor screen; such a monitor might be important to providing care for the critically ill patients. Alternatively, a note in a child's medical record that documents suspected sexual abuse might only be accessible to providers on a domestic violence team who have specific authentication credentials.

Control

- A pediatric hospitalist has access to a standard list of antibiotics in the hospital's CPOE system. In order to prescribe a new, restricted antibiotic, the hospitalist consults an infectious disease specialist about a patient. The infectious disease specialist agrees with the appropriateness of the antibitiotic and orders the medication from a restricted antibiotics order menu in the CPOE system that is not available to the pediatric hospitalist.
- A surgery department billing staff person reviews a patient's visit history while substantiating a claim to Medicare for a recent procedure. The Finance Information System restricts her from seeing that the patient receives substance abuse counseling at the health system, as the staff person does not need this information to process the Medicare claim.
- A patient experiences an adverse reaction to a medication and a nearby physician is asked to assist. The physician opens the patient's record in the EHR, and because the patient is a local celebrity, the physician is prompted with a warning that reads:

  > *You are not part of the patient's medical team. Do you want to "Break the Glass" on this record? Doing so in a non-emergency violates the hospital's security policy and may be cause for disciplinary action.*

- An Infection Control Officer frequently reviews reports and patient information from home with his hospital laptop and a secure Internet connection. He is able to save aggregate reports with de-identified patient data to the laptop but not files that include identifiable patient information; such files only exist on the hospital's servers.

Once a user has been identified, provisioned, and authenticated, the user's actions within an information system must still be controlled. Different individuals within a health system need to enter, access, and use patient information differently. Technologies offer many controls: applications define individual roles with different privileges and capabilities, such as access to restricted antibiotic medications or the ability to sign off on test results; devices allow for configuration settings that expand or restrict functions, such as a laptop that can be used to view patient information remotely via a hosted application but cannot be used to download patient information, or a mobile phone that does not display a physician's number when calling a patient.

Audit

- The nightly news reports on a subway accident and mentions a victim by name who is hospitalized at a local trauma center. Many clinicians and administrative staff appropriately access the patient's information during her course of treatment. The hospital's security department reviews a daily audit log and identifies an entire office group that has accessed the record without any professional need.

- The pitcher for a nearby major league baseball team, a recent patient at the hospital, requests a list of all hospital staff who have accessed his medical record. System audit logs report that only one nurse accessed the patient's ECG during a 6-hour stay in the Emergency Department, but the nurse reviewed the ECG 28 times and printed 15 paper copies; the audit also reveals that this nurse was logged on to ECG system for 6 days continuously, despite only working three 12-hour shifts that week.
- A new compliance policy requires that all information system accounts must be tracked in a database of health system personnel, both employed and affiliated. Annual audits will be required to assure that accounts are appropriately deprovisioned when individuals no longer are affiliated or employed with the health system.

Audits in healthcare frequently require answers to six basic questions:

- *Who* had access to patient information?
- *What* information did the person access?
- *Where* was the person when accessing the information?
- *When* did the person access the information?
- *How* did the person access the information?
- *Why* did the person access the information?

A health system might perform an audit of information systems for a variety of reasons: to affirm or refute a violation of an identity management policy or process; to create reports for staff training, reinforcing that audits are possible and that violations of identity management policies and processes will be detected; to perform routine surveillance of access to records of VIPs treated by the health system, as such individuals are at high risk of confidentiality breaches; or to respond to an individual request by a patient. Audits identify violators of policies as well as weaknesses in processes and technologies, involving Identification, Provisioning, Authentication, and Control. An identity management system is only as strong and complete as the processes in place to support the system and the staff who implement the policies.

Recognizing that no identity management system is foolproof, audits provide a means of performing continuous quality monitoring of the identity management system in place and the compliance of the staff it governs. Because audits are retrospective, any transgression that is identified by an audit has already occurred and if not addressed appropriately could be repeated. Health systems should create policies and procedures to address identity management transgressions prior to performing audits and prior to initiating identity management programs. Such policies and procedures must comply with oversight regulations but also must be understood and supported by patients and staff. Lastly, but of the highest importance, the policies and procedures should be designed to support the care of patients by clinicians.

HEALTHCARE DIFFERENTIATORS: PATIENTS, STAFF, WORKFLOW, AND CULTURE

The Patients

In healthcare, unlike other industries, all standards, regulations, practices and policies are often put aside for the benefit of an individual patient. While such deviations of standard practice should only occur in extraordinary circumstances involving life and death situations, such circumstances occur on a regular basis in hospitals, emergency departments and even ambulatory care sites. A physician can often gain approval for a desired medication for a specific patient, regardless of cost; policies about the delivery of care, such as whether or not a procedure must be done in an operating room or at a patient's bedside, may be modified in cases of emergency. Similarly, identity management policies and procedures may need to be disregarded if there is an urgent need for an individual to gain access to a patient's record without the time to navigate official pathways. Such realities require that many policies and procedures in healthcare are crafted with flexibility and appropriate exceptions for emergencies. Any audit results must be screened for transgressions that are actually workarounds to care for patients appropriately. Policies and procedures should be created to address such circumstances in a manner that enables proper and timely patient care. Similarly, true transgressions must be identified, addressed and communicated to both patients and staff. Only then will patients and staff understand both the risks and consequences of such transgressions.

The Staff

Health systems depend on employed staff (e.g., nurses), affiliated staff (e.g., physicians), volunteers (e.g., transport staff) and others (e.g., students) for many tasks. Usually, multiple offices maintain independent databases to track these varied individuals, which impedes the monitoring of all persons who deliver care and access patient information at a given health system. Additionally, some staff are only present occasionally (e.g., the physician who admits a patient to a hospital a few times each year), some staff may be transient (e.g., students and residents in training) and some staff may start on minimal notice (e.g., agency nurses). The continued flux of individuals adds another level of complexity to any identity management system. The existence of non-employed staff, whether affiliated or volunteer, often prevents the hospital from enforcing policies that create inefficiencies for such staff. An identity management system must be flexible enough to support the staffing requirements of health systems, easy enough to be used by transient staff, yet robust enough to be effective.

The Workflow

Unique workflows are the failure point for many health IT projects. The workflow in healthcare is fast, and providers are frequently intolerant of even small delays and inefficiencies; after all, patients do not wait to become sick, more complex or even critical. To complicate technology deployments in healthcare, providers usually share computers that are distributed throughout a hospital or ambulatory care environment, as opposed to having a personal device that is only used by one individual. For example, the description that follows illustrates how an individual computer might be used in a busy emergency department:

- 10:00 AM—Dr. Branford checks a patient's laboratory test results
- 10:03 AM—Nurse Glick documents a patient's blood pressure reading
- 10:06 AM—Dr. Maxfield orders a portable chest x-ray
- 10:10 AM—Dr. Kent checks the status on a previously entered blood bank order
- 10:14 AM—Nurse Glick logs the administration of medication to a patient

In a hospital that has implemented an EMR for clinical documentation, order entry and results reporting, each provider often signs on and off the computer, a desktop, and various applications throughout the day in order to perform professional tasks. In *no other industry* do so many different users share computers to the extent of healthcare staff; it is common in certain locations in hospitals for more than 50 individuals to use a single computer during a 24-hour period. "Fast user switching," or the ability for sequential users to quickly access a shared computer resource to perform individual tasks, is now a requirement for most identity management solutions for healthcare settings.

In addition to healthcare providers' need to rapidly access computers, signing on and off different computers throughout the delivery of care, these same providers often access multiple applications in order to review a patient's complete medical record. Although most health systems select a core clinical information system to support the majority of information-based workflows, there are almost always additional self-standing information systems, or applications. The typical reason for these self-standing applications is that a unique workflow or environment, such as the provision of care in an ICU or the presentation of laboratory results or radiology studies, requires a specialized application for optimal efficiency and quality of care. Just as a physician reviews laboratory results, diagnosis lists, medication records, and other information in a paper chart prior to treating a patient, the physician needs to review the broad information available about a patient when the patient's record is computerized. However, signing on to multiple information systems, waiting for applications to launch, and navigating multiple systems to review the information about a patient could require a clinician to spend several minutes every time a new computer is used. In order to save time, the busy clinician will often choose to use only a few applications, possibly omitting the review of important patient data, or to use an application that another clinician has already signed on to, disregarding the identity management policy violation that occurs.

"...[T]here is something about the ability of computers to disrupt rather than improve the workflow of people who are very busy," comments Edward Shortliffe, MD, an internationally reknowned leader in the field of computers and medicine.[5] Physicians and nurses want fast access to information in an easy manner not for the sake of reviewing the information but rather to treat patients best. To complicate the healthcare workflows, within most healthcare settings exist different subworkflows—physicians in an ambulatory diabetes center use different workflows than physicians in an ICU, and nurses in an emergency department use different workflows than nurses in a neurology service. Therefore, all healthcare identity management systems must maintain sufficient flexibility to function effectively across a health system, with different technologies, controls or features deployed in different settings.

The Culture

The focus on providing patient care and the close working relationships that develop between providers contribute to a culture of tolerance for "shared access" to a patient's record. Physicians and nurses, as part of a care team, often feel comfortable sharing user names and passwords for application accounts because they share the same information about the patient under normal circumstances; additionally, people have difficulty remembering their multiple usernames and passwords needed for secure access to these information systems, so sharing is viewed as the only means of accessing important patient information. The combination has produced an abundance of workarounds to address forgetting a username or password at most health systems. Physicians and nurses write down their multiple usernames and passwords on cards, keyboards, monitors, and other locations; additionally, they store them in smart phones or elsewhere.

Recent regulations, including audit requirements under HIPAA and HITECH, require that health systems address this culture of information access sharing and even open information sharing. However, no identity management solution will be successfully implemented without the end users, including clinical staff, accepting that past practices about sharing patient information and access to patient information are no longer appropriate. The most successful identity management solutions will show end users that compliance with identity management policies and processes not only complies with regulatory oversight but also enables more efficient access to patient information and more effective care.

SOLUTIONS TO THE PROBLEMS OF IDENTITY MANAGEMENT

Technologies will continue to evolve and improve to meet the identity management challenges of healthcare, but several key solutions have matured and are being deployed widely. Examples include single sign-on, strong authentication, password synchronization, context management, system auditing and user provisioning. This section will review some of the more commonly deployed identity management technologies used in healthcare today.

Facilitating Access to Information

Username/Password Synchronization: The ability to standardize a single username and password across multiple information systems. Simply synchronizing usernames and passwords to require the same username and password of an individual across all information systems would be far easier for users and would dramatically streamline password management. Anecdotal information reports that several U.S. health systems have initiated password synchronization projects, but it is unknown if any health system has been able to standardize all usernames and passwords for an individual, and, due to the unique username and password formats often required by different information systems, it is unlikely that this is achievable (i.e., alphanumeric requirements, number of characters, and symbol requirements vary across systems). However, depending on an individual health system's needs, the information systems involved and resources available, password synchronization might offer sufficient value to justify the approach.

Single Sign-on (also known as simplified sign-on): The ability to access any combination of applications as authorized by a secure credential repository with only one single set of credentials (i.e., one username/password used one time to access all appropriate applications). Password management is streamlined as the user only has one set of credentials to remember; workflow is streamlined as a user is only prompted one time to present credentials and afterwards simply accesses the information systems and information that are necessary. Single sign-on solutions leverage both technology standards (see following section on technology standards) and custom software adapters to sign-on an authenticated user to applications. Additionally, single sign-on applications single sign-*off* users from their applications. Proper sign-off of applications maintains smooth technical transitions between users and ensures that the next user of a computer does not have access to the prior user's patient information.

Strong Authentication: Requiring a user to present a token, "something you have," during the authentication process is often combined with requiring a user to present "something you know." The following technologies are being deployed in health systems with varying success:

- **Smart cards** have embedded chips that identify an individual and might include encrypted information about the individual's role in an organization; a physician or nurse could be required to swipe a smart card through a card reader and then input a password to authenticate that "they are who they say they are" in order to access information systems.
- **RFID cards** are used to identify an individual and are usually coupled with another form of authentication. Common examples of passive RFID proximity cards are the passes used in many industries to access employee-only parking lots. When a user places the card in front of a reader at the entrance to the parking lot, a small signal is stimulated and released from the card, identifying the user and opening the parking lot gate. Passive RFID cards are rapidly being deployed in healthcare settings due to convenience, low cost, and ease of implementation. Second authentication steps (i.e., password, biometric authentication, etc.) must be combined for security purposes; otherwise, anyone who picked up a dropped card could access patient information—again, "something you have and something you know".
- **Number-generating tokens** generate and display changing numerical codes that can be assigned to a specific individual and digital certificate. The nature of the changing codes, plus the addition of a password or other authenticating information, limits the ability for a shared or stolen code to be used by someone other than the assigned user. The most common use of such tokens in healthcare is for authentication to applications outside of an institution, whether for individual health systems or governmental programs.
- **Biometric scanners** and readers verify that a presenting body part (e.g., fingerprint, iris, etc.) has the same features as a stored reference file previously identified as being that of a specified individual. While passwords and tokens

can be shared, forgotten, and lost, unique body parts are not as transferable between users. Many technologies have been developed to leverage the uniqueness of fingerprints, irises, retinas, ear pinnae, and even pictures of a person's face. Fingerprint biometric readers appear to be the most commonly deployed in healthcare. Two main types of fingerprint readers exist—those that match a scanned fingerprint to an actual image of the user's fingerprint and those that perform minutiae sampling and match a number of small points of a scanned fingerprint to a mathematical formula of the ridges of the user's fingerprint. In both cases, a reference database stores a file for comparison with that of the finger placed in the reader. Biometric scanners have remained expensive and difficult to maintain compared to other strong authentication technologies; additionally, biometric scanners have not been widely accepted for use by healthcare providers. New computing devices are incorporating fingerprint readers directly which should make such technologies easier to deploy and better integrated into existing IT infrastructure.

IMPROVING NAVIGATION THROUGH SYSTEMS: CONTEXT MANAGEMENT

Context management is the ability for a clinician or other computer user to select a patient or other information focal point (e.g., billing visit code) in one information system and have all other applications synchronize on the same patient (or code). Context management is a navigational tool, decreasing the complexity of using multiple information systems to access a comprehensive view of a patient. If a physician prescribes a new medication for a patient with asthma, the following information systems might be needed:

- EHR to electronically prescribe the medication.
- Billing system to check that the medication is on the patient's insurance formulary.
- ECG system to screen the patient for pre-existing cardiac rhythm abnormalities.

Just as single sign-on facilitates accessing these systems, context management facilitates accessing one patient's information within these systems, enabling a clinician or other user to easily view an integrated health record.

Context management originated with the development of the HL7-CCOW standard (see following section on technology standards) but is now implemented with and without this standard at many health systems. Context management technologies, like single sign-on solutions, function with information systems that are not compliant with the HL7-CCOW standard through software adapters custom built for each application. Combining single sign-on with context management provides an effective visual integration tool for different information systems, while preserving the department-specific functionality that a specialty information system provides.

KNOWING WHO REVIEWED THE PATIENT'S INFORMATION: AUDIT REPORTS

A complete audit report states who accessed which information from which patient, including the time, date, and location (or computer) of access. Whether an audit is required for regulatory compliance, patient-centered customer care (i.e., a specific request by a patient for a report of who has viewed that patient's files) or another cause, such as suspected transgression of a health system's security policy, the audit might require information to be gathered about information systems, technology hardware and even personnel. As health systems deploy more and more information systems, broader reaching audit systems that report activity in all potential information systems in a health system quickly and efficiently must be developed. Due to the number of information systems in healthcare, most health system IT staff will not have the time or the capacity to review all information systems to determine whether a patient's record has been accessed, but rather will require a global approach to review a patient's record and the access that occurred. Audit reports could be generated from individual information systems and then integrated into a single report, or an integrated identity management solution can enable all information systems to be audited as one system. Such evolving auditing systems are becoming more appealing to health systems as the issues of patient confidentiality become a higher priority, and the need to audit all information systems becomes more commonplace. The security and privacy requirements of the ONC's Meaningful Use criteria will accelerate the routine auditing of information systems and access.

CREATING, MAINTAINING AND REMOVING ACCESS TO INFORMATION: PROVISIONING SYSTEMS

Provisioning systems automate and streamline the creation and management of user identities and their corresponding application accounts. Advanced solutions use messaging systems, workflow engines, and customizable rules to automate and expedite the approval processes and workflows which accompany these tasks. Also, these processes must be able to be audited in an automated and efficient manner, just as the target information systems themselves. The decision processes for awarding professional privileges and information access in healthcare is usually decentralized and delegated across multiple departments, possibly involving a credentialing office, human resources, and even a clinical or academic division; provisioning solutions that streamline such processes and automate communications and escalations of each step in the creation of user accounts eliminate great inefficiencies and inaccuracies.

Provisioning systems can provision, or deprovision, a user into an information system automatically with minimal manual data entry tasks, eliminating the potential for human error and, more importantly, decreasing the workload on all involved departments; in order to perform such tasks, these systems leverage technology standards for system integration, software connectors and adapters, and messaging protocols. Provisioning system implementation projects have the potential to be extremely complex organizational change efforts, just as an enterprise resource planning (ERP) system or a CPOE system implementation. A large number and variety of human tasks usually exist in a health system to provision users into information systems, and the individuals who perform these tasks are often located in different organizational departments and/or even different geographical locations. Automation of provisioning processes requires the transformation of these tasks and increases the accountability of all provisioning processes. Similar to the automation of ordering processes with CPOE or materials-tracking processes for ERP, baseline provisioning practices cannot be, nor should they be, completely duplicated in an automated environment.

VISUAL INTEGRATION: A WORKFLOW SOLUTION AND AN IT STRATEGY

Visual integration of information systems uses single sign-on and context management to present multiple information systems as one. Visual integration is not a replacement for integrated repositories of information, but rather a complementary solution to a related problem. Population-based reporting and analytics requires integrating patient information from multiple information systems on a single large database, but large databases are not always appropriate or necessary for individual patient care. When a physician needs information about one patient, or needs to order medication for one patient, he requires fast transactions between his computer and the supporting application's database. Individual patient decisions by a provider do not require database integration from multiple applications, either, if the information can be visually integrated and easily accessed.

For example, a physician may want to review a patient's ECG prior to changing the patient's blood pressure medication. To do so, the physician needs to review the patient's ECG and the existing medication list. The physician performs the "analytics" once the ECG and medication list are reviewed and prescribes a desired medication. The ECG and the medication list may be most effectively presented to the physician from individual, separate information systems that have been specifically designed for these tasks. Visual integration with single sign-on and context management enables the physician to easily access this information in a seamless manner and to take advantage of the specialized design of the independent systems.

Also, visual integration enables a health system to present not only specialized information systems to users in an integrated manner, but also new and old systems. All hospitals today periodically replace information systems while trying to maximize value from existing legacy systems. Visual integration provides a platform upon which old systems and new ones can be integrated and continually changed, with the least amount of disruption to the end-user experience. The physician signs on to all systems using single sign-on and navigates all systems using context management; the only change remains that functionality within the applications.

TECHNOLOGY STANDARDS IN HEALTHCARE IDENTITY MANAGEMENT

Identity management technologies in healthcare often leverage existing standards for identity management, such as SAML (Security Assertion Markup Language) and SPML (Service Provisioning Markup Language) supported by OASIS (Organization for the

Advancement of Structured Information Standards[6] or Integrated Windows Authentication (IWA) by Microsoft. However, due to the unique workflows of healthcare, such as the need to for many clinicians to share a single computer and the need for context management across multiple applications, the HL7 Context Management Standard was established. This HL7 standard is often referred to as CCOW (Clinical Context Objects Workgroup), the name of the workgroup within HL7 that maintains the HL7 Context Management Standard. The mission of HL7-CCOW is to:

> ...define standards that enable the visual integration of healthcare applications.... [which] work together in ways that the user can see in order to enhance the user's ability to incorporate information technology as part of the care delivery process.[7]

In doing so, CCOW defines standards that enable a software application to provide single sign-on and context management to other applications that contain patient or other relevant information and are compliant with the standard. Like other technology standards, CCOW was created to decrease the complexity of linking information systems into a single patient record and maintaining the system integration because vendor applications are pre-built to function in compliance with the standard. Standards-based integration allows a health system information technology team to focus on application deployment, technology, and platform support; user training; process redesign; and other critical roles without having to focus on developing the technology integration. Because the security and patient selection protocols within CCOW are ratified by the HL7-CCOW committee, a highly expert level of scrutiny and open development minimize the risk to an individual health system which integrates systems using the standard.

In the past few years, information technology vendors have developed non-HL7-CCOW-based software connectors that enable applications to be visually integrated *as if* compliant with the standard. Such technologies have extended much function of the HL7-CCOW standard to non-HL7-CCOW compliant applications. The flexibility of these custom connectors is sometimes easier for a health system to manage than testing and implementing the standard HL7-CCOW integration. One potential trend may be that the HL7-CCOW standard becomes less important as a true standard but remains a guiding model for custom application integration.

SUCCESSFUL DEPLOYMENT STRATEGIES FOR HEALTHCARE IDENTITY MANAGEMENT SOLUTIONS

Implementing identity management solutions in healthcare is similar to implementing change and technology in other environments—the likelihood of success is directly related to the end user awareness of the problem with the original processes and workflows, as well as to the value perceived in the technology and new processes being introduced. Everett Rogers, in his classic text *Diffusion of Innovation*, identified five key properties that determine how rapidly a new innovation is adopted by a social system:[8] relative advantage, compatibility, complexity, trialability, and observability. Workflows and processes vary within a single health system, which can affect each of the five key properties listed by Rogers. Non-modifiable circumstances such as the sterile environment of an operating room, the inability for a wireless network to be deployed in a particular building, or the mobility requirements of respiratory therapists may affect these properties. A biometric fingerprint reader technology may work effectively in one environment, but a token with a changing numerical display might be better suited to another environment.

Successful identity management solution implementations may vary in the specific technologies deployed, but the overall strategy of protecting the confidentiality of patient information while supporting an effective workflow for clinicians must remain. Pilot implementations that provide flexibility to identify and select different implementation strategies and technology solutions are best suited to health systems with a wide range of environments. Pilots can be used to demonstrate *relative advantage*, prove workflow and cultural *compatibility*, allow for full preparation to address issues of workflow and technology *complexity*, provide opportunities for *trialability* of the new technologies and workflows, and allow for *observability* that the new approach will be successful in a specific health system.

THE FUTURE—HEALTH INFORMATION EXCHANGES, CONNECTING COMMUNITIES, AND THE NATIONWIDE HEALTH INFORMATION NETWORK

The future of healthcare depends on effectively coordinated patient care across the spectrum of acute and chronic disease management and preventative care, which requires connected healthcare providers who routinely exchange patient information. The future of identity management will be to enable such exchanges to occur in a secure and efficient manner. Having the right information at the right place at the right time so that a person receives the right care also requires safeguarding the information from the wrong people. Health systems are just beginning to effectively address identity management issues within their own organizations. Policies, processes and technologies for identity management must develop further if we are to effectively protect patient information while making it available across a community or the Nationwide Health Information Network.

> To accomplish this, standardized technologies and methodologies coupled with mandatory business practices are necessary to provide sufficient security systems that track user identities and only permit authorized access to health data for all NHIN related and connected entities, including RHIOs [Regional Health Information Organizations]. NHIN user identities must be tracked and maintained in a directory or database. Systems must be protected from unauthorized access. Data within systems must be protected from unauthorized modification and review.
>
> ...The backbone of achieving such protections is the ability to create electronic identities for all people known to the NHIN and to manage the set of inter-relationships and associated data access permissions that would be granted to each person. People include not only the clinical users of the NHIN, but the people about whom health information is exchanged.

People also include friends and family who presently care for, or may someday be caring for, another person.[9]

As health systems become more sophisticated in identity management and technologies to support identity management continue to evolve, the driving issues of *security*, *privacy*, and *efficiency* will remain critical to healthcare. The push by the CMS and ONC for broad adoption of health IT across the health delivery systems in the United States will only drive further the attention paid to privacy and security.

ACKNOWLEDGMENT

The author would like to thank Robert Seliger for his contributions to content included in this chapter.

REFERENCES

1. Nationwide Privacy and Security Framework for Electronic Exchange of Individually Identifiable Health Information. Office of the National Coordinator for Health Information Technology, U.S. Department of Health & Human Services, Dec. 15, 2008.
2. Council on Scientific Affairs, American Medical Association: Feasibility of ensuring confidentiality and security of computer-based patient records. *Arch Fam Med.* 1993:2-5.
3. Leiderman E. AMDIS Physician Computer Symposium. July 2005
4. Federal Register. *U.S. National Archives and Records Administration.* 44328; July 28, 2010.
5. Austen I. For the doctor's touch, help in the hand. *The New York Times.* Aug. 22, 2002: G:1.
6. Available at: www.oasis-open.org. Last accessed December 2010.
7. Available at: http://www.hl7.org/Special/committees/visual/overview.cfm. Last accessed September 2010.
8. Rogers E. *Diffusion of Innovation.* 5th ed. New York, NY: Simon and Schuster; 2003.
9. Hannet F, Hiscock J, Leviss J et al. Development and Adoption of a National Health Information Network. RFI Response. January, 2005.

Chapter 10

Clinical Decision Support

Ken Ong, MD, MPH

DECISION SUPPORT: AN EVERYDAY THING

You use or see decision support every day.

With more than a quarter million motor vehicles on our nation's roads, it is likely that most of us have seen a car dashboard.[1] If you have seen a car dashboard, you have seen decision support.

A typical dashboard has a speedometer, tachometer, odometer, engine thermometer, battery and fuel gauges, and indicators for gear shift position and the turn signal, as well as visual and audio alerts that tell us if the seat belts are fastened, the parking brake is on or when the engine needs maintenance. Newer cars have an indicator for low tire pressure and even have an indicator to tell you if the indicator itself is broken (tire pressure monitoring system). The dashboard has controls for heating, ventilation, lighting controls, turn signals, sound system and—for a little more money—a GPS (global positioning system).[2]

The dashboard brings together the myriad of data the driver needs to get where he or she wants to go safely and efficiently. No doubt without these decision support tools, there would be many more than the 10.6 million motor vehicle accidents and 43,100 traffic fatalities that occur each year.[3]

A dashboard with decision support is critical to driving safely. In turn, an EHR with clinical decision support is necessary for safer, more efficient and effective healthcare.

INFORMATION OVERLOAD

The amount of information that exists in modern healthcare can be dizzying.

The National Center for Health Statistics lists and updates more than 68,000 diagnoses and complications in the newest version of the International Classification of Diseases (ICD-10-CM).[4] The U.S. Food and Drug Administration (FDA) has approved more than 3,903 drugs, and that does not even include the many food supplements or herbal medications that are clinically relevant.[5]

Keeping up is a challenge. With the number of articles published in the medical literature, a recent medical school graduate who reads two articles every day would be 1,225 years behind at the end of the first year.[6]

The sheer growth of medical knowledge prolongs the time it takes for clinical research to effect clinical practice. One study calculated that the average time from discoveries made at the bench to reach the bedside is 17 years.[7]

Yet, there is little time in the day to browse the recent literature. The old saw that there just aren't enough hours in the day applies doubly to the average physician. If a physician followed all the recommendations from national clinical care guidelines for preventive services and chronic disease management and added the time needed to answer phone calls, write prescriptions, read laboratory and radiology results and perform other tasks for a typical patient panel of 2,500, she would need 21.7 hours per day.[8]

Couple that with the reality that only 55 percent of Americans receive recommended care,[9] and the information overload and paucity of time suggest the value of not only more team-based care but the need for the EHR and clinical decision support.

WHAT IS CLINICAL DECISION SUPPORT (CDS)?

> CDS provides clinicians, staff, patients and other individuals with knowledge and person-specific information, intelligently filtered at appropriate times, to enhance health and health care. CDS encompasses, but is not limited to, computerized alerts and reminders to care providers and patients, methods to bring care into compliance with clinical guidelines; condition-focused order sets, patient data reports and summaries, and documentation templates; advice to promote more accurate and timely diagnoses; and other tools that enhance decision making in clinical workflow.[10]
>
> —*American Health Information Community*

The most frequently cited example of CDS is a drug-allergy interaction alert to a physician at time of order entry. Drug-drug, drug-allergy, and drug-food interaction alerts are indeed prototypical examples of clinical decision support, but there are others that are no less useful.

The CDS toolbox is a compendium of technologies, each with a different use case, appropriate target audience, and particular point in the clinical workflow (see Table 10-1). For example, a reminder for colorectal cancer screening could be sent to a physician, practice office staff, and the patient via his or her personal health record (PHR).

The order set is one of the more powerful and adaptable CDS tools. The modern electronic order set has a proud lineage whose progenitor is the paper checklist.

The checklist was a product of the analysis of the fatal crash of an experimental aircraft during a test flight in 1935. The test pilots made this first checklist, a step-by-step list for takeoff, flight, landing and taxiing, short enough to fit on an index card. After this modest, paper-based innovation was implemented, the aircraft that inspired it flew another 1.8 million miles without another accident.[14]

Table 10-1: Clinical Decision Support Tools[11,12,13]

- Alerts and reminders
- Clinical guidelines
- Clinician patient assessment forms
- Data flow sheets
- Diagnostic support and suggestions
- Smart documentation forms or documentation templates
- Extended-time guideline and protocol followers
- Order facilitators (order sets, order consequents, order modifiers)
- Patient data reports and dashboards
- Patient self-assessment forms
- Patient summaries for hand-offs between clinicians
- Performance dashboards with prompts for areas needing attention
- Procedure refreshers, training, and reminders
- Protocol/pathway support
- Reference information delivered
- Relevant data displays
- Targeted reference, including contextually relevant medical references or info buttons
- Task assistants for tasks such as drug dosing and acknowledging laboratory results
- Tracking and management systems that facilitate task prioritization and whole-service management

This checklist technology has crossed over into healthcare. Peter Pronovost, MD, an intensivist from Johns Hopkins University School of Medicine, partnered with the World Health Organization (WHO) to promote the Surgical Safety Checklist to prevent surgical complications and deaths. The 19-item surgical safety checklist improves team communication and consistency of care (see Figure 10-1).[15] Eight hospitals around the globe participated in a study with an outcome of a nearly halved death rate and a significantly reduced complication rate post-surgery.[16,17]

A Sampler of CDS Tools

If a checklist on paper can generate so much value, imagine what can be done with an electronic checklist. The enhanced EHR order set is such a checklist but with bells and whistles. An order set can offer functionality that would either be difficult or impossible with paper.

An example of an admission order set for congestive heart failure (CHF) enables the following features:

- Links to evidence
- Reminders for preferred diagnostic or therapeutic interventions
- Icons to indicate order items recommended by government or quality organizations, e.g., CMS, The Joint Commission, Institute for Healthcare Improvement (IHI), or the American College of Obstetrics and Gynecology
- Preferred medications with recommended dosing, frequency and route
- Relevant laboratory results or other patient information, e.g. serum creatinine for aminoglycosides, patient weight for pediatric dosing

Before Induction of Anaesthesia (Present: at least nurse and anaesthetist)	Before Skin Incision (Present: nurse, anaesthetist and surgeon)	Before Patient Leaves Operating Room (Present: nurse, anaesthetist and surgeon)
Has the patient confirmed his/her identity, site, procedure, and consent? _Yes Is the site marked? _Yes _Not applicable Is the anaesthesia machine and medication check complete? _Yes Is the pulse oximeter on the patient and functioning? _Yes Does the patient have a: **Known allergy?** _Yes _No **Difficult airway or aspiration risk?** _No _Yes, and equipment/assistance available **Risk of >500ml blood loss (7ml/kg in children)?** _No _Yes, and two IVs/central access and fluids planned	_Confirm all team members have introduced themselves by name and role. _Confirm the patient's name, procedure, and where the incision will be made. Has antibiotic prophylaxis been given within the last 60 minutes? _Yes _Not applicable **Anticipated Critical Events** **To Surgeon:** _What are the critical or non-routine steps? _How long will the case take? _What is the anticipated blood loss? **To Anaesthetist:** _Are there any patient-specific concerns? **To Nursing Team:** _Has sterility (including indicator results) been confirmed? _Are there equipment issues or any concerns? **Is essential imaging displayed?** _Yes _Not applicable	**Nurse Verbally Confirms:** _Name of the procedure _Completion of instrument, sponge and needle counts _Specimen labeling (read specimen labels aloud, including patient name) _Whether there are any equipment problems to be addressed **To Surgeon, Anaesthetist and Nurse:** _What are the key concerns for recovery and management of this patient?

Adapted from http://whqlibdoc.who.int/publications/2009/9789241598590_eng_Checklist.pdf. © WHO, 2009.

Figure 10-1: WHO Surgical Safety Checklist 2009 edition

Zynx (Los Angeles, California) is a leading provider of order sets. It offers order sets that cover the most common diagnoses and procedures for both inpatient and ambulatory care. A panel of clinical subject matter experts (SMEs) updates the order sets as needed. Order items recommended by a national professional or quality organization are indicated with a blue ribbon icon. A bell icon precedes reminders. A blue "Z" icon links to evidence compiled by the Zynx expert panel. A prescription slip icon links to drug information details. See Figure 10-2 for a sample Zynx order set and Figure 10-3 for a sample of Zynx evidence for ACE inhibitors for CHF.

Angiotensin Receptor Blockers

An ARB should be given to patients who are intolerant to ACE inhibitors (except when intolerance is due to renal insufficiency or hyperkalemia)

The evidence for administering the combination of an ACE inhibitor plus an ARB is conflicting

candesartan

- [ ] 4 milligram orally once a day
- [ ] 8 milligram orally once a day

losartan

- [ ] 25 milligram orally once a day
- [ ] 50 milligram orally once a day

valsartan

- [ ] 20 milligram orally 2 times a day
- [ ] 40 milligram orally 2 times a day

Angiotensin-Converting Enzyme Inhibitors

An ACE inhibitor should be used; for pati... n ARB should be given in the absence of contraindications

The evidence for administering the combi...

National Quality Forum–Endorsed Performance Measure
AHA/ASA Get With The Guidelines Core Measure
Hospital Quality Alliance–Endorsed Quality Measure
CMS National Hospital Inpatient Quality Measure
CMS Premier Hospital Quality Incentive Demonstration Measure
IHI 5 Million Lives Campaign Performance Measure
The Joint Commission National Hospital Inpatient Quality Measure
ACC/AHA Clinical Performance Measure

captopril

- [ ] 6.25 milligram orally 3 times a day

enalapril

- [ ] 2.5 milligram orally 2 times a day

Figure 10-2: Sample of Zynx CHF Order Set
Source: ZynxHealth. Reprinted with permission.

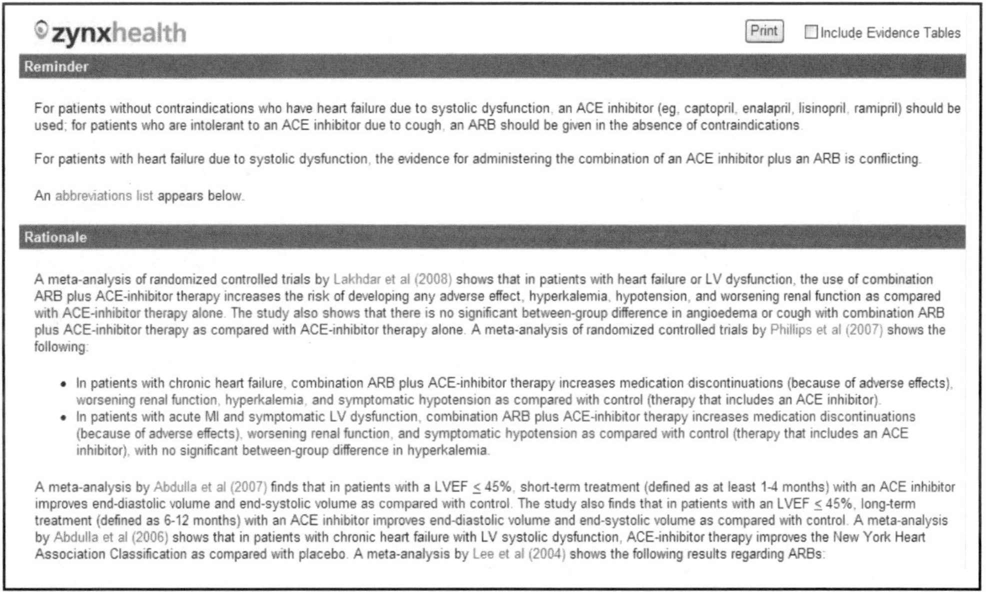

zynxhealth

Print | Include Evidence Tables

Reminder

For patients without contraindications who have heart failure due to systolic dysfunction, an ACE inhibitor (eg, captopril, enalapril, lisinopril, ramipril) should be used; for patients who are intolerant to an ACE inhibitor due to cough, an ARB should be given in the absence of contraindications.

For patients with heart failure due to systolic dysfunction, the evidence for administering the combination of an ACE inhibitor plus an ARB is conflicting.

An abbreviations list appears below.

Rationale

A meta-analysis of randomized controlled trials by Lakhdar et al (2008) shows that in patients with heart failure or LV dysfunction, the use of combination ARB plus ACE-inhibitor therapy increases the risk of developing any adverse effect, hyperkalemia, hypotension, and worsening renal function as compared with ACE-inhibitor therapy alone. The study also shows that there is no significant between-group difference in angioedema or cough with combination ARB plus ACE-inhibitor therapy as compared with ACE-inhibitor therapy alone. A meta-analysis of randomized controlled trials by Phillips et al (2007) shows the following:

- In patients with chronic heart failure, combination ARB plus ACE-inhibitor therapy increases medication discontinuations (because of adverse effects), worsening renal function, hyperkalemia, and symptomatic hypotension as compared with control (therapy that includes an ACE inhibitor).
- In patients with acute MI and symptomatic LV dysfunction, combination ARB plus ACE-inhibitor therapy increases medication discontinuations (because of adverse effects), worsening renal function, and symptomatic hypotension as compared with control (therapy that includes an ACE inhibitor), with no significant between-group difference in hyperkalemia.

A meta-analysis by Abdulla et al (2007) finds that in patients with a LVEF ≤ 45%, short-term treatment (defined as at least 1-4 months) with an ACE inhibitor improves end-diastolic volume and end-systolic volume as compared with control. The study also finds that in patients with an LVEF ≤ 45%, long-term treatment (defined as 6-12 months) with an ACE inhibitor improves end-diastolic volume and end-systolic volume as compared with control. A meta-analysis by Abdulla et al (2006) shows that in patients with chronic heart failure with LV systolic dysfunction, ACE-inhibitor therapy improves the New York Heart Association Classification as compared with placebo. A meta-analysis by Lee et al (2004) shows the following results regarding ARBs:

Figure 10-3: Sample of Zynx Evidence for ACE Inhibitors for CHF
Source: ZynxHealth. Reprinted with permission.

The Zynx product provides a ready starting point for customization and ongoing updates as evidence evolves. The final order set can then be built with or without links to evidence into an EHR for CPOE.

Order sets *do* work. Santolin et al. reported that a higher percentage of patients whose physicians initiated hospital therapy with standardized order sheets, which follow American Heart Association/American College of Cardiology Guidelines for acute coronary syndrome, received appropriate medications in a timely fashion.[18]

Other CDS technologies have proven beneficial.

Infobuttons are context-specific links that provide connection to resources that relevant to particular diagnoses or conditions.[19] The evidence links in the previous order set example are infobuttons.

Risk assessment tools can target patients at risk for given conditions and recommend focused treatment. An Agency for Healthcare Research and Quality (AHRQ)-funded study at the Children's Hospital of Philadelphia demonstrated that a pediatric asthma-control tool in the ambulatory EHR improved compliance with National Asthma Education Prevention Program guidelines.[20]

The Jesse Brown Veterans Affairs Medical Center created and implemented a standardized deep vein thrombosis (DVT) risk assessment program in their electronic medical record (see Figures 10-4 and 10-5.[21] With implementation of the DVT risk assessment program, the number of patients receiving the recommended pharmacologic prophylaxis preoperatively more than doubled, and use of sequential compression devices (SCD) increased 40 percent. The percentage of at-risk patients receiving

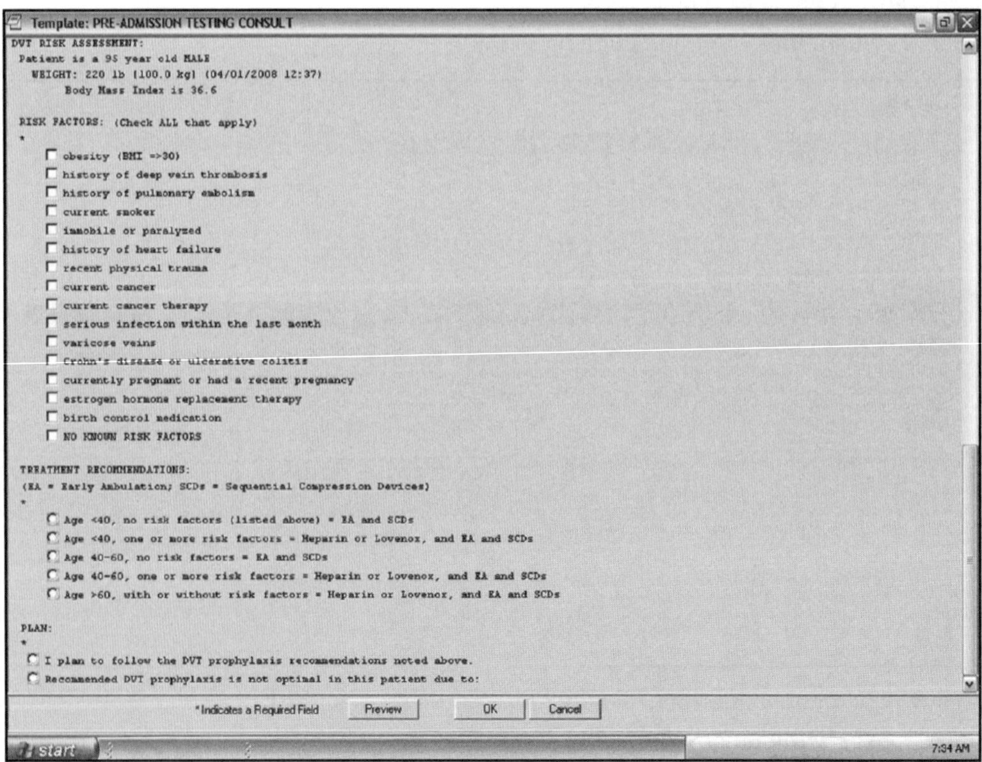

Figure 10-4: Screenshot of the Electronic DVT Risk Assessment (part of the mandatory Pre-Admission Testing that must be completed for all patients undergoing surgery). Reprinted from *Journal of Vascular Surgery*, Volume 51, Issue 3, March 2010, Sarah Jane Novis, et al. Prevention of thromboembolic events in surgical patients through the creation and implementation of a computerized risk assessment program, pp. 648–654, 2010, with permission from Elsevier.

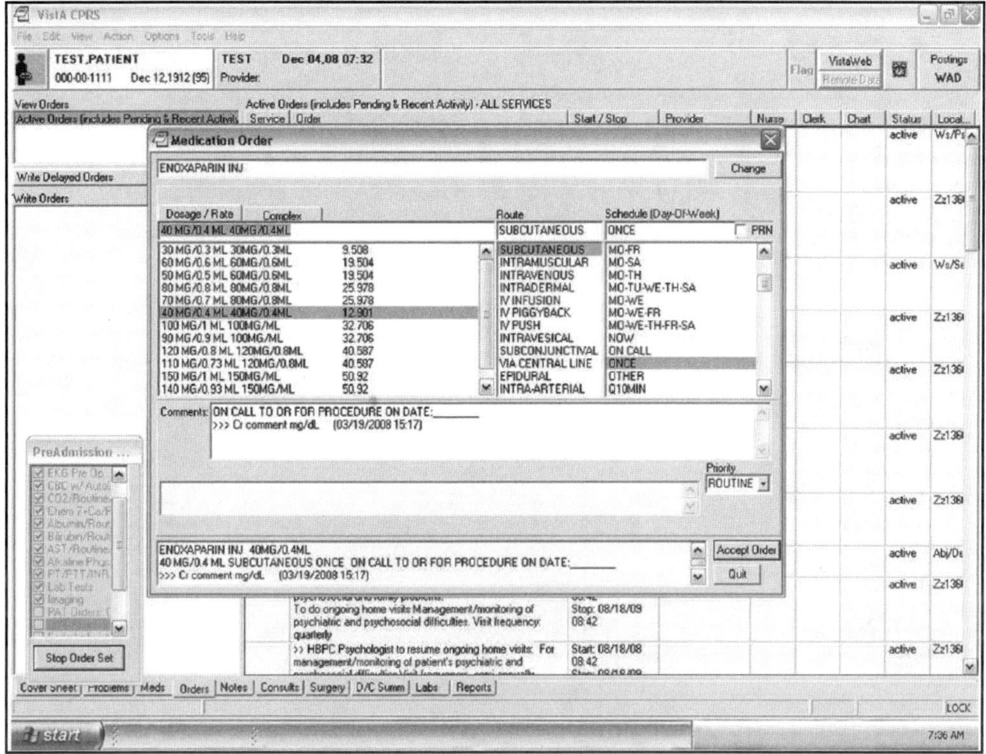

Figure 10-5: Screenshot of Automatic Orders Generated by the DVT Risk Assessment Program Based on the Different Risk Categories
Reprinted from *Journal of Vascular Surgery*, Volume 51, Issue 3, March 2010, Sarah Jane Novis, et al. Prevention of thromboembolic events in surgical patients through the creation and implementation of a computerized risk assessment program, pp. 648–654, 2010, with permission from Elsevier.

the recommended combined DVT prophylaxis of SCD and pharmacologic prophylaxis increased nearly seven-fold.

An active problem list records the diagnoses and conditions necessary to treat a patient in the hospital, physician's office and elsewhere. An active problem list for patients is also a measure for meaningful use of the EHR. However, problem list maintenance is often problematic because updating the list falls outside the clinician's workflow. Galanter et al. at the University of Illinois Medical Center developed a CDS tool that suggests adding the appropriate diagnosis to a patient's problem list by the medications ordered.[22] An example of a levothyroxine order that prompts the addition of goiter or hypothyroidism to the problem list is shown in Figure 10-6. Other medication-diagnosis associations created are shown in Table 10-2.

CDS is not for healthcare providers alone. CDS is for patients and informed consumers, as well. Mt. Sinai Hospital (New York, NY) observed significant improvement in medication adherence and a reduction in rejection episodes with text messaging reminders for pediatric recipients of liver transplants.[23]

iTriage is another example of a patient-centered CDS technology. Patient self-management is a key component of the Patient Centered Medical Home and mean-

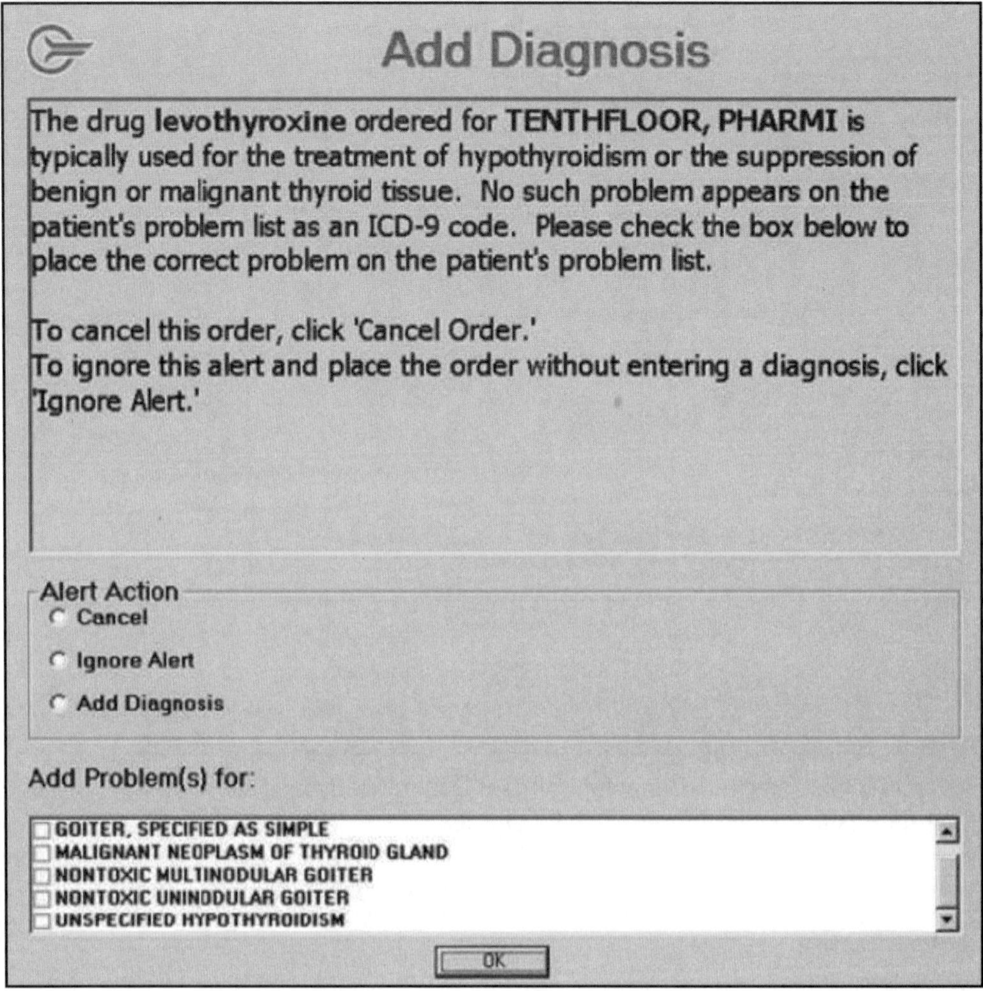
Add Diagnosis

The drug **levothyroxine** ordered for **TENTHFLOOR, PHARMI** is typically used for the treatment of hypothyroidism or the suppression of benign or malignant thyroid tissue. No such problem appears on the patient's problem list as an ICD-9 code. Please check the box below to place the correct problem on the patient's problem list.

To cancel this order, click 'Cancel Order.'
To ignore this alert and place the order without entering a diagnosis, click 'Ignore Alert.'

Alert Action
- Cancel
- Ignore Alert
- Add Diagnosis

Add Problem(s) for:
- GOITER, SPECIFIED AS SIMPLE
- MALIGNANT NEOPLASM OF THYROID GLAND
- NONTOXIC MULTINODULAR GOITER
- NONTOXIC UNINODULAR GOITER
- UNSPECIFIED HYPOTHYROIDISM

OK

Figure 10-6: Example of a Medication-diagnosis Link Alert. The alert is for an order for levothyroxine in a test patient.

Reprinted from *International Journal of Medical Informatics*, Volume 79, Issue 5, May 2010, William L. Galanter, et al. Computerized physician order entry of medications and clinical decision support can improve problem list documentation compliance, pp. 332–338, 2010, with permission from Elsevier.

ingful use, as well. iTriage is a free iPhone application developed by Healthagen. The app assists with patient self-diagnosis prior to a physician visit. In addition to medical information, iTriage has a 911 function for iPhone users.[24]

Implementing CDS

As ingenious and as much as CDS technology appears, getting user adoption can be much harder than expected. No matter how cool the tool, if it is not used, it is worthless.

Some remarkable work has explored why CDS works or does not work.

Investigators from the Veterans Heath Administration, Regenstrief Institute, and Partners HealthCare System examined provider perceptions of colorectal cancer screening CDS (CRC CDS) at their facilities. They conducted interviews, focus groups,

Table 10-2: Target Diagnosis Groups and Medication Triggers Used in the CDS Intervention

Target diagnosis group name	All ICD-9 diagnoses in group	Medication triggers
Diabetes mellitus (DM)	Diabetes mellitus (250.00) polycystic ovarian syndrome (256.4)	Exenatide, meglitinides, metformin, pioglitazone, rosiglitazone, *sulfonyluria*
Hypothyroidism	Goiter (240.0) Hypothyroidism (244.9) Multinodular goiter (241.1) Solitary thyroid nodule (241) thyroid cancer (193)	Levothyroxine
Hyperlipidemia, Coronary atherosclerosis	Unspecified hyperlipidemia (272.4) coronary atherosclerosis (414.00)	Niacin, cholestyramine, colesevelam, colestipol, ezetimibe, fenofibrate, gemfibrozil, HMG-CoA reductase inhibitors
Human immunodeficiency virus (HIV)	Human immunodeficiency virus [HIV] disease (042)	Combination medications, fusion inhibitors, nucleoside reverse transcriptase inhibitor, non-nucleoside reverse transcriptase inhibitor, protease inhibitors.
Asthma, chronic obstructive pulmonary disease	Asthma unspecified (493.90) asthma unspecified with exacerbation (493.92) obstructive chronic bronchitis without exacerbation unspecified (491.20) obstructive chronic bronchitis with exacerbation unspecified (491.21)	Fluticasone inhaled, fluticasone/salmeterol inhaled, tiotroprium inhaled
Ischemic stroke, transient ischemic attack (TIA)	Cerebral thrombosis with cerebral infarction (434.01) cerebral embolism with cerebral infarction (434.11) cerebral thrombosis without mention of cerebral infarction (434.00)	Dipyridamole/aspirin (*aggrenox*)

More then one diagnosis could be proposed for each medication and a diagnosis could be associated with more than one medication.

Reprinted from *International Journal of Medical Informatics*, Volume 79, Issue 5, May 2010, William L. Galanter, et al. Computerized physician order entry of medications and clinical decision support can improve problem list documentation compliance, pp. 332–338, 2010, with permission from Elsevier.

and used direct observation to better understand barriers to adoption of CRC CDS. Six common barriers were described from the primary care providers from all institutions: receiving and documenting exam results from outside the facility, inaccuracy of the CDS, compliance issues, poor usability, lack of coordination between primary care and gastroenterology and the need to attend to more urgent patient issues.[25]

One physician reported: "One patient was sent to GI three times for a colonoscopy. Each time they told him he wasn't due. But the reminder keeps coming up. He had a colonoscopy recently, so I don't know why the reminder doesn't turn off."

Kawamoto et al. from Duke University systematically reviewed the literature in order to determine why some CDS systems succeed while others fail. They identified 22 technical and nontechnical factors in the literature as important determinants of a system's ability to improve clinical practice. Of that number, they found four of the features were significantly correlated with system success, and one feature just over the 0.05 significance level. The four features strongly associated with a CDS's ability to improve clinical practice were as follows: decision support provided automatically as part of clinician workflow, decision support delivered at the time and location of decision making, actionable recommendations provided, and computer based.[26]

Bates and Kuperman are two of the nation's thought-leaders in CDS and have done some of the seminal and groundbreaking work in CPOE and CDS. They have created the Ten Commandments for Effective CDS (see Table 10-3).[27]

Table 10-3: Ten Commandments for Effective Clinical Decision Support[27]

1. Speed is everything—this is what information system users value most.
2. Anticipate needs and deliver in real time—deliver information when needed.
3. Fit into the user's workflow—integrate suggestions with clinical practice.
4. Little things can make a big difference—improve usability to "do the right thing."
5. Recognize that physicians will strongly resist stopping— offer alternatives rather than insist on stopping an action.
6. Changing direction is easier than stopping—changing defaults for dose, route or frequency of a medication can change behavior.
7. Simple interventions work best—simplify guidelines by reducing to a single computer screen.
8. Ask for additional information only when you really need it—the more data elements requested, the less likely a guideline will be implemented.
9. Monitor impact, get feedback, and respond—if certain reminders are not followed, readjust or eliminate the reminder.
10. Manage and maintain your knowledge-based systems—both use of information and currency of information should be carefully monitored.

Reproduced from *Journal of the American Medical Informatics Association*, David W. Bates, et al. Ten Commandments for Effective Clinical Decision Support: Making the Practice of Evidence-based Medicine a Reality, Volume 10, Issue 6, pp. 523–530, 2003, with permission from BMJ Publishing Group Ltd.

The Institute for Safe Medication Practices (ISMO) has released its Guidelines for Standard Order Sets.[28] While its focus is on medications, many of its guidelines apply to other order items.

The guidelines encompass:

- Format
  - Layout and directions for use
  - Font style and type
  - Prompts for patient information
  - Use of symbols, abbreviations, dose designations, punctuation, and Tall Man Letters[29,30]
- Content
  - Content development
  - Content of medication orders
- Approval and Maintenance
- Specific criteria
  - For IV/epidural solutions/medications
  - For electrolytes and compounded products
  - For doses that include fractional amounts
  - For chemotherapy orders
  - For analgesics
  - For pediatric medications dosed according to weight
  - For all medications dosed according to weight
  - For medications intended for patients older than 65 years
  - For paper-based preprinted order sets

On a given project level, an AHRQ-funded study by Das and Eichner found challenges and barriers on the nontechnical, project level:[31]

- The management of the design of clinical decision support interventions takes considerable time and effort.
- Lack of alignment with an organization's overall goals and incentives can affect CDS projects.
- Clinicians do not agree on how prescriptive the CDS application should be.
- Local institutions and providers chose to "customize knowledge."
- Written guidelines are ambiguous and unclear, making it difficult to translate them to computable code.
- Terminology and data exchange standards are still maturing and lack constrained implementation specifications (e.g., the mapping of diagnosis codes used locally at a particular healthcare organization to SNOMED).
- Suboptimal EMR usage by clinicians diminishes the impact of CDS interventions.

For an in-depth guide for how address very real problems like these in implementing medication CDS, see *Improving Medication Use and Outcomes with Clinical Decision Support: A Step-by-Step Guide.*[12] The guide is the product of a unique collaboration of quality organizations, providers, a government agency and EHR vendors: Scottsdale Institute,[32] Epic Systems Corporation,[33] Advocate Health Care,[34] Eclipsys Corporation,[35] Memorial Hermann Health System,[36] CPSI,[37] and the Agency for Healthcare Research and Quality.[38]

The guide includes chapters on optimizing governance structures and management processes, defining outcome improvement opportunities and baselines; setting up interventions in key clinical information systems and for specific targets; deploying CDS interventions to optimize acceptance and value; measuring results and refining the program; and approaching CDS knowledge management systematically.

The guide shares practical pearls like the CDS Five Rights model. The model espouses five critical success factors for CDS improvement:

1. The right information: evidence-based, suitable to guide action, pertinent to the circumstance.
2. To the right person: considering all members of the care team, including clinicians, patients and their caretakers.
3. In the right CDS intervention format: such as an alert, order set or reference information to answer a clinical question.
4. Through the right channel: for example, a clinical information system (CIS) such as an EMR, PHR, or a more general channel such as the Internet or a mobile device.
5. At the right time in workflow: for example, at time of decision/action/need.

WATCH OUT FOR THAT OIL SPILL

When an oil worker told investigators on July 23 [2010] that an alarm to warn of explosive gas on the Transocean rig in the Gulf of Mexico had been intentionally disabled months before, it struck many people as reckless. Reckless, maybe, but not unusual. On Tuesday, the National Transportation Safety Board said that a crash last year on the Washington subway system that killed nine people had happened partly because

> train dispatchers had been ignoring 9,000 alarms per week. Air traffic controllers, nuclear plant operators, nurses in intensive-care units and others do the same. Mark R. Rosekind, a psychologist who is a member of the National Transportation Safety Board, said the cases had something in common. "The volume of alarms desensitizes people," he said. "They learn to ignore them."[39]

We have all done it. An alert or alarm (read "decision support") goes off and we ignore it. Maybe it is jaywalking against a red walk signal on New Year's Day with no cars in sight. Maybe it is driving your car with the empty fuel icon lit trying to see how far you can drive before stopping at the next gas station.[40] We have all succumbed at one time or other to alert fatigue.

Alert fatigue is a loathsome barrier to CDS adoption and success. When the noise-to-signal ratio becomes unbearable, we ignore that annoying alert. Unfortunately, with too many false alarms, the one true alarm can be too easily overlooked.

Van der Sijs et al. reviewed the literature on physician response to drug safety alerts. In the 17 studies they reviewed, drug safety alerts are overridden by clinicians in 49 to 96 percent of cases. The authors recommended that a distinction between appropriate and useful alerts should be made. The alerting system may contain error-producing conditions, such as low specificity, low sensitivity, unclear information content, unnecessary workflow disruptions, and unsafe and inefficient handling. These may result in active failures of the physician, such as ignoring alerts, misinterpretation and incorrect handling.[41]

At Partners Healthcare, Paterno et al. analyzed 71,350 drug-drug interaction (DDI) alerts, of which 39,474 occurred at a site with non-tiered alerts and 31,876 at a site with tiered alerts. There were 3 grades of tiered alerts: least serious (Figure 10-7), more serious (Figure 10-8) and most serious (Figure 10-9). Compliance with DDI alerts was higher at the site with tiered DDI alerts compared to the non-tiered site (29 vs. 10 percent, p=0.001). At the tiered site, 100 percent of the most severe alerts were accepted, versus only 34 percent at the non-tiered site; moderately severe alerts were also more likely to be accepted at the tiered site (29 vs. 10 percent). Tiered alerting by severity was associated with higher compliance rates of DDI alerts in the inpatient setting, and lack of tiering was associated with a high override rate of more severe alerts.[42]

George Reynolds, MD, a pediatric intensivist and chief medical informatics officer at Children's Hospital Medical Center in Omaha, Nebraska, remarks "I don't want alerts to fire at all. I want the order sets to be written well enough that they steer doctors to the right choices." Using a business intelligence application and 300 order sets, he's driven down the rate that CPOE triggers an alert to 6.6 percent of orders. Even with that alert rate, only 22 percent of the alerts result in a physician changing his behavior.[43]

CDS technology is not (yet) standardized. What has been coded at one hospital may not work at another hospital even if they have the same EHR vendor. If they have different EHR vendors, the CDS tool will have to be recreated (if the hospital has the staff to help develop it and the EHR vendor is willing).

As an expert panel from the American Medical Informatics Association opined: "Such multiple 'reinventing-the-wheel' processes limit the availability of good CDS tools, as each manufacturer and implementer of such systems struggles to develop the

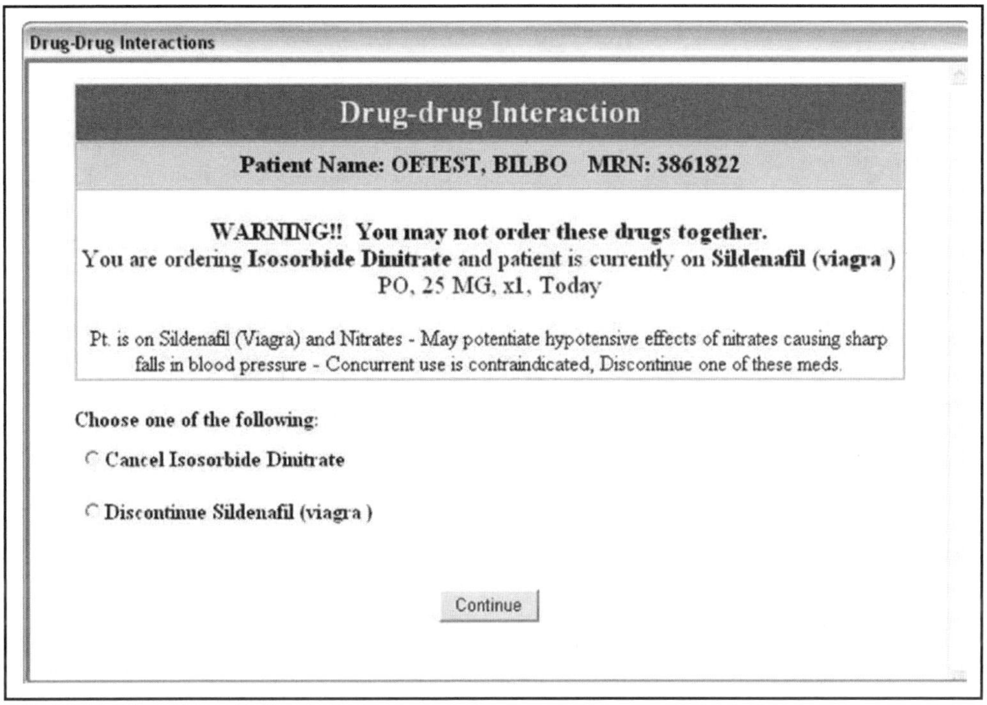

Drug-Drug Interactions

Drug-drug Interaction

Patient Name: OETEST, BILBO MRN: 3861822

WARNING!! You may not order these drugs together.
You are ordering **Isosorbide Dinitrate** and patient is currently on **Sildenafil (viagra)** PO, 25 MG, x1, Today

Pt. is on Sildenafil (Viagra) and Nitrates - May potentiate hypotensive effects of nitrates causing sharp falls in blood pressure - Concurrent use is contraindicated, Discontinue one of these meds.

Choose one of the following:

○ **Cancel Isosorbide Dinitrate**

○ **Discontinue Sildenafil (viagra)**

Continue

Figure 10-7: Level 1 Alert

Reproduced from *Journal of the American Medical Informatics Association*, Marilyn D. Paterno, et al. Tiering Drug–Drug Interaction Alerts by Severity Increases Compliance Rates, Volume 16, Issue 1, pp. 40–46, with permission from BMJ Publishing Group Ltd.

Drug-Drug Interactions

Drug-related Alerts

Patient Name: OETEST, BILBO MRN: 3861822

You are ordering: **WARFARIN SODIUM.** Click here to
Cancel Warfarin Sodium

To keep the WARFARIN SODIUM order, you must respond to each of the interaction alerts below.

Drug-drug Interaction Alerts	Action
Patient is currently on: **Fluconazole** PO, 400 MG, QD, Begin day before transplant and continue QD Pt. on Warfarin and Azole Antifungal : Potentiation of warfarin - Recommend to avoid concurrent use but if co-therapy is warranted, Rec. to reduce warfarin dose by 33-50 % and follow pt closely.	○ Discontinue Fluconazole **Reason for override** ☐ Will adjust dose as recommended ☐ Will monitor as recommended ☐ Patient has already tolerated combination ☐ No reasonable alternatives ☐ Other

Continue (Keep WARFARIN SODIUM)

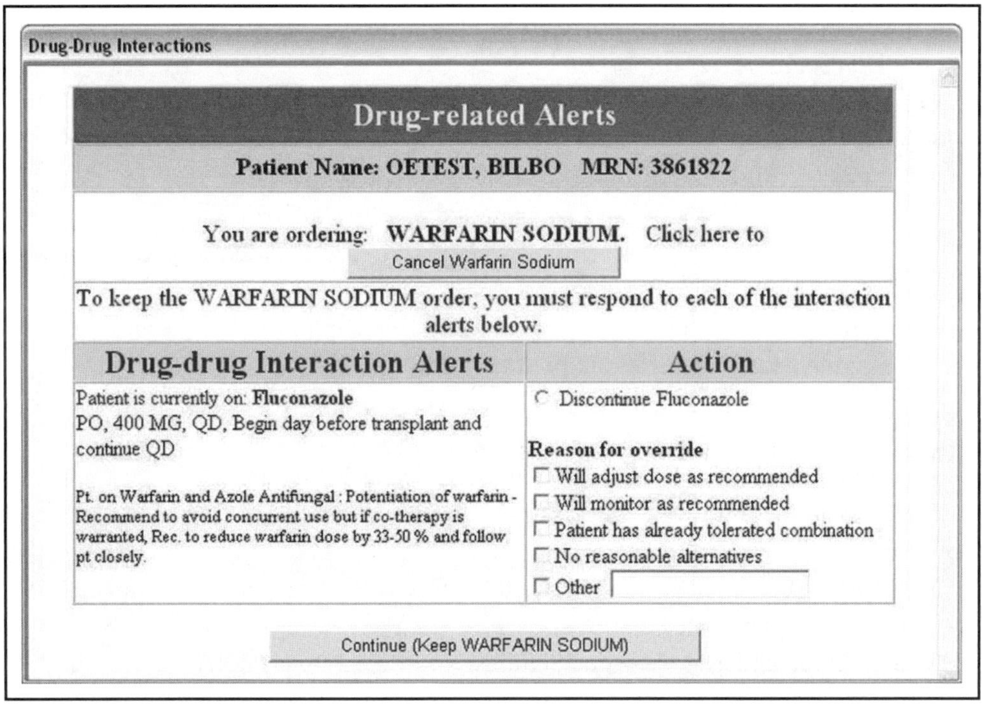

Figure 10-8: Level 2 Alert

Reproduced from *Journal of the American Medical Informatics Association*, Marilyn D. Paterno, et al. Tiering Drug–Drug Interaction Alerts by Severity Increases Compliance Rates, Volume 16, Issue 1, pp. 40–46, with permission from BMJ Publishing Group Ltd.

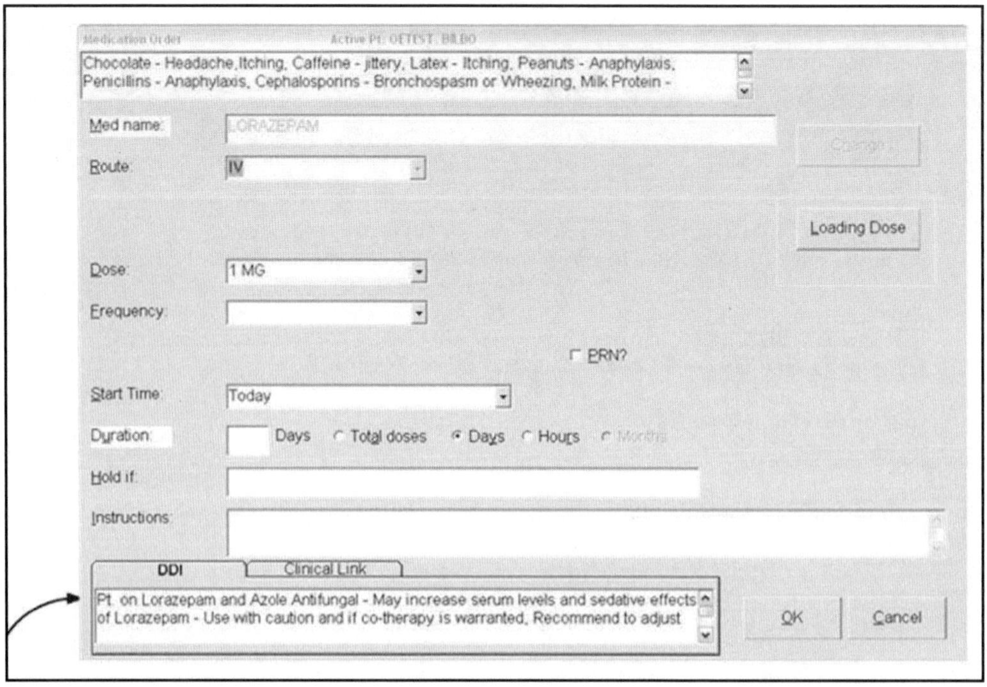

Figure 10-9: Level 3 Alert

Reproduced from *Journal of the American Medical Informatics Association*, Marilyn D. Paterno, et al. Tiering Drug–Drug Interaction Alerts by Severity Increases Compliance Rates, Volume 16, Issue 1, pp. 40–46, with permission from BMJ Publishing Group Ltd.

same interventions, or, for lack of time and ability to do so, simply leaves out CDS interventions that could deliver important benefits.[44]

Sittig et al. advocate a national repository for CDS interventions would mitigate the following problems:[45]

- Difficulty translating medical knowledge and guidelines into a form usable by EHRs.
- Technical challenges in developing a standard representation for CDS content that could be shared across sites.
- Absence of a central knowledge repository where human readable and executable guideline knowledge can be shared and stored.
- Challenges integrating decision support into clinical workflow and other barriers to IT adoption.
- Limited capabilities for CDS in commercially available EHRs.

They recommend the following preliminary standards for creating such a national repository:

- **Step 1:** Access to high-quality, standardized, syntactically and semantically encoded patient data.
- **Step 2:** A standard for encoded clinical knowledge that is both human- and machine-readable.
- **Step 3:** A set of standard CDS intervention types (drug-drug interaction alerts or condition-specific order sets).

- **Step 4:** A set of standard locations within clinicians' electronically enabled clinical workflow at which CDS interventions can be presented to clinicians, and the requisite EMR functionality for the CDS intervention. For example, when selecting a medication from a list, the clinician is told that the current patient has an allergy to a particular medication.
- **Step 5:** A standard method for either requesting patient data in a standard format or having these data automatically sent to an application that is separate from the EMR (perhaps as a service on the Internet, for example).
- **Step 6:** A validated, open-access, CDS knowledge base that contains at least a starter set of standard, high-quality, clinically evaluated CDS interventions that can be downloaded and utilized, or perhaps accessed over the Internet as a service, by any CCHIT-approved EMR system.
- **Step 7:** Agreement on and development of a set of clinical quality measures that can be used to measure and monitor the effectiveness of the CDS interventions previously described.

CMS-certified EHRs and the meaningful use measures provide an opportunity to standardize and require CDS that works. Public comments from a recent ONC workshop on CDS illustrate how the current national discussion on CDS can guide its future development.[13]

- CDS should support team-based care: New audiences for CDS over time may well be expected to include patients, case managers, and others as new models of team-based, information-driven care emerge to achieve high-value, accessible, affordable care for all Americans.
- A culture of quality improvement is important to effective use of CDS.
- Clinician engagement in CDS planning and implementation is critical to success.
- User adoption depends upon implementation of highly usable systems.
- Greater CDS specificity can reduce alert fatigue: Multiple participants noted that the knowledge base for DDIs is such that if you turn on "all" alerts, so many alerts fire that it grinds clinical workflow to a halt. Discussions noted that there is not yet an easy or clear way to identify a subset of highest-value, highest-priority rules that will improve patient safety without impeding workflow. If a provider office or hospital chooses not to turn on all DDI alerts in order to decrease the number of alerts that do not need to be acted upon, there is concern that this may lead to increased liability exposure. Discussions noted that it would be helpful to specify the top drug-drug and drug-allergy interactions, as well as the top drug dosing guidelines, for use within CDS in the meaningful use matrix.
- Other fields offer computer interaction principles that can be leveraged, e.g., nuclear power, space aviation.
- Promote collaborations among stakeholders that can support effective use of CDS.
- Including CDS in the definition of meaningful use of EHRs is important.
- Meaningful use should allow for variations in CDS techniques, objectives and localization of goals.
- Specialties and different practice types must not be overlooked.

- Provide effective guidance and best practice examples.
- Incentives and drivers can promote CDS adoption.
- Providing liability protection or advantage may speed CDS adoption.
- Patients have a role to play in CDS.
- Translating guidelines into CDS is complex, so we should be able to leverage collective efforts.
- Opportunities for data standardization.
- Translation of knowledge into codified structures and mechanisms for dissemination of codified knowledge are key to sharing and reuse of CDS interventions.
- CDS & quality need to quickly incorporate evolving evidence.
- Specific ideas that stakeholder groups may consider for focused development/action.
- Identify a "short list" of the most important drug-drug, and drug-allergy interactions to support with CDS. This will necessitate the development of a model for rule creation/review/editing.
- Develop a reference of best CDS practices and exemplary implementation sites:
  - Build a library of CDS reference implementations, by practice type, as a starting point that others could emulate.
  - Develop a "usability checklist" that identifies standard wait times of no longer than X seconds, etc.
  - Collect good practices and exemplars associated with incorporating a computer into the exam room during ambulatory patient visits.
  - Build a national health IT simulation lab, similar to the national driving simulator, to help providers assess the functionality and usability of EHR and CDS systems. Products could be configured to address specific patient scenarios, and users could "test drive" them to assist vendors in improving their products while giving providers information on which systems are the most functional and usable.
  - Develop a vendor-independent certification for "expert implementers of Health IT systems"—similar to a Good Housekeeping seal or Angie's List.
  - Develop an accreditation for guideline developers to ensure that they follow required principles in translating guidelines into codified knowledge and CDS interventions.
  - Develop a robust set of use cases to test the hypothesis that a common data set could service both CDS and quality measurement.
  - Develop a list of CDS intervention types with key parameters as a first step in standardization and sharing of CDS across disparate EHR systems.

Clearly, we have much work to do in developing and standardizing CDS to optimize meaningful use of the EHR. Nevertheless, one day CDS in health IT will be as ubiquitous as the dashboard in our cars.

REFERENCES

1. For the year 2007. U.S. Department of Transportation. Available online at: www.bts.gov/publications/national_transportation_statistics/html/table_01_11.html. Last accessed August 2010.

2. Available online at: http://en.wikipedia.org/wiki/Dashboard. Last accessed August 2010.

3. Table 1067. Motor Vehicle Accidents—Number and Deaths: 1980 to 2007. Available online at: www.census.gov/compendia/statab/2010/tables/10s1067.pdf. Last accessed August 2010.

4. Barta A et al. ICD-10-CM Primer. *Journal of AHIMA*. 79, no.5 (May 2008): 64-6. Available online at: http://library.ahima.org/xpedio/groups/public/documents/ahima/bok1_038084.hcsp?dDocName=bok1_038084. Last accessed August 2010.

5. National Drug Code Database File Available online at: http://www.fda.gov/downloads/Drugs/DevelopmentApprovalProcess/UCM070838.zip. Last August 2010.

6. Stead WW, Kelly BJ, Kolodner RM. Achievable steps toward building a national health information infrastructure in the United States. *JAMIA*. 2005;12(2):113–120.

7. Balas EA. Information systems can prevent errors and improve quality. *JAMIA*. 2001;8(4):398-9.

8. Yarnall KSH, Ostbye T, Krause KM et al. Family physicians as team leaders: "Time" to share the care. *Preventing Chronic Disease*. April 2009;6(2):1-6. Available online at: www.cdc.gov/pcd/issues/2009/apr/08_0023.htm. Last accessed August 2010.

9. McGlynn EA, Asch SM, Adams J et al. The quality of health care delivered to adults in the United States. *N Engl J Med*. 2003;348:2635-45.

10. Recommendations to HHS By the American Health Information Community Clinical Decision Support Ad Hoc Planning Group April 22, 2008. Available online at: www.hhs.gov/healthit/documents/m20080422/6.2_cds_recs.html. Last accessed August 2010.

11. Clinical Decision Support (CDS) Fact Sheet. HIMSS, 2009. Available online at: www.himss.org/content/files/CDSFactSheet3-17-09.pdf. Last accessed August 2010.

12. Osheroff JA (ed). *Improving Medication Use and Outcomes with Clinical Decision Support: A Step-by-Step Guide*. Chicago: HIMSS; 2009.

13. Clinical Decision Support Workshop Meeting Summary, August 25 – 26, 2009. Office of the National Coordinator for Health Information Technology Available online at: http://healthit.hhs.gov/portal/server.pt/gateway/PTARGS_0_11113_898639_0_0_18/ONC%20CDS%20Workshop%20Meeting%20Summary_f.pdf. Last accessed August 2010.

14. Gawande A. *The Checklist Manifesto*. New York City: Metropolitan Books, 2009.

15. Available online at: http://whqlibdoc.who.int/publications/2009/9789241598590_eng_Checklist.pdf. Last accessed August 2010.

16. Haynes AB, Weiser TG, Berry WR et al. A surgical safety checklist to reduce morbidity and mortality in a global population. *N Engl J Med*. 2009;360:491-9.

17. Gawande A. The Checklist: If something so simple can transform intensive care, what else can it do? *The New Yorker*, December 10, 2007. Available online at: www.newyorker.com/reporting/2007/12/10/071210fa_fact_gawande. Last accessed August 2010.

18. Santolin CJ, Boyer LS. Change of care for patients With acute myocardial infarctions through algorithm and standardized physician order sets. *Crit Pathways in Cardiol*. 2004;3: 79–82.

19. Cimino JJ. Use, Usability, Usefulness, and Impact of an Infobutton Manager. *AMIA Annual Symp Proc*. 2006;151-5.

20. Bell LM et al. Electronic health record based decision support to improve asthma care: A cluster-randomized trial. *Pediatrics*. 2010;125;e770-7. Available online at: www.pediatrics.org/cgi/content/full/125/4/e770. Last accessed August 2010.

21. Novis SJ et al. Prevention of thromboembolic events in surgical patients through the creation and implementation of a computerized risk assessment program. *J Vasc Surg*. 2010;51:648-54.

22. Galanter WL, Hier DB, Jao C et al. Computerized physician order entry of medications and clinical decision support can improve problem list documentation compliance. *Int J Med Inform.* 2010;79(5):332-8.

23. Miloh T, Annunziato R, Arnon R et al. Improved adherence and outcomes for pediatric liver transplant recipients by using text messaging. *Pediatrics.* 2009;124;e844-50.

24. Available online at: www.itriagehealth.com/. Last accessed August 2010.

25. Saleem JJ et al. Provider Perceptions of Colorectal Cancer Screening Clinical Decision Support at Three Benchmark Institutions. *AMIA 2009 Symposium Proc.* 558-62.

26. Kawamoto K, Houlihan CS, Balas A et al. Improving clinical practice using clinical decision support systems: a systematic review of trials to identify features critical to success. *BMJ.* 2005; doi:10.1136/bmj.38398.500764.8F.

27. Bates DW, Kuperman GJ, Wang S et al. Ten commandments for effective clinical decision support: making the practice of evidence- based medicine a reality. *JAMIA.* 2003;10:523–30.

28. Available at: www.google.com/url?sa=t&source=web&cd=1&ved=0CBUQFjAA&url=http%3A%2F%2Fwww.ismp.org%2FTools%2Fguidelines%2FStandardOrderSets.pdf&ei=ugZfTJm6NoWKlwfw7PEM&usg=AFQjCNF4DkkPOsd_ANUUugcEW-L89FVGGg&sig2=KLjWB80zRsbcgKtCAOv5bQ. Last accessed August 2010.

29. Available online at: www.ismp.org/tools/tallmanletters.pdf. Last accessed November 2010.

30. Available online at: www.ismp.org/tools/errorproneabbreviations.pdf. Last accessed November 2010.

31. Das M, Eichner J. Challenges and Barriers to Clinical Decision Support (CDS) Design and Implementation Experienced in the Agency for Healthcare Research and Quality CDS Demonstrations (Prepared for the AHRQ National Resource Center for Health Information Technology under Contract No. 290-04-0016.) AHRQ Publication No. 10-0064-EF. Rockville, MD: Agency for Healthcare Research and Quality. March 2010.

32. Available online at: www.scottsdaleinstitute.org. Last accessed November 2010.

33. Available online at: www.epicsystems.com. Last accessed November 2010.

34. Available online at: www.advocatehealth.com. Last accessed November 2010.

35. Available online at: www.eclipsys.com. Last accessed November 2010.

36. Available online at www.memorialhermann.org. Last accessed November 2010.

37. Available online at: www.cpsinet.com. Last accessed November 2010.

38. Available online at: www.ahrq.gov. Last accessed November 2010.

39. Wald ML. For No Signs of Trouble, Kill the Alarm. *New York Times.* July 31, 2010.

40. The Dealership, Seinfeld episode first broadcasted on January 8, 2998. Available at: www.seinfeld-scripts.com/TheDealership.htm. Last accessed August 2010.

41. Van der Sijs H, Aarts J et al. Overriding of drug safety alerts in computerized physician order entry. JAMIA. 2006;13:138–47. DOI 10.1197/jamia.M1809.

42. Paterno M, Maviglia S, Gorman P et al. Tiering drug–drug interaction alerts by severity increases compliance rates. *JAMIA.* 2009;16:40–46. DOI 10.1197/jamia.M2808.

43. Avoiding Alert Fatigue. Health Data Management Magazine, October 1, 2009. Available at: www.informationmanagement.com/news/data_management_health_care_information_entry-10016200-1.html. Last accessed August 2010.

44. Osheroff JA, Teich JM, Middleton BF et al. A Roadmap for National Action on Clinical Support *JAMIA.* 2007;14(2):141-5. Epub 2007 Jan 9.

45. Sittig DF, Wright A, Ash JS et al. A Set of Preliminary Standards Recommended for Achieving a National Repository of Clinical Decision Support Interventions. *AMIA 2009 Symposium Proc.* 614-618.

CHAPTER 11

Project Management: Lessons from the Primary Care Information Project

Mytri Pritam Singh, MPH

INTRODUCTION

The Primary Care Information Project (PCIP) is a community EHR extension project founded by the New York City Department of Health and Mental Hygiene (NYC DOHMH). Since July 2007, the PCIP has implemented a commercially available EHR, eClinicalWorks (eCW), at more than 460 practices and with 2,200 providers in private physician offices, health centers, and hospital out-patient departments (OPDs).

Small practices typically include between one and five providers' offices, whereas large practices can vary between five and a few hundred providers spread over numerous sites and can include many medical specialties. Even though the practices we work with are typically already using some kind of practice management system, they require significant assistance preparing and transforming their practice to a fully integrated EHR. Our implementation success rate is over 99 percent, with less than 1 percent of our providers reverting back to paper.

Some of the reasons for this success are:

- PCIP's role as a neutral third party that can advocate for the practice and EHR vendor as needed
- Hands-on support provided by our team of PCIP Project Managers (called Implementation Specialists) who work closely with the vendor and practice project managers (PMs)
- A close monitoring of the implementation process and slippage using high-level project milestones
- Weekly status meetings with the eCW PMs to touch base on practices and problem-solve through any challenges, the eCW support account managers to escalate practice issues, and the two executive teams to discuss high-level strategy
- Enterprise-wide solutions to systemic challenges, such as creating a separate project management pathway for tracking reference lab implementations

- A prerequisite set of utilization and quality measures that demonstrate a practice's comprehensive use of their EHR
- Leveraging the ability of the DOHMH to connect practices to hardware subsidy programs and bulk discounts, making EHR implementation affordable to providers serving the medically underserved patients in New York City

This chapter will describe how best-practice project management concepts can be applied to EHR implementation. The key players in this process are the PMs from the physician practice, the EHR vendor, and PCIP. The usual mechanism of engagement is one in which a practice contracts with the EHR vendor and relies on them for implementation and post go-live support. In this case, PCIP was funded to not only subsidize the cost of the EHR, but also to provide additional project management and wraparound support to practices who serve medically underserved patients in New York City. This is the model being used by Regional Extension Centers to help support and serve healthcare providers to become adept and meaningful users of EHRs.

One definition of Project Management is "the discipline of planning, organizing, and managing resources to bring about the successful completion of specific project goals and objectives."[1] In addition, it seeks to apply the "techniques and systems to the execution of a project from start to finish to achieve predetermined objectives of scope, quality, time and cost,"[2] which are the critical constraints of any project. Project Managers can obtain Project Management Professional certification from the Project Management Institute (PMI) and join a network of over 300,000 professionals in the field.[3] This certification provides a strong foundation in the principles of project management methodology and enhances a PMs marketability.

PROJECT STAFF ROLES

Sponsor

The Project Sponsor is the "senior executive responsible for the project. The sponsor has authority over both the project team and the customer and makes sure that all the resources necessary to succeed are available to the team. The sponsor kicks off the project at the initial meeting, promotes the project at the highest level of the organization, receives regular status reports, and intervenes when necessary to remove roadblocks for the project team."[4] The Sponsor is also responsible for selecting the PM and signing off on the Project Charter.

The Project Sponsors for PCIP were Commissioner Thomas R. Frieden, MD, MPH, and Assistant Commissioner Farzad Mostashari, MD, MSPH, both of whom provided significant oversight of the project. Dr. Mostashari met with various PCIP project teams on a daily basis, and Dr. Frieden met with PCIP's Executive team twice a month. For small practices, the Sponsor will predominantly be the lead physician—and in health centers and hospital OPDs, the CEO, CMO, or CIO. Some projects have suffered greatly due to inadequate support from the Sponsor who was faced with competing priorities and let the EHR implementation take a backseat to others. There is a dramatic difference in implementations that have strong sponsor support and presence, especially as the team faces challenges along the way. It is the role of the PM to ensure that Sponsors receive adequate feedback at the appropriate frequency and in sufficient detail, so they can provide optimal assistance in clearing any obstacles. Providing too little detail might obscure important points, whereas giving too much detail might waste time and energy.

The role of the Sponsor is absolutely essential in the rollout of a large multi-site implementation. The Sponsor can help facilitate the rollout discussions with the site-level leaders to determine the best sequence and speed for the project. Sometimes external determinants, such as the need to spend down allocated resources within a fiscal year, can determine the parameters of a project, but site-specific needs must also be taken into account to allow for the best possible results.

In the Planning phase, the Project Team must work closely with the Sponsor to take into account various factors such as:

- The presence of key opinion leaders among the early adopters who can weather the initial hurdles experienced by going first. These early adopters must also serve as super users for those that follow.
- The effect of other internal or external competing priorities, such as upcoming construction, annual reporting deadlines for health centers, the start of the school year for pediatricians, planned vacations, etc.
- The hardware preparedness of a site—the better equipped and more tech-savvy, the easier their implementation.
- The computer skills of all staff including those at the front desk, billing department, clinical support staff and providers.
- The number of external interfaces required, such as with reference labs, diagnostic imaging and billing companies.
- The number of PM staff available to assist each practice adequately through all phases of the project, including preparing for the implementation, execution and post go-live support.
- The number of staff at the site, as well as the mix of full-time and part-time staff, residents, specialists, etc.

Once the decision about the rollout schedule has been determined, it is the role of the Sponsor to help launch the project, build buy-in, and provide ongoing support and momentum to the team. The Sponsor will need to engage the necessary leaders to ensure that the sites are on board with the project and the PM team does not experience push back from sites that seek to slow down or resist their implementation. The PM team must engage the Sponsor as soon as there is project slippage, as this is a shared responsibility. This allows the PM to focus on the rollout without engaging in combative discussions with resistors. There should also be periodic celebrations that recognize the achievement of interim or significant milestones. Large institutions can undergo projects that last over several years, so it is critical to support and celebrate the successes of the team along the way.

Project Manager

Some of the key skills necessary for a PM include the following: communication, organization and planning, budgeting, conflict management, negotiation and influencing, leadership, and team building and motivating.[5] PMs need to have sufficient depth and breadth of knowledge in order to be effective. They need to understand the needs of the project in sufficient detail and be able to keep track of all its moving parts. In health

IT projects, "Project managers are expected to possess more of an understanding of technology than a command of technology."[6] In addition to having the training and background in the principles and tools necessary to manage this process, PMs must possess the intangible drive and "can-do" attitude that provides them with the fortitude to overcome obstacles and continuously be a few steps ahead of the rest of the team. The PM is ultimately accountable for the success and quality of the project and must mobilize all necessary resources to accomplish their tasks.

In the case of the PCIP, this role is shared between all three, but ultimately the PMs from PCIP and the vendor have the shared goal of bringing approximately 100 providers live per month. This allows the PMs the flexibility to modify individual project plans for struggling practices while keeping the overall project goals on track.

Project Team

As shown in Table 11-1, a project team is "comprised of the project manager, project management team, and other team members who carry out the work but who are not necessarily involved with the management of the project. The team is comprised of individuals from different groups with knowledge of a specific subject matter or with a specific skill set who carry out the work of the project."[7]

The PCIP PM (or Implementation Specialist) serves as the main point of contact during the project implementation. Additional teams are mobilized based on the stage of implementation and size of the practice. As seen in Table 11-1, in a small practice, the Provider or Office Manger can play multiple roles (including that of a PM), which may be outside of his or her typical field of expertise. This can cause significant delays

Table 11-1: Makeup of an EHR Implementation Team

Task [PCIP Team Member]	EHR Vendor	Small Practices	Large Practices
Implementation Project Management [Implementation Specialist]	Project Manager, Support Manager, Trainer	Project Manager, Provider, Office Manager	Project Management Team
Infrastructure [IT Coordinator]	Technical Specialist	IT Consultant	IT Department
Interfaces: labs, billing, immunization registry, diagnostic imaging [Systems Integration team]	Interface team External vendors (reference labs, billing company, Health Department, DI companies)	Providers, Office Managers	IT Department, Hospital or in-house lab
Billing [Billing Specialist]	Billing Specialist	Provider, Office Manager, Biller	Financial Department
Privacy and Security [Privacy and Security Consultant]	Trainer	Provider, Office Manager, IT Consultant	IT Department, Legal Counsel
Quality Assurance [Development team]	Trainer	Provider, Office Manager	Site Administrators, QI Unit
Quality Improvement [Super User, Quality Improvement Specialist]	Data Reporting team	Provider, Office Manager, Panel Manager	Quality Improvement Unit, Data Analysis Department

in the time line and in the speed at which the project gets implemented. Some practices function at such a small profit margin that the provider will allocate time during the day to see some walk-in patients rather than complete necessary project tasks, such as filling in clearinghouse information necessary to start their practice enrollment. In this scenario the provider is performing the function of a Provider, Project Manager, and biller. In the long run, providers may need to find a part-time biller who can dedicate time and energy to the billing setup and testing rather than trying to do it all themselves.

One solution that was used by a few collaborating neighborhood practices was to share a PM who was just dedicated to their EHR implementations, thereby allowing the providers to see patients with minimal interruptions. The PM spent 1–2 days per week at each practice, facilitating quicker dissemination of new learning between the practices, sharing resources, enabling greater flexibility in training schedules, sharing templates between specialists, and negotiating a bulk discount for hardware.

The PMs should ensure that they learn the privacy and security settings of the EHR to protect the patients and practice. They should work with the trainers, IT or legal departments to sign off on the default settings that force password resets, time out for sessions, and set up role-based access. Practices must also ensure that Quality Assurance measures that existed on paper are adapted to the EHR and that Site Administrators configure the system appropriately so that they are able to run their QA and QI reports once the project is complete and the data are captured in the EHR.

Table 11-1 also shows the range of tasks that need to occur, sometimes concurrently during the months of implementation. For example, a PM will need to engage the Interface team at the start of the process to ensure that all interfaces are set up at the time of go-live. Inadequate interface testing can cause some of the most significant delays in the implementation time line, and its importance can never be underestimated. Therefore, engaging the right team members at the right time and with the correct frequency is a crucial part of the process.

Larger practices have different teams that handle the different tasks of Project Management, external interfaces, billing, and IT support, so they are able to dedicate a significantly large amount of resources to the overall project. Ideally, having strong teams dedicated to various aspects of the project should lead to a more coordinated and smoother implementation process, but often challenges inherent to every organization rise to the surface. The PM has the formidable task of coordinating conflicting schedules, juggling multiple team priorities, addressing organizational politics, and addressing entrenched resistance to change. The process of EHR adoption can often exacerbate any pre-existing issues that exist at a practice and must be dealt with deftly. A skilled PM can help facilitate such resolution with the help of the Sponsor.

The interplay of multiple teams in a large practice, if managed well, can work to create a matrix organization that can be a powerful vehicle for change. One large health center in PCIP created such a structure for their EHR rollout, and it remains a focal point from which new initiatives are launched. The project team has proven itself to be well respected, talented, empowered, resourceful and visionary. They have demonstrated project success and have the full support of their senior leadership.

Customers

In the context of an EHR Implementation, the customers can be the providers, ancillary practice staff, patients, families, caregivers and health plans. Patients are important stakeholders in this process, as they are dramatically affected by the short-term upheaval the practice is undergoing during this significant project and are often provided no roadmap for what to expect. Practices forget to communicate to the patients how they are the ultimate beneficiaries of this practice transformation. The end point of the project may be limited to the practice going live on the EHR, but the goal for the providers to start using the EHR as a tool to improve the quality of care they provide through the use of clinical decision support, point of care alerts, population management, medication reconciliation tools, and the other features of the EHR. However, the immediate experience of the patient is not an understanding of how they will ultimately receive better preventive care, but rather one of longer wait times, less quality time with the provider and a repetition of their medical history that is no longer accessible to the provider. This is a very real concern of both provider and patient and must be addressed.

A key role of the PM is to help the provider engage patients in this transformative process from the start. Putting up signs in the waiting room that have an upbeat description of the stages of the project and its current status will go a long way in empowering the patients. Showing patients what they stand to gain through this process is also critical in having them be active participants in their healthcare. Encouraging them to sign up for the patient portal at an early stage can yield some early benefits, such as getting them immediate access to their lab results. The PCIP also made use of our Department of Health's public health detailing campaigns[8] (modeled after the pharmaceutical model) to deliver brief health messages and materials that focus on key clinical areas. The PCIP campaign encouraged providers to adopt an EHR and also marketed the benefits to the patients.[9] These materials were distributed to the entire care team at a practice and attractively displayed in waiting rooms for patients to read. When the full care team is engaged, members see their own role in the newly enhanced workflows. For example, instead of just having the patient sign a check-in sheet and sit in the waiting room, the front desk staff can now educate the patient about the patient portal, obtain their consent and e-mail address, and queue them up for a conversation with the provider.

Stakeholders

Stakeholders can be internal (such as board members, the legal department, site administrators, medical directors and providers) or external (such as patients; federal, state, or local government funders; Public Health reporting agencies; quality improvement organizations; and banks). Engaging and communicating with all stakeholders is a key aspect of the PM's task, especially as organizations stand to lose considerable funding if they fall behind in their loan repayment plan or have a disruption in their mandatory reporting requirements. Obtaining funding for the purchase of hardware has been increasingly challenging for practices, such that PMs must adjust their schedules to accommodate a bank's requirement of matching the release of funds with proof of work completed. Similarly, all Federally Qualified Health Centers (FQHCs) have a Quarter 1 deadline for completing their Uniform Data System (UDS) data such that all available resources will be mobilized to help compile these reports. The PMs must plan for and adjust their expectations during the first quarter of the year to accommodate this critical stakeholder.

A key stakeholder and partner for PCIP has been the Medical Independent Practice Associations (IPAs) that have negotiated rates with EHR vendors, provided support to members implementing an EHR, built a network of shared resources, facilitated group training and other activities critical to adoption. Their role in mobilizing their affiliated community providers (often affiliated based on geography, ethnicity or hospital affiliation) has been extremely beneficial.

Vendors

Prior to the start of the project, the Sponsor must engage and line up contracts with multiple vendors or subcontractors to ensure that services and deliverable deadlines are coordinated and met. Some of the critical contracts are with the EHR vendor, reference laboratories, radiology and diagnostic imaging centers, pharmacies, the E-prescribing company, IT consultants, Internet providers, hardware retailers, clearinghouses, and billers. The role of the PM is to ensure that all necessary contracts are in place and monitored over the course of the project. Holding all vendors accountable and coordinated is essential, especially as delays with one may significantly affect other interdependent entities.

PROJECT LIFECYCLE

There are typically five phases to a project's lifecycle: concept, definition, planning, execution and closeout.[10] The Concept or Initiation phase involves conducting a review of the market and an articulation of the problem. The Definition phase involves developing a mission and vision for the project and outlining what is included and excluded from the scope. Spending sufficient time in the Definition phase is essential, as it determines the ensuing success of the project. Planning is an absolutely critical phase, as poorly planned projects have a greater likelihood of failure. This is the time to think through all the possible challenges and impediments, as it is considerably cheaper to solve them in this early phase than during execution. Planning the implementation pathway and all possible risk management strategies is also important so that they seamlessly lead into the execution phase. This phase also includes control because mid-course corrections must be reflected in the revised plan, which then serves as the new roadmap.

Finally, closing an EHR Implementation Project can be challenging, as the scope of the project can continue to expand due to technological advances and changes in the industry. For example, there can be significant "add-ons" that were not part of the original scope or not developed at the time of implementation, such as the patient portal, connectivity to an HIE and bi-directional lab or immunization registry. Therefore, a project can be coming to a close but may need to be expanded if a significant set of additions needs to be implemented. This can also be addressed by creating multi-phase projects with staggered time lines.

In addition, a project may need to be halted due to unforeseen or unavoidable conditions, at which point all concerns and accomplishments must be documented with the appropriate level of detail.[11] There have been cases in which practices halt their implementation midway through due to budgetary concerns or a change in leadership. Having appropriate archival documentation will help the next team pick up where the first one left off.

PROJECT MANAGEMENT TOOLS

Numerous tools can be used for tracking during the cycle of the project. Those which end up being used are typically dictated by the budgetary restrictions or by the level of sophistication of the project staff. IT consultants and EHR vendors typically use Visio[12] or MS Project[13] to create floorplan recommendations and project plans. They serve not only as implementation documents but also as reference guides for their policy and procedure manuals. Providers can also be given access to the vendor's project management and support portals so they can stay current with the latest project plans, add in key provider- and practice-level information, make requests for additional training dates, schedule times for software installation, and other project tasks. When all else fails, making detailed plans using Excel[14] can be just as effective and easy to use.

PROJECT MANAGEMENT KNOWLEDGE AREAS

According to the Project Management Book of Knowledge (PMBOK), there are nine knowledge areas that a Project Manager must master:[7]

Project Integration Management

The activities of Integration Management include creating the project charter, scope, project plan, project management plan, managing the execution of the project, monitoring and controlling the work, performing integrated change control, and closing out the project or phase.[7] A creative PM will use different strategies to get to the end result and ensure that all components are coordinated.

Project Scope Management

Defining and controlling what is within or external to the scope of the project is critical along with its associated work breakdown structure. A common example for large multi-site practices is that they add new practice sites over a period of years and face a significant challenge of integrating and supporting a variety of legacy practice management systems. This makes the task of data integration and migration challenging, and it requires developing detailed scope documents with each of their existing vendors. Managing the scope and sequence of these interfaces is critical, especially as it relates to time and cost management of the project. Therefore, an IT team should spend a significant amount of time conducting assessments with each site and involving employees at all levels in this discussion. The risk of forgetting a key part of the data chain is that something essential will be left out, leading to cumbersome and inefficient workarounds.

Decisions about the scope of a project sometimes need to be modified along the way. For example, a practice that was staffed mostly by primary care providers had a small ophthalmology practice that was not part of the original scope for implementation. At some point during implementation, the EHR vendor developed a vision module that was available for immediate deployment, and the practice had to make a decision if it was worth adjusting the scope to add in the ophthalmologists or leave it until a later date. The practice considered the cost of gathering the necessary team members and resources in the future and decided to approve the change request even though it lengthened their implementation slightly. Therefore, they were able to fully implement the entire practice at one time and added to their quality goals of improving care coordination between their primary care providers, podiatrists, and ophthalmologists treating patients with diabetes.

Project Time Management

Large hospital outpatient practices are especially dependent on external vendors to set up interfaces with their hospital scheduling and billing systems. This task of coordinating between the various teams is formidable and is the foremost cause of implementation delays in large practices. Slippage in this area has significant impact on keeping the project on schedule. It is useful to assume that there will be delays and build in sufficient float to ensure that there are dedicated resources set aside to work solely on interfaces.

A common challenge for small practices is that they have fewer backup staff members, such that when one leaves for month-long vacation, his/her tasks must be distributed to others, thereby causing disruption to time lines. While vacation schedules can be adjusted slightly, there are some hard deadlines to which providers, such as pediatricians, must adhere, so any implementation that overlaps with a September deadline is sure to be delayed. Setting up realistic expectations and commitment required from the entire team is important at the start of the project so that staff can adjust vacation schedules and work hours as needed.

The PCIP PMs use a customer relationship management tool to track the overall project time lines, time allocation, and slippage. Keeping individual projects as close to schedule as possible allows for the best allocation of resources and maintains our capacity to continuously assist new practices.

Project Cost Management

Unrealistic and unplanned costs are one of the top causes of project failures. It is important to plan budgets thoroughly so that all parties have an accurate estimate of their ability to carry out the project according to the scope, time and budget. Providing updated budgets and interim analyses, including reviewing planned versus actual costs, can also dramatically increase success.

At PCIP, the Outreach team and Infrastructure Coordinator conduct a cost analysis for practices at the start, so they have an estimate of the cost of purchasing new hardware for their office. In addition, they must be prepared for a loss of productivity during their training phase, as well as decreased revenue after they go live. Not only must PMs budget for these known costs, they must also keep vigilant track of unexpected costs and plan for some reserves to address any IT emergencies that may necessitate some consultant time.

Health centers that typically serve as safety-net providers experience significant budgetary and personnel challenges. Some have had turnover of key staff and have had to place their projects on hold until they hired new CMOs or CIOs. As a result, they wasted significant resources and were in danger of falling behind on their deliverables for their stakeholders, especially for their funders. The cost of maintaining the salaries of a full Project team given these setbacks can be very expensive. A PM may need to shift his or her attention to other duties in the practice until the project is back on track. The danger of this delay is not just additional costs but a decreased sense of urgency to advance the project. This can lead to a loss of focus which is hard to undo when the project resumes.

Project Quality Management

Performing thorough quality assurance and control checks is essential to maintaining a standard for the project. In EHR implementation, this can be achieved by developing and disseminating best practice guides and checklists that have demonstrated success. Large practices often capitalize on this transition as an opportunity to standardize the methodology used between sites and create institutional quality management plans. The process of EHR implementation is often a golden opportunity for a practice to redesign its inefficient processes, and the PM can help facilitate these discussions.

Quality management applies not just to the steps of hardware and software deployment, but also to the migration of medical data into the EHR. Providers are faced with the burdensome task of accurately transferring key patient information, such as problem lists, medication history, and allergies from thick medical charts into structured data fields in the EHR. As providers switch from paper to an EHR, they are afraid of losing tried-and-tested methods of conducting their own quality checks. PMs must make sure that quality processes are recreated in the EHR so that critical patient events are given priority. For example, providers typically want abnormal results scanned in so that they can conduct the appropriate level of follow-up based on the severity of the diagnosis. Each practice must make a strategic decision about the length of time it will devote to preloading historical data and ensuring it follows extensive quality assurance procedures. After the initial practice management data migration is complete and basic patient demographic data has been imported, the PM must work with the internal practice resources to create a systematic process for reviewing, flagging and entering key data elements based upon a set of predetermined criteria. It is important to involve the Quality Assurance team so that data checks are performed with regular frequency until a certain quality of work is observed and maintained.

Project Human Resource Management

The Project Sponsor and PM must make decisions about how many team members will be selected from within or from the outside the organization. If considering team members from within, they should determine if they currently possess the necessary skills or if they need additional training in advance of the project's start. External hires may not know the key players, and therefore it may be harder to garner support or work through the politics associated with the organization. On the other hand they may provide objective guidance that can cut across unproductive political divisions.

Teams should be augmented as needed with subject matter experts. The role of these experts can be temporary and time-limited. PMs should not be afraid to pull in additional help, as it will prove to be cost-effective in the long run; failure to incorporate some key input may result in costly delays later on. Finally, periodic assessments of team performance should be conducted along the way to make sure staff is performing up to standards. Underperforming members should be replaced if remediation efforts fail. Efforts should also be made to find a good fit for staff members, and attention should be given to group dynamics to ensure the group is functioning optimally and there is cooperation and communication between members.

The initial structure of the PCIP team did not include any super users, but we soon realized that our providers were struggling with templates and system customization soon after they went live. Pediatricians who used to capture immunization history within a matter of minutes were spending an inordinate amount of time documenting during their visits. We responded to this unexpected and urgent need by hiring a group of technically-skilled super users to provide on-site assistance to tailor the EHR to the provider. By the time the super user arrives at the practice, the provider is versed on the basic functionality of the EHR and is ready for training on its advanced features.

Project Communications Management

The goals and mission of the project should be clearly communicated from the start and maintained throughout the project. Insufficient information leads to a feeling of disempowerment and can be a setback for the project. PMs should continuously communicate the progress of the project, changes in time lines and challenges experienced to the appropriate stakeholders and project staff. They should also keep an open process for communication so that all project staff feels comfortable sharing their concerns.

Providing interim progress data back to all stakeholders is critical for building buy-in and significantly affects adoption when people feel they have an impact on the project. The success of the EHR project will be significantly affected by the empowerment of the care team, and failure to engage these key stakeholders can be disastrous. One practice did not communicate the project implementation phase to their end users and, as a result, were not prepared for their final training and go-live. They lost credibility with their staff and later had to spend unnecessary resources to pay for additional training days.

The PCIP relies on open and frequent communication between all members of its project team. The weekly meetings with the vendor teams help to build strong partnerships between different staff members so that we can all provide coordinated assistance and communication to our practices.

Project Risk Management

PMs should conduct periodic qualitative risk assessments to gauge the perceived and actual risks by stakeholders. A process should be established for identifying, addressing, and communicating responses to the survey. The "first step in risk planning is risk assessment, which is a matter of turning uncertainty into risk."[4] Through this process, we are able to identify and prepare for potential future challenges.

For example, losing a PM midway through a project is a significant risk for each medical practice. The PM in most small practices is typically not a full-time person and is expected to maintain his or her existing workload in addition to managing the extensive task of the EHR implementation. This has led to staff burnout and turnover, causing a significant setback to the team. Since budgets are tight and finding another full FTE is improbable, practices can assist PMs by spreading some of the sub-tasks among other staff. This creates a layer of redundancy and the project learning is shared. It is also critical to have clear and meticulous documentation of the project management process and progress at all times so that should there be turnover a new PM can pick up where the last one left off.

A significant risk for EHR implementations is that a bi-directional lab interface is often not completed by the time the practice goes live so that orders and results are not entered electronically. The practice PM must work actively with the lab company and EHR vendor to ensure that contracts are signed at the start of the project and that the lab tasks are built into the work breakdown structure (WBS)[15] in sufficient detail. There is a risk this may still not occur, and workarounds need to be in place should the practice need to go live on paper. Thinking through the two sets of workflows for paper and an electronic interface are essential so that the end user has clear instructions of the contingency plan. The benefit of being part of a large-scale implementation such as PCIP is that some of these predictable risks have been mitigated, and the best practices can be disseminated.

Project Procurement Management

Procurement issues can derail a project's scope, time, and budget and can be avoided with careful planning of purchases, especially of hardware. A PM must ensure all contracts are in place at the start of the project and identify a set of resources that can help expedite approvals and procurement if needed in an emergency.

CASE STUDY OF A SMALL PRIVATE PRACTICE

The case study is of a solo provider practice in Staten Island (New York) that started its implementation in 2004 and went live in four months. The practice has been live on a fully integrated EHR for the past six years and serves predominantly working class families, civil servants and small business owners, many of whom are on Medicare or are uninsured. This is an example of a small scale implementation and is a realistic model for the majority of practices at PCIP.

The project team consisted of:

- A full-time physician who is board certified in Internal Medicine, Pediatrics and Geriatrics. The physician was the Sponsor of the project as well as the part-time PM. The responsibilities of Project Management were shared between him and the Office Manager. This practice implemented their EHR using many part-time staff and performed Project Management on a budget.
- An Office Manager (OM) who functioned as the part-time Project Manager during implementation, as well as a Medical Assistant (MA) and front desk receptionist. Her key role was to coordinate all activities within the office and with external vendors. She was the main point of contact with external groups

such as IT consultants, EHR vendor, lab companies, hardware vendor, etc. She mapped out the current state workflows for the practice and worked with the provider and staff to modify the future state workflows. She also created policies and procedures and made sure they were being followed and adapted as necessary. She became an adept EHR user and proficient with IT issues, such that over time she provided the first-line IT support for simple issues such as password resets, rebooting the server, etc. She served as a liaison between the staff and provider, communicating next steps in the project time line and bringing back concerns to the provider. Her role facilitated dialogue between staff members and addressed issues so they did not escalate.

In addition, staff included:

- A full-time Medical Assistant (MA) who divided her time between prepping the patients for the provider and tending to the front desk.
- A half-time biller who had to learn billing for an EHR.
- A part-time assistant who helped with basic clerical work, made appointments, coordinated referrals, and handled the phones.
- A part-time IT consultant whose primary role was coordinating between the hardware and software vendors during implementation and was used on an ad-hoc basis during the rest of the year. The OM functioned as the first line of support, and the physician served as the second line of support so the IT consultant costs were kept to a minimum. He was brought in approximately twice a year for hardware issues that could not be managed internally.

The entire team added up to approximately one provider FTE and three "part-time" FTEs. This is an example of a lean implementation team in which members took on multiple roles based on the stage of implementation and on the needs of the practice and patients during different times of the day. This flexible arrangement allowed for a cross-training of staff and shared the burden of implementation between the team members.

Planning

The most critical piece of the project was planning for the budget. The physician and the OM created a projected budget for the EHR implementation that was outside their standard operating budget for the year. They projected the cost of hardware, software, and loss of revenue during implementation and for the subsequent six months. This came to approximately $30,000. The costs were based on a client server model, with one application/database server, one back-up server, one scan server, three client machines, one fax server, two printers and one scanner.

The physician had to take into account not just his business expenses, but also make cuts in his private life to meet the needs of this expansion. He was able to get a line of credit from his bank, setting aside some of the profits for 12 months, cutting back on family vacations for two years, reducing dinners at restaurants and factoring an overall reduction on living expenses. This took a significant amount of management and planning to keep it as close to budget as possible. It took approximately 6–8 weeks post-implementation before productivity went up to the pre-EHR level. At the end of one year, the practice began to experience a *recurring ROI* through a combination of decreased FTE staff and improved billing coding. This provider later chose to join PCIP even though he was already live on eCW because he stood to benefit from all the wrap-around services we had to offer, including systems integration support, assistance with upgrades, updated lab compendiums, access to pilot programs, free basic and advanced EHR training for new staff, access to a wider provider community, etc. Providers can now benefit from the Meaningful Use incentives to offset the cost of EHR.

EHR Vendor Selection

The physician conducted an extensive vendor selection process and investigated approximately 12 EHR vendors before making the final selection. He viewed vendor product demos at IT conferences and medical society events and followed the online User's Forum for the vendor he ultimately chose. He had also assisted a colleague with his vendor selection process, so he was somewhat familiar with the products. His final EHR selection was based on the best value for price.

Scope of Project

The scope of the project had to be scaled back due to cost constraints. While the project goal was to go live on the integrated EHR, the practice recognized that, given the rapid changes in technology, they would need to continuously adapt and modify the practice and, therefore, followed more of a staged implementation approach. For example, a bi-directional lab interface was out of the scope of the initial project because very few labs had the necessary technology in place at that time. The practice still submitted lab requisitions on paper and scanned results into the EHR. Setting up the bi-directional lab interfaces occurred only two years later when it became the norm and was not cost prohibitive. The provider also ended up modifying the scope of the project because of cost overruns. The initial goal was to give tablet PCs to the MAs so they could review the status of referral appointments with patients as they waited to see the provider, but they had to design a different workflow once the cost of the hardware became prohibitive.

Communications

The project staff recognized that the lines of communication had to be kept open at all times for the project's success. In a small office, this was easier to do as staff worked in adjoining rooms within earshot of each other. It was still important keep protected time for the provider and PM to communicate regularly, as well as for the PM to meet with the entire staff. They reserved one weekend a month for all staff to come in for a breakfast meeting so that they could get updates on the next month's plans. This was their chance to give input into the planning process and share any concerns that had not been addressed. This process is especially important to influence members who may still be skeptical or nervous about the transformation that accompanies such a project.

Project Tools

The tools available to PMs are extensive and sophisticated. For this small practice, Excel was sufficient for planning and monitoring the budget. The physician and OM used it to create a spreadsheet to plan and track their budget and checked it on a weekly basis for the length of the project. They also used the DOQ-IT[16] toolkit to map out their current and future state workflows. This served as a training tool for new employees, as well as a means for conducting workflow redesign, making enhancements to the practice and increasing efficiencies.

Vendors

The primary vendor the practice had to negotiate with was the reference lab company. This is another example of a staged approach in which the provider had to first focus on interfacing with their primary lab company and then moved on to the secondary lab company and finally worked on an interface with his referring hospital. In the future, the practice would like to work with its diagnostic and imaging company and, with the help of the RHIOs, connect to other providers and specialists in the community.

Workflows

The OM created a problem log book in which all tickets opened were logged along with their solution. This became the reference manual and training log for new staff. It also provided the continuity for staff that were out and helped with the resolution of issues. An example of a recurring issue was the fax server would go down periodically and the solution was to reboot and perform manual instead of automatic Windows updates.

Lessons Learned

- Successful EHR implementations require the judicious deployment of PM best practices and the full backing of senior sponsors. If you have one without the other, the project will falter.
- Empower the practice to succeed by sharing best practices from other implementations and develop the role of a Project Manager. This person can oversee the overall implementation or can work closely with the external PM to ensure a smooth rollout. Ideally the PM should be someone who has good organizational skills and is naturally adept at problem-solving and creative thinking. They can also become the first line of support for simple IT issues, thereby reducing the reliance on an IT consultant and helping to keep the project within budget.
- Make sure that both the project and the practice review their respective budgets carefully and check their progress on a weekly or monthly basis. Cost overruns are a common cause of project failures during implementation, especially for small physician offices.
- Participate in other online forums and user groups that are hosted by EHR vendors, professional organizations such as HIMSS[17] and the PMI.

The case study described above took place prior to the passage of ARRA/HITECH and the creation of the Regional Extension Centers (RECs). There are now 60 RECs that provide assistance with implementation and getting the practice to meaningful use.[18] The RECs engage the collective bargaining power of the group in negotiations with lab companies, software and hardware vendors; encourage collaboration with the local Department of Health for mandatory disease reporting; and connecting to RHIOs and other enablers of meaningful use. A PM can get significant assistance by joining the larger community to build on the experience of the experienced.

ACKNOWLEDGEMENTS

The author wishes to thank the entire PCIP Implementation, Infrastructure and Systems Integration teams for their hard work and dedication these past three years, as well as the co-founders of PCIP, Dr. Farzad Mostashari and Mat Kendall, for their leadership and guidance. Our success would also not have been possible without our strong collaboration with eCW—especially the Project Managers and Strategic Account Managers, who have helped serve the unique needs of our providers in NYC. Of course, special thanks go to each of our PCIP providers who have partnered with us to form a community of 2,200 users spread throughout the five boroughs. Dr. Salvatore Volpe is one of these providers who contributed greatly to the development of our new EHR functionality. He shared lessons learned right from the start and is the contributor of the small practice case study.

REFERENCES

1. Available at: http://en.wikipedia.org/wiki/Project_management. Last accessed December 2010.
2. Available at: http://cio.osu.edu/projects/framework/glossary.html. Last accessed December 2010.
3. Available at: http://www.pmi.org. Last accessed December 2010.
4. Kemp S. *Project Management Demystified.* New York: McGraw-Hill; 2004.
5. Heldman K. *PMP: Project Management Professional Study Guide.* 3rd ed. Hoboken, NJ: Wiley Publishing; 2005.
6. Kerzner H, Saladis FP. *What Executives Need to Know about Project Management.* Hoboken, NJ: John Wiley & Sons; 2009.
7. *A Guide to the Project Management Body of Knowledge (PMBOK Guide).* 4th ed. Newtown Square, PA: Project Management Institute; 2008.
8. Available at: http://home2.nyc.gov/html/doh/html/csi/csi-detailing.shtml. Last accessed December 2010.
9. Available at: www.nyc.gov/html/doh/downloads/pdf/csi/ehrkit-patient_info.pdf. Last accessed December 2010.
10. Lewis JP. *Fundamentals of Project Management.* 3rd ed. New York: AMACON; 2007.
11. Kendrick T. *The Project Management Tool Kit. 100 Tips and Techniques for Getting the Job Done Right.* New York: AMACON; 2010.
12. Available at: http://office.microsoft.com/en-us/visio/. Last accessed December 2010.
13. Available at: www.microsoft.com/project/en/us/default.aspx. Last accessed December 2010.
14. Available at: http://office.microsoft.com/en-us/excel/. Last accessed December 2010.
15. Available at: http://en.wikipedia.org/wiki/Work_breakdown_structure. Last accessed December 2010.
16. Available at: http://www.masspro.org/HIT/PFQ/docs/tools/DOQIT%20WB%20for%20WEB.pdf. Last accessed December 2010.
17. Available at: www.himss.org/ASP/index.asp. Last accessed December 2010.
18. Available at: http://healthit.hhs.gov/portal/server.pt?open=512&objID=1495&parentname=CommunityPage&parentid=58&mode=2&in_hi_userid=11113&cached=true. Last accessed December 2010.

CHAPTER 12

Quality and Health IT

Joseph Conte, MPA

INTRODUCTION

Does health IT provide a return on investment (ROI), both in terms of quality and health outcomes? Up until quite recently the jury has been out. According to an independent analysis, the Veterans Administration's $4 billion healthcare information technology investment has answered the question.[1] In fact, when the team from Partners Healthcare from Massachusetts Center for Information Technology Leadership finished its analysis, it found that the reduction in expenses approached nearly $3.1 billion in eliminated duplicate tests, reduced medical errors, medication errors, workloads for order entry, imaging and laboratory costs. What is clear from this review is that on a nationwide scale, with a well-funded budget, health IT may be the magic bullet to bend the cost curve in healthcare. Has this effort improved quality? That depends on how you define quality.

The domain of "business quality" has evolved significantly since the early 1920s when statistical theory was first applied in a product quality control context. The pioneers of quality by design transformed the manufacturing sector and paved the way for the industrywide focus on quality in healthcare. Since that time, the implications of quality and the consequences of its absence have changed drastically. Many industries have witnessed the transformation from quality as an exception to an expectation.

Quality in a given industry or service implies excellence in design, performance, and outcome. Attributes like durability, affordability, customer satisfaction, and value are also often associated with quality. In healthcare, other terms used to describe quality have evolved from stakeholders, such as the Institute of Medicine (IOM), National Quality Forum (NQF), American Hospital Association (AHA), and Agency for Health Care Research and Quality (AHRQ). These aspects, described in detail in the IOM report, *Crossing the Quality Chasm: A New Health System for the 21st Century,*[2] include safety, effectiveness, patient centeredness, timeliness, efficiency and equity. From a performance improvement perspective, quality is defined as consistently superior performance in both process and outcome measured against a benchmark or gold standard.

Influencing improvement in healthcare quality is a complex balancing act. External forces that have been used to influence quality include regulation, legislation, and compensation while internal forces are innovation, training paradigms, and medical and IT. It would be remiss to leave out litigation and enforcement as adversarial processes utilized in efforts, mostly unsuccessful, to improve quality.

In an interesting and perhaps long overdue turn of events, consumerism in healthcare is shaping the next evolution in quality initiatives. What is important to the patient as a consumer is replacing professional society standard setting in shaping quality priorities. The national effort to eliminate hospital-acquired infections, prevention of the 27 "never events"[3] identified by NQF and publicly reporting healthcare performance, also known as the transparency movement, are all examples of quality initiatives driven by consumerism. Consumers do not expect to pay a premium for services that are ineffective or wasteful. In a strange paradigm, institutions and providers have been reimbursed equally, whether they succeed or fail, heal or harm.

In this regard, perhaps understanding what quality is *not* should also be stated. While much of this is obvious, as an industry, healthcare has been slow to adopt and adapt when confronted with the stark realities of its failures. Patient harm in healthcare is not a characteristic of quality, but is a very real phenomenon. For many decades a "white wall of silence" met many patients and families when adverse outcomes occurred. The 1999 IOM report, "To Err is Human,"[4] estimated that between 44,000 and 98,000 Americans die in healthcare institutions each year as a result of medical errors, with many more being transiently or permanently harmed. Many well-publicized safety lapses spurred the changes discussed later in this chapter. Even today, more than 10 years later, high-profile medical errors abound. In 2007, the prematurely born twins of the actor Dennis Quaid were nearly killed as a result of a medication error in a Neonatal Intensive Care Unit at one of the country's finest hospitals.[5] This case revealed that the error may have occurred due to the similarity of label and design packaging of the adult and infant versions of the drug. The Quaids subsequently sued the drug manufacturer and settled with the hospital for $750,000 in damages. A point-of-care, integrated electronic medication prescribing system might have prevented this near-tragic event.

Another glimpse of what quality is not is the provision of service that is not consistent with the current medical evidence also known as "standard of care." While this does sound somewhat elementary, the evidence from multiple studies is somewhat shocking. In the results illustrated in Table 12-1, Mc Glynn et al.[6] demonstrated that for common conditions including diabetes management, heart failure, asthma, and community-acquired pneumonia, Americans only receive about half of the recommended medical care processes. One suspect in this poor performance is the fact that only 15 percent of hospitals nationwide provide electronic medical record support to their practitioners. This technology gap is one of the fundamental barriers to closing the quality "chasm" identified by the IOM.

In 2009, healthcare costs consumed a staggering $2.47 trillion, nearly 17 percent of our gross domestic product. This calculates to $7,681 for every citizen, which is nearly double the next highest expenditure of any industrialized nation. The return on this huge investment has been disappointing. Outcomes of care illustrated in Table 12-2 shown next suggest we spend more and get less than nearly every nation in the comparison.

Table 12-1: Adherence to Quality Indicators, According to Condition[6]

Condition and Number of Indicators	Number of Eligible Participants	Number Of Times Eligibility Was Met	Percentage of Recommended Care Received (95% CI)*
Senile cataract – 10	159	602	78.7 (73.3-84.2)
Breast cancer – 9	192	202	75.7 (69.9-81.4)
Prenatal care – 39	134	2920	73.0 (69.5-76.6)
Low back pain – 6	489	3391	68.5 (66.4-70.5)
Coronary artery disease – 37	410	2083	68.0 (64.2-71.8)
Hypertension – 27	1973	6643	64.7 (62.6-66.8)
Congestive heart failure – 36	104	1438	63.9 (55.4-72.4)
Cerebrovascular disease – 10	101	210	59.1 (49.7-68.4)
Chronic obstructive pulmonary disease – 20	169	1340	58.0 (51.7-64.4)
Depression – 14	770	3011	57.7 (55.2-60.2)
Orthopedic conditions – 10	302	590	57.2 (50.8-63.7)
Osteoarthritis – 3	598	648	57.3 (53.9-60.7)
Colorectal cancer – 12	231	329	53.9 (47.5-60.4)
Asthma – 25	260	2332	53.5 (50.0-57.0)
Benign prostatic hyperplasia – 5	138	147	53.0 (43.6-62.5)
Hyperlipidemia – 7	519	643	48.6 (44.1-53.2)
Diabetes mellitus – 13	488	2952	45.4 (42.7-48.3)
Headache – 21	712	8125	45.2 (43.1-47.2)
Urinary tract infection – 13	459	1216	40.7 (37.3-44.1)
Community-acquired pneumonia – 5	144	291	39.0 (32.1-45.8)
Sexually transmitted diseases or vaginitis – 26	410	2146	36.7 (33.8-39.6)
Dyspepsia and pectic ulcer disease – 8	278	287	32.7 (26.4-39.1)
Atrial fibrillation – 10	100	407	24.7 (18.4-30.9)
Hip fracture – 9	110	167	22.8 (6.2-39.5)
Alcohol dependence – 5	280	1036	10.5 (6.8-14.6)

Note: CI denotes confidence interval.

Adapted from: McGlynn EA, Asch SM, Adams J et al. The Quality of health care delivered to adults in the United States. N Engl J Med. 2003;348:2635-45.

Fortunately, there are many examples of improvement in care and outcome that suggest these international comparisons, while troubling, do not represent the full picture of healthcare in America. The following sections will introduce national agencies responsible for healthcare quality, as well as the private organizations that are involved in the quality effort. Likewise, we will review the history of some of the common performance improvement methodologies being used in healthcare today, such as Six Sigma

Table 12-2: Overall Ranking (2010)[7]

Overall Ranking

Country Rankings
1.00–2.33
2.34–4.66
4.67–7.00

	AUS	CAN	GER	NETH	NZ	UK	US
OVERALL RANKING (2010)	3	6	4	1	5	2	7
Quality Care	4	7	5	2	1	3	6
Effective Care	2	7	6	3	5	1	4
Safe Care	6	5	3	1	4	2	7
Coordinated Care	4	5	7	2	1	3	6
Patient-Centered Care	2	5	3	6	1	7	4
Access	6.5	5	3	1	4	2	6.5
Cost-Related Problem	6	3.5	3.5	2	5	1	7
Timeliness of Care	6	7	2	1	3	4	5
Efficiency	2	6	5	3	4	1	7
Equity	4	5	3	1	6	2	7
Long, Healthy, Productive Lives	1	2	3	4	5	6	7
Health Expenditures/Capita, 2007	$3,357	$3,895	$3,588	$3,837*	$2,454	$2,992	$7,290

Note: * Estimate. Expenditures shown in $US PPP (purchasing power parity).
Source: Calculated by The Commonwealth Fund based on 2007 International Health Policy Survey; 2008 International Health Policy Survey of Sicker Adults; 2009 International Health Policy Survey of Primary Care Physicians; Commonwealth Fund Commission on a High Performance Health System National Scorecard; and Organization for Economic Cooperation and Development, *OECD Health Data, 2009* (Paris: OECD, Nov. 2009).

and Lean and then examine case studies in which the contributions of multiple stakeholders and quality initiatives have resulted in substantial improvements in outcomes. First, a history of the development of the quality movement is important.

HISTORY LESSON IN QUALITY

Without understanding our heritage in healthcare quality, it is easy to lose our way among the "flavor of the month" quality methods that are marketed to institutions, providers and consumers. The legacy of the giants in the quality movement does not have its origin in healthcare at all.

W. Edward Deming, Joseph M. Juran and Walter A. Shewhart are the three most significant names in quality. They made their mark during the 1920s to the 1940s, when the application of their work to healthcare could not have been contemplated. In fact, industrial manufacturing is where they made their initial impact. Today, however, their contributions remain foundational. For example, many performance improvement initiatives are based on Shewhart's "Plan, Do, Check, Act" or PDCA model (see Figure 12-1). Coming from industrial manufacturing, their focus on structure, process, and outcome had a unique application to healthcare, yet it took decades before its adoption. Deming likewise exerted great influence once the healthcare industry realized that improving outcomes relied on improving systems and not simply focusing on flawed individual performance. Deming's philosophy can be summed up as follows:

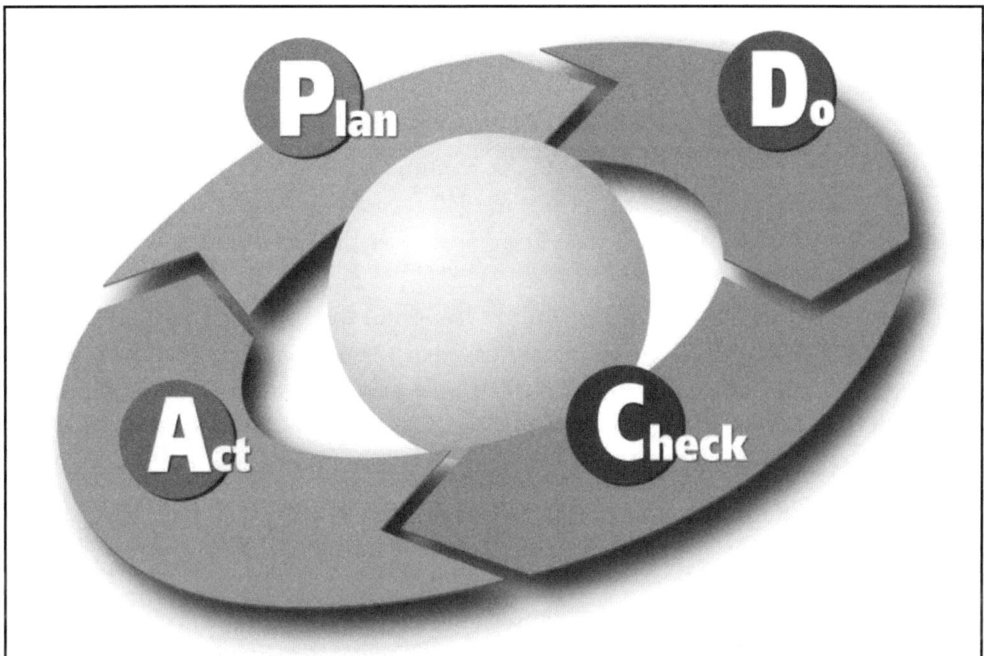

Figure 12-1: PDCA Cycle[9]

> By adopting appropriate principles of management, organizations can increase quality and simultaneously reduce costs (by reducing waste, rework, staff attrition and litigation while increasing customer loyalty). The key is to practice continual improvement and think of manufacturing as a system, not as bits and pieces.[8]

The Shewhart PDCA Cycle

Shewhart and Juran were both working at Bell Telephone Laboratories to achieve higher levels of quality and less variation in manufacturing. It was here that Shewhart developed the first control charts in the 1920s, marking the first use of statistics to formally manage process variability. The control chart signaled the beginning of the age of statistical quality control. The original control chart allowed an inspector to document the percentage of defective product in both a tabular and a time ordered graphic format. As data collection progressed, statistically computed limits could be drawn to identify the expected range of defective products. This focus on defects was the foundation of Six Sigma.

Shewhart showed that Three Sigma, or three standard deviations from the mean, is the point at which a process is said to be out of control and requires correction. This helped alert the operator to problems in the process sooner than was previously possible. Motorola, followed by General Electric, both industry leading giants, adopted Six Sigma as their respective industry operational models. It has grown remarkably in the healthcare industry as the quest for zero defects to both reduce cost of care and harm from medical errors is paramount. The current head of The Joint Commission, Mark Chassin, MD, has now adopted Six Sigma at The Joint Commission.

In 1939, Shewhart published a book entitled *Statistical Method from the Viewpoint of Quality Control*, which firmly established the concept of statistical process control, or SPC, to monitor process quality. The editor was his friend and colleague, W. Edwards Deming, another recognized expert in sampling and applied statistics in quality who was working for the U.S. Department of Agriculture. During this time, Deming demonstrated to the U.S. Census Bureau (for the 1940 census) that quality and productivity can also be improved in non-manufacturing processes, thus broadening the scope and use of these quality tools.

Deming and Juran both found great inspiration in the work of Shewhart. During World War II, Deming used Shewhart's control charts to improve the quality of American war production while a member of the Emergency Technical Committee. Juran, meanwhile, served in the Lend-Lease Administration and Foreign Economic Administration. In 1941, Juran came across the work of the Italian industrialist of the late 1800s, Vilfredo Pareto, and began to apply the Pareto principle, which espouses that 80 percent of a problem is caused by 20 percent of the causes to quality issues. This principle is also known as "the vital few and the trivial many" or as Juran preferred "the vital few and the useful many" as a reminder that the 80 percent of causes should not be totally ignored. Though extremely successful during those years, the use of statistical tools in industry faded in the United States after the war ended, and ironically, the importance of quality and cost reduction started to take hold in a defeated Japan.

Out of the ashes of World War II, Japan was compelled to change its focus from being a military power to becoming an economic one. Despite Japan's ability to compete on cost, its products suffered from a long-established reputation of being shoddy and cheap. While in Japan, Deming's teachings of quality control techniques caught the attention of the Japanese. Deming went on to train hundreds of engineers and managers in SPC and other concepts of quality. Deming's message to Japan's chief executives can be summed up as follows: improving quality will reduce expenses while increasing productivity and, most importantly, market share.[10]

Japanese manufacturers applied Deming's teachings diligently and achieved unprecedented levels of quality and productivity in the following decades. The improved quality, productivity and lower costs were a perfect match for American and international demand.

Through the 1970s until his death in 1993, Deming continued his consulting throughout the U.S., Japan and internationally. Although he still advocated SPC and quality, he also focused about the importance of management and company culture. This evolution led to the conclusion that when people and an organization's culture focuses primarily on quality, quality tends to improve and costs fall over time. However, when people and organizations primarily focus on costs, costs tend to rise and quality declines over time. Deming claimed that many companies cannot perform well from a long-term perspective because their managers do not know what to do. He was fond of repeating "There is no substitute for knowledge!" Deming's management philosophy is directed toward managers asking the right questions. Throughout the years, Deming promoted the use of the Plan, Do, Check, Act (PDCA) cycle of continuous improvement and later changed it to the Plan, Do, Study, Act or PDSA cycle, a forerunner of Six Sigma.

Juran is widely credited for adding the human dimension to quality management. Resistance to change or cultural resistance is at the root cause of the majority of quality issues. For Juran, human relations were the ones to isolate. Juran's vision of quality management extended outside the walls of the factory to encompass nonmanufacturing processes, and his work found a home in healthcare. He developed "Juran's trilogy," an approach to cross-functional management that is composed of three managerial processes: quality planning, quality control, and quality improvement. His concept of integration was known as "Big Q" or quality through management's active involvement and ownership.

In 1986, an engineer named Bill Smith at Motorola first formulated the particulars of a "new" methodology called Six Sigma, referred to earlier in mention of Motorola and GE. It originated as a set of practices designed to improve manufacturing processes and eliminate defects—a defect being defined as any process output that does not meet customer specifications. Its application has been successfully extended to other types of business processes, such as healthcare and the service industry. Its success lies in its rigorous linear application of many of the statistical tools and management philosophies set forth and developed over the past seven decades by giants such as Shewhart, Deming, Juran, as well as their predecessors. The Six Sigma methodology might be only 25 years old, but at its foundation, it encompasses more than 70 years of quality innovations and a relentless focus on measurement.

MEASUREMENTS

At the foundation of all good performance improvement efforts is the often thorny issue of measurement. Confounding issues in healthcare measurement strategies include proper definitions, what to include and exclude, risk adjustment for complexity of care, and attribution of outcome to individuals, groups or organizational accountability.

The availability of accurate, reliable, and valid performance measures has been a limiting step in moving the quality agenda forward. Despite the critical importance of having valid, timely and actionable information about quality and performance, development of standard quality measures remains a work in progress. Even common measures, such as infection rates, mortality, prevalence of medication errors, incidence of pressure ulcers and fall frequency are all subject to interpretation and engender lively debate when definitions are considered.

The National Quality Forum, or NQF, has created the most consistent and reliable measurement development process in the United States. The Consensus Development process is designed to elicit peer input, public comment and includes an appeal mechanism before final approval. Many of the measurement strategies approved by various agencies for public reporting are founded on the NQF process. These indicators tend to be condition-specific and are very focused on process measures.

An area of interest that is attracting growing attention is the "all or none" measurement strategy. It is often difficult to parse out from series of care processes, which have the greatest impact on outcome. Some professional societies like the American Heart Association Stroke Division now include an "all or none" method for performance measurement. All or none measures encourage healthcare providers to act as a team in providing services. This concept is the foundation for the patient accountable care organization codified into law under the health insurance reform of 2010, the Affordable Care Act.

Health IT is an enabler of effective measurement but, perhaps more importantly, it offers clinical reminders and evidence-based recommendations for care at patients' point of care, whether it be the bedside, office, ED or even in their home.

The PDSA process remains at the foundation of healthcare quality efforts nationally, crossing boundaries from private physician practices to multistate health systems. A practical application of this method applied to a vexing clinical problem, such as hospital-acquired infection, described next, illustrates how it can save lives and reduce cost.

The Institution for Healthcare Improvement (IHI) described later in this chapter is a progressive, privately funded organization that focuses on quality and safety in healthcare. In 2004, IHI, utilizing classic principles of reducing variability and thinking of the intervention as a system of care that utilizes defined processes and careful outcomes measurement, developed a quality initiative known as the Central Line Bundle. What that particular IHI team learned was that organizations with the lowest central line infection rates consistently followed the same processes of care when inserting and maintaining a central line, over and over again.[11] The results were remarkable compared to the undisciplined approach most organizations followed until that point.

Richard Shannon, MD, and his colleagues from Alleghany Hospital in Pennsylvania responded to the IHI challenge. In 2005, they published their findings on "Using Real-Time Problem Solving to Eliminate Central Line Infections." In an adaptation of classic quality management principles, Shannon not only demonstrated its impact on outcomes but in another analysis from the same data titled, "Economics of Central Line–Associated Blood Stream Infections" also illustrated one of its key tenets—high quality is associated with lower cost. As Shannon pointed out, however, "The business case for such an assertion is lacking in healthcare." This was true until this study was published.

INITIATIVE SUMMARY

Central line–associated bloodstream (CLAB) infections occur throughout the hospital, most often in critical care units. They arise from insertion of catheters, which are long tubes inserted through the carotid or femoral arteries for the delivery of medications or monitoring of vital physiological parameters, such as blood pressure and cardiac output.

At Alleghany, Shannon's team adopted a modified version of Shewhart's PDSA cycle that had its roots in Toyota's Production System called LEAN. This method was influenced by none other than Deming himself.[12] The five steps were:

1. Establish the true dimension of the problem by retrospective data analysis and chart review.
2. Observe actual work processes.
3. Analyze concurrent data and move quickly to actionable solutions.
4. Solve problems as close to the actual process as possible.
5. Provide continuous feedback and education.

The simplified CLAB Bundle Process Flow is listed as:[13,14]

1. Appropriate hand hygiene
2. Standard line insertion kit
3. Full barrier precautions for the staff
4. Maintaining sterile field with draping of the patient
5. Systematic daily monitoring of site and removal as soon as possible

A checklist was created and adopted by the clinical team to support documentation and statistical measurement. Outliers in terms of process adoption were identified and remediated by peer counseling and direct observation of process compliance and subsequent change in clinical practice. The focus was the system of care, with each process broken down into its most basic elements.

New processes were implemented within 90 days. Within one year, CLAB infections decreased from 49 to 6 (10.5 to 1.2 infections/1,000 line-days), and mortalities from 19 to 1 (51% to 16%), despite an increase in the use of central lines and number of line-days. These results were sustained during a 34-month period. The baseline year showed an infection rate of 10.5 per 1,000 line-days. The ensuing three years showed rates of 1.2, 1.6 and 0.39, respectively, approximately a 90 percent improvement. Deaths, perhaps the ultimate outcome measure, declined from 19 to 1 in the base year, to 2 in year two and then to zero in year three. From a severity adjustment standpoint, the patients were slightly older in the post-study group and ranked as higher acuity using the Atlas severity grade. This was a resounding success in outcomes.

To further close the loop on the initiative, Shannon examined the economic impact of these infections, also categorized as adverse events. As stated earlier, Shannon examined the economics of the "defects" in care. The study encompassed 54 cases of CLAB confirmed in the medical ICU at Alleghany Hospital between July 2002 and June 2005. Remarkably the average expense for these cases was $91,733, but the reimbursement was $64,894. The hospital lost an average of $26,839 per case and over $1.45 million more than the three years studied. As Shannon pointed out, "The elimination of these preventable infections constitutes not only an opportunity to improve patient outcomes but also a significant financial opportunity." Unfortunately, 22 of these patients died, and only 9 were discharged to their homes. Sixty-five percent of payments were provided via a government-funded program (Medicare 43 percent and Medicaid 22 percent).

Further emphasizing Shannon's point has been the implementation of a CMS policy called hospital acquired conditions (HACs) more commonly referred to as "Never Events." Effective 2009, when one of these events is identified, no additional payment will be made to a hospital. In Shannon's study, the cost of a CLAB to the payer of services was on average $40,179—a large price for poor quality!

REGULATORS: QUALITY STAKEHOLDERS

Defining quality is not simply an academic exercise. It is an evolving process in which stakeholders participate through their respective spheres of influence. Regulation, standard setting, accreditation, reimbursement and consumer advocacy are significant power bases from which stakeholders attempt to influence the quality paradigm.

Described below are some major stakeholders that influence quality and are reshaping how care is delivered in the United States and to some extent throughout the world.

Institute of Healthcare Improvement (IHI)

IHI is an independent nonprofit organization dedicated to improving healthcare quality. IHI does not participate in the accreditation process but rather seeks to promote change through collaboration, prioritization of initiatives, convening of industry experts, and development of tools and mobilizing other stakeholders. One such tool is the IHI Improvement Map to help hospitals identify priority improvements or Impacting Cost + Quality to help reduce waste.

IHI defines quality by the standards set out by the Institute of Medicine (IOM) in its report *Crossing the Quality Chasm: A New Health System for the 21st Century.*[2] The report focuses on care that is safe, effective, patient-centered, timely, efficient and equitable. They use these principles to define a "no-needless list":

- No needless deaths
- No needless pain or suffering
- No helplessness in those served or serving
- No unwanted waiting
- No waste
- No one left out

The Institute's definition of quality includes not just high performance but an absence of undesirable health outcomes (death, pain, suffering), undesirable healthcare delivery processes (waiting, waste), and social outcomes (helplessness, patients left out). IHI also recognizes that there are many social determinants of health and that improving healthcare quality effectively requires addressing issues within *as well as* outside of the healthcare delivery setting.

IHI also includes in its mission, improving the skills, knowledge, and satisfaction of the healthcare workforce—those who are truly instrumental to healthcare quality. Several programs are also focused on patients and their interface with the healthcare system.

Centers for Medicare & Medicaid Services (CMS)

The mission of CMS is, "To ensure effective, up-to-date health care coverage and to promote quality care for beneficiaries." In accomplishing this mission, CMS works on five strategies: developing a capable, committed workforce; providing accuracy in reimbursement; realizing effective and efficient care; equipping consumers with information; and fostering collaboration. Within CMS, there is an Office of Clinical Standards and Quality and a Quality of Care Center, under which are several quality initiatives, such as home health and nursing home quality initiatives. Medicaid and CHIP also have several Web pages devoted to quality, with topics ranging from evidence-based care to patient safety to value-driven healthcare.

Quality as defined by CMS is, "The right care for every person every time." Some of the additional criteria mentioned in the same breath with quality include safety, effectiveness, efficiency, patient-centeredness, timeliness and equity. In the Office of Clinical Standards and Quality, which is part of the CMS Leadership, there are five groups that govern the functional activities of the Office: Clinical Standards; Coverage & Analysis; Information Systems; Quality Improvement and Quality Measurement; and Health Assessment.

Under the auspices of the CMS, the federal government spends nearly $500 hundred million annually on the nation's healthcare bill. A large portion, 50 percent, of these expenditures are accounted for by hospital-related care. CMS, therefore, has a great influence over healthcare providers not only because of it regulatory authority but because of its control over the monetary flow. CMS not only influences hospitals via regulations, it also has the authority to grant or exclude both hospitals' and physicians' participation in the CMS program. Since the program controls nearly two-thirds of healthcare spending, CMS has a powerful stick when it comes to enforcement.

The Conditions of Participation (COP) is the regulatory code identifying the requirements that institutions must follow to remain in compliance with CMS. There are over 470 requirements, and each major subcategory of institutional care providers has its own rules. Examples include hospitals, long-term care/nursing homes, and dialysis facilities among others. The Joint Commission described in the next section is the surveyor and "deeming agent" on behalf of CMS as it relates to an organization's compliance with the COP. Exclusion from the Medicare program due to a failure to comply is essentially a closure threat for any organization or provider.

For a long period of time, CMS was a sleeping giant paying for the lion's share of care and demanding little more than regulatory compliance. However, CMS has taken aggressive steps, beginning in 2000, to improve quality. The transparency movement, public reporting of hospital outcomes, is one such effort. Today every hospital, except the VA-supported network has outcomes of care posted on the site.[15] Consumers are able to evaluate the process and outcomes of care in more than 10 common conditions, as well as evaluate the patient experience scores including the "likelihood to recommend" ranking of a hospital. These rankings are also linked to hospital finances. Organizations performing in the bottom quartile of the nation's hospitals have had a portion of the annual Medicare (market basket update) increase withheld, while top performers have received bonuses.

The Joint Commission

The Joint Commission is a quasi governmental agency comprised of representatives of the ACS, AHA, and other national healthcare associations and professional organizations. A standard setting body, The Joint Commission is an independent, not-for-profit agency that evaluates, accredits and certifies more than 18,000 healthcare organizations and programs in the United States. The Joint Commission is governed by a 29-member Board of Commissioners, which includes physicians, administrators, nurses, employers, a labor representative, health plan leaders, quality experts, ethicists, a consumer advocate and educators. The Joint Commission's corporate members are the American College of Physicians, the American College of Surgeons, the American Dental Association, the American Hospital Association, and the American Medical Association. The Joint Commission's hospital accreditation program has held deeming authority since the inception of the Medicare program in 1965. It has the authority to conduct on-site surveys of institutions that seek to participate in government-funded programs, such as

Medicare/Medicaid. This authority is granted by Congress and has positioned The Joint Commission to become a powerful voice in the quality movement. The Joint Commission establishes standards based on professional and peer society consensus groups whose members are assigned sections from their recognized areas of expertise. In addition to hospitals, The Joint Commission has federal deeming authority for ambulatory surgery centers, critical access hospitals, durable medical equipment suppliers, home health organizations, hospices, and laboratories.

Joint Commission standards address the organization's level of performance in key functional areas, such as patient rights, patient care and treatment, medication safety and infection control. The standards focus on setting expectations for an organization's actual performance and assessing its ability to provide safe, high-quality care. Standards are used to set performance expectations for activities that impact the safety and quality of patient care. One of the most far-reaching efforts to accomplish this mission is the ongoing development of patient safety initiatives, including National Patient Safety Goals, Sentinel Event Policy and Alerts, development of a medication abbreviation "Do not use" list, and patient safety-related accreditation standards and survey techniques called tracer methodology.

Information technology plays a major role in improving healthcare quality and safety. Any form of technology may adversely affect the quality and safety of care if it is designed or implemented incorrectly. This point has not only been recognized by The Joint Commission but continues to be a major focus of its initiatives.

Standards. The Joint Commission has developed standards that include specific requirements for accreditation or certification for each of the eligible areas. Joint Commission standards specify requirements to ensure care is provided in a safe and effective manner and in a secure environment. The Joint Commission develops its standards in consultation with healthcare and measurement experts, providers, purchasers and consumers. The Joint Commission incorporates IT-related standards into both Leadership and Information Management chapters of required standards.

National Patient Safety Goals. The Joint Commission's National Patient Safety Goals were developed to promote specific improvements in patient safety. The goals are derived primarily from patient safety literature, *Sentinel Event Alert*, and sentinel events reported to The Joint Commission.

The goals highlight problematic areas in healthcare and describe evidence- and expert-based solutions to these problems. Organizations are then evaluated on their compliance with the goals. The Advisory Group, The Joint Commission's Board of Commissioners, reviews and approves existing and new goals and requirements.

Sentinel Event Policy and *Sentinel Event Alert*. A sentinel event is an unexpected occurrence involving death or serious physical or psychological injury, or the risk thereof. Serious injury specifically includes loss of limb or function. The phrase, "or the risk thereof" includes any process variation for which a recurrence would carry a significant chance of a serious adverse outcome. Such events are called "sentinel" because they signal the need for immediate investigation and response.[16]

In support of its mission to improve the quality of healthcare provided to the public, The Joint Commission includes the review of organizations' activities in response to sentinel events in its accreditation process.

The Joint Commission publishes a *Sentinel Event Alert* which identifies specific sentinel events, describes their common underlying causes, and recommends steps to prevent occurrences in the future. Accredited organizations should consider information in an *Alert* when designing or redesigning relevant processes and consider implementing relevant suggestions or reasonable alternatives.

The effectiveness and safety of technology in healthcare ultimately depends on the proper design and implementation of electronic systems. Previous issues of *Sentinel Event Alert* have addressed specific technology-related safety issues: infusion pumps (issue 15), ventilators (issue 25) and patient-controlled analgesia (issue 33).

"Never Events"

Hospitals and their staff are under increasing pressure to avoid "Never Events," situations that should never happen in a hospital. In 2002, the NQF published a report, *Serious Reportable Events in Healthcare*, which identified and endorsed as "never events" 27 preventable adverse health events that are clearly identifiable, largely preventable and serious in their consequences. These include serious problems that nearly always can be avoided, such as surgery on the wrong body part, death or disability from a medication error at a healthcare facility and discharging an infant to the wrong parents.

In 2000, a coalition of major employers and public purchasers founded the Leapfrog Group in an attempt to consolidate the purchaser voice and engage consumers and clinicians in improving healthcare quality. In response to these never events, the Leapfrog Group asked hospitals to report the never event to a state agency, a patient safety organization, or The Joint Commission. As of 2009, more than 650 hospitals across the U.S. have signed on to the Leapfrog Initiative.

In recognition of the need for transparency of hospital performance, The Joint Commission began publishing hospital performance data in 2000. Their website[17] is an example of how The Joint Commission is moving toward a consumer-oriented model of hospital performance that is available for the public's review. The site allows consumers, insurance companies and other interested parties to evaluate process and outcome measures on several common conditions. The most widely used conditions for comparison are heart failure, heart attack (myocardial infarction), joint replacement, cardiac bypass surgery and pneumonia.

Some professional groups have disputed the value and accuracy of these measurements. Others have gone so far as to say these measurements actually are harmful to patients because of the lack of hard scientific evidence as to whether compliance with individual steps or processes in care improves overall outcomes. While the jury may be out, the following case study strongly suggests improvement in overall compliance with process measures has been positively associated with reduced mortality, readmission and overall cost of care.

ECONOMIC INCENTIVES AND THE QUALITY AGENDA

Linking incentive payments to improved outcomes is a time-honored tradition in business. Marketplace incentives have not been well aligned and therefore have been ineffective in advancing the overall quality outcomes agenda in healthcare. Linking incentive payments to improved outcomes is also a time-honored tradition in for-profit business. This so-called "pay for performance" concept was not initially well received by healthcare providers, as concerns regarding how and by whom the indicators and achievement levels are selected, identifying appropriate incentive amounts, and importantly, the potential to shortchange (ration) patient services to reduce cost and earn a bonus. The professional concern over bureaucratic interference between the physician-patient relationship is another prevalent issue. Perhaps at a deeper level is the most often heard complaint from practitioners, "My patients are sicker" or "noncompliant," so I cannot achieve high-performance outcomes.

At some level, all of these concerns are somewhat valid. Over time, the ability of biostatisticians to develop more sophisticated risk adjustment has "leveled the playing field" as it relates to risk adjustment. Numerous innovative providers have demonstrated that noncompliance can be modified by case management and technology. The Affordable Care Act of 2010 promotes the promise of coverage for the previously uninsured 40 million Americans who were underserved in terms of access and ability to afford basic healthcare coverage. The potential for all providers to earn significant bonus income is growing.

The most successful pay-for-performance program to date has been the CMS/Premier project known as Hospital Quality Improvement Demonstration project or HQID. Defining success is tricky business in healthcare. Success in reducing cost that comes at the expense of patient outcome is clearly not a victory for quality of care. Balancing cost and outcome, the value equation that Porter and Teisberg[18] so elegantly described in *Redefining Healthcare*, is rapidly being identified as the holy grail of quality. Realigning incentives for providers, payers, and the public is an enormous undertaking. Some of the work involves substantial cultural reorientation that may take a generation (or two), while a restructuring of medical training paradigms, outcome monitoring, and elimination of provider sensitive care that researchers at Duke University, led by John Wennberg, MD,[19] have clearly identified is implemented. Their work suggests that mis-use, underuse and overuse are all significant drivers of both the unsustainable cost curve and the quality concerns found in healthcare.

In spite of these concerns, some initiatives have been successful. The CMS/Premier project has demonstrated the efficacy of pay-for-performance as an incentive program to adopt effective care process.

HQID was designed to provide financial rewards and positive public reinforcement to hospitals achieving high-quality performance in select inpatient care conditions. Launched in 2003, HQID enrolled 278 hospitals across 38 states with the promise of participating in a unique initiative. The underlying premise was that rewarding organizations to provide top-quality care and receive bonus payments from a pool of nearly $10 million annually would spur innovation and investment in quality processes.

The program was organized in a stringent research-based model. Tight statistical controls, well-defined clinical parameters defined by peer experts, risk adjustment modeling and data validation characterize HQID. For the first time, an initiative focusing on process measures balanced with objective outcomes of care to create a composite score linked to bonus was implemented on a nationwide scale.

This is an important departure from other initiatives in which the focus had only been on processes of care. In HQID, hard outcome measures such as mortality rate, readmission rate, postoperative hemorrhage, and postoperative complications were combined to create a "composite quality score." This is an adaptation of Deming's and Shewhart's work focusing on structure-process-outcomes.

The results were impressive. In the first year of the project, of the 33 quality measures, 22 achieved statistically significant improvement (p<.05) and 10 improved but did not attain statistical significance. The hospital shaved nearly $9 million in bonus payments. Overall, bonuses averaged $71,960 per year and ranged from $914 to more than $847,000. Perhaps more significantly, by the end of year two, the improvement continued. In fact, in each of the 33 quality measurements being evaluated, results from the 8th quarter compared to the first quarter, demonstrated significantly higher performance, p<001; based on paired t-test of means.

Further confirming the value of pay-for-performance was a study by Lindenauer et al. on public reporting and pay-for-performance in hospital quality improvement.[20] Published in *The New England Journal of Medicine*, this study systematically analyzed HQID hospital performance compared to "non-incentivized" hospitals that were used as a control group. They found that, "As compared with the control group, pay-for-performance hospitals showed greater improvement in all composite measures of quality, including measures of care for heart failure, acute myocardial infarction, pneumonia, and all composite measures."

This study did not close the chapter on the value of pay for performance. Much more structuring of the programs needs to be undertaken. Important questions need to be answered on whom to incentivize, i.e., those with the greatest overall improvement from baseline measures or those with the highest scores? Which conditions should be focused on for improvement remains a contentious issue. Should diabetes or cardiovascular disease be a priority? What about screening for breast or prostate cancer? Some suggest incentives to help bend the cost trajectory of care by focusing on misuse or overuse of services as a target for incentives. Other questions concern how much is the right amount to incentivize change in performance, and importantly, where should the funds come from? Is it fair to penalize underperformers? Some theorize that funds should be estimated from the financial benefits from improved care such as cost avoidance for readmissions and that those monies should be used as bonus pools.

This approach to improving quality addresses the issue of ameliorating the phenomenon identified as underuse. If the issue of underuse were the root cause of the quality conundrum United States' healthcare faces, we would be well on our way to improving outcomes and reducing costs. Unfortunately, underuse is only the tip of the iceberg in improving quality. Misuse and overuse, both very real phenomenon explored by Wennberg and his colleagues at Dartmouth, remain persistent offenders in the misaligned incentives of the present health care system. The use of healthcare IT to bring evidence-based decision making to the bedside remains one of the prime solutions on the horizon as the VA experience has demonstrated.

CONCLUSION

Transformational quality management systems in healthcare are those which are designed to address the issues identified by the IOM in *Crossing the Quality Chasm*.[2] They are transformational because they shift the paradigm improvement from narrow measurement and focus on individual performance to global metrics capturing population-based indicators. This evolution is perfectly timed to mesh with the needs of the Accountable Care Organization concept.

There remains a place—and a significant one—for condition specific metrics and peer performance analytics. After all, the whole is the sum of its parts. The critical aspect for the quality movement of the future is to continue to develop broad initiatives with actionable metrics that will guide effective improvement efforts without excessive burden on data collection. At the same time, these efforts need to be concurrently included into patient care workflows. This critical aspect drives improvement to the patient's bedside and allows for immediate translation into improvement in care and outcome with specific emphasis on safety.

Healthcare IT is the backbone of this type of transformational effort. By design, health IT brings decision support to the bedside, improves safety at the point of care, and enhances workflow. Importantly from a data management standpoint, it captures each step, process, and intervention in a data warehouse capable of providing advanced analytics. This database specifically responds to the need to continually evaluate efficiency, efficacy and timeliness, the ingredients to improved value and reduced cost.

The health IT platform of the future promises to fill many functional and operational gaps in the current healthcare delivery system. One thing that it cannot achieve is consensus for the prioritization of national improvement efforts across our delivery system that serves over 330 million people. This change needs to be driven by the stakeholders described earlier in this chapter. The Joint Commission, CMS, National Healthcare Improvement, Consumer Advocates and professional societies all have a significant role to play.

Perhaps one of the biggest obstacles to overcome is consensus around the improvement paradigm. Pay-for-performance cannot be effective if the goals are misaligned with priority conditions. The ACO concept will be insufficient if the outcomes to be achieved are ill-defined, poorly constructed, and not consistent with achieving value. Value perhaps oversimplified is outcome over cost. As Porter and Teisberg[18] point out, if we cannot reform the delivery system to achieve value, the cost trajectory will continue unchecked.

Building stakeholder consensus is difficult but achievable. The crisis in the economy of 2010 may create an opportunity for the various stakeholders to find common ground before the system collapses under the staggering weight of cost, access, overheated utilization, safety concerns and misaligned incentives.

ACKNOWLEDGMENTS

I would like to recognize the contributions of my colleagues, Joseph Marcone, MS, CNMT, RT (N), Certified Six Sigma Black Belt and Mary Marino, MS for their contributions to the development of the Six Sigma and Joint Commission sections of the chapter. I would also like to thank my proofreader and sister, Lisa Conte-Preston.

REFERENCES

1. Byrne CM, Mercincavage LM, Pan EC et al. The Value From Investments In Health Information Technology at the U.S. Department of Veterans Affairs. 10.1377/hlthaff.2010.0119. *Health Affairs* 29, No. 4 (2010):629–38.
2. Committee on Quality of Health Care in America, Institute of Medicine. *Crossing the Quality Chasm: A New Health System for the 21st Century.* The National Academies Press 2001. Available at: www.nap.edu/catalog.php?record_id=10027. Last accessed September 2010.
3. Serious Reportable Events in Healthcare: A Consensus Report. National Quality Forum. 2002. Available at: www.qualityforum.org/Publications/2002/06/Serious_Reportable_Events_in_Healthcare.aspx. Last accessed September 2010.
4. *To Err Is Human: Building a Safer Health System.* Kohn LT, Corrigan JM, Donaldson MS, eds. Institute of Medicine, 2000. Available at: www.nap.edu/openbook.php?record_id=9728. Accessed September 2010.
5. Parker-Pope T. A Hollywood family takes on medical mistakes. *New York Times,* March 17, 2008. Available at: http://well.blogs.nytimes.com/2008/03/17/a-hollywood-family-takes-on-medical-mistakes/?scp=1&sq=dennis%20quaid%20cedars%20sinai%20hospital&st=cse. Last accessed September 2010.
6. McGlynn EA, Asch SM, Adams J et al. The Quality of health care delivered to adults in the United States. *N Engl J Med.* 2003;348:2635-45.
7. Available at www.commonwealthfund.org/Content/Charts/Report/Mirror-Mirror-on-the-Wall-2010-Update/Overall-Ranking.aspx. Accessed on September 25, 2010.
8. Deming's Philosophy of Quality Management by Terry Halwes. Available at: www.dharma-haven.org/five-havens/deming.htm. Accessed September 26, 2010.
9. Available at http://en.wikipedia.org/wiki/File:PDCA_Cycle.svg. Accessed on September 25, 2010.
10. Available at http://en.wikipedia.org/wiki/W._Edwards_Deming#cite_note-lecture-0. Accessed on September 25, 2010.
11. Griffin FA. 5 Million Lives Campaign. Reducing methicillin-resistant Staphylococcus aureus (MRSA) infections. *Jt Comm J Qual Patient Saf.* 2007 Dec;33(12):726-31.
12. Shannon RP, Patel B, Cummins D et al. Economics of central line-associated bloodstream infections. *Am J Med Qual.* 2006;21(6 Suppl):7S-16S.
13. Available at www.ihi.org/IHI/Topics/CriticalCare/IntensiveCare/Changes/ImplementtheCentralLineBundle.htm. Accessed September 25 2010.
14. Shannon RP, Frndak D, Gunden N et al. Using real-time problem solving to eliminate central line infections. The Joint Commission. *J Qual Patient Saf.* 2006;32(9):479-87.
15. Available at: www.hospitalcompare.hhs.gov. Last accessed December 2010.
16. Available at: www.jointcommission.org/SentinelEvents/. Last accessed September 2010.
17. Available at: www.jointcommission.org/performancemeasurement/performancemeasurement/current+nhqm+manual.html. Last accessed December 2010.
18. Porter ME, Teisberg EO. Redefining competition in health care. *Harv Bus Rev.* 2004;82(6):64-76, 136.
19. Wennberg JE. Practice variation: implications for our health care system. *Manag Care.* 2004;13(9 Suppl):3-7.

20. Lindenauer PK, Remus D, Roman S et al. Public Reporting and Pay for Performance in Hospital Quality Improvement. *N Engl J Med.* 2007;356:486-96.

CHAPTER 13

Software Selection

Ken Ong, MD, MPH

Time for a pop quiz. Not to worry, you already know the answers.

Question 1: Is your desired software an electronic health record (EHR) or a related module?

- If yes, answer question 2.
- If not, you can skip the EHR sections and move on to the next.
- If you are unsure, see the Centers for Medicare & Medicaid Services (CMS) website (http://www.cms.gov/EHRIncentivePrograms/).[1]

Question 2: Are you shopping for an ambulatory EHR?

- If yes, read "Selecting an Ambulatory EHR" and call your local health information technology regional extension center (REC).
- If not, feel free to skip that section.

SELECTING AN AMBULATORY EHR

> "You're going to see a shake-out after a year or two if some of the major vendors don't have a lot of client base hitting stimulus dollars. You'll see a shift in the market if a vendor can say it has 30 organizations that hit meaningful use in 2011 and will have 40 in 2012, and another vendor can only say they have two. That's going to be a selling point."
>
> — *Brian D. Patty, MD*
>
> *Vice President and CMIO at HealthEast Care System*[2]

Practically speaking, there are just two kinds of ambulatory EHRs: those that are CMS-certified and those that are not.

To qualify for the CMS EHR incentive program (before 2015) and to avoid the CMS payment penalties (after 2015), a physician practice will need a CMS-certified EHR to achieve meaningful use.

Even if a physician practice has chosen to forego the incentives and suffer the penalties, they will probably get a better value for their dollar if they purchase an EHR certified by CMS than one that is not.

Here is why a CMS-certified EHR is better. Providers and patients want to be sure that the EHRs can (1) share patient information securely and confidentially with other IT systems and (2) provide the functionality required to generate safety, quality and efficiency. Through a rigorous review process, CMS has defined standards to ensure both.[3]

Selecting, implementing and maintaining an EHR is expensive and difficult. Help is available at your local health information technology regional extension centers (RECs). The American Recovery and Reinvestment Act of 2009/Health Information Technology for Economic and Clinical Health Act of 2009 has appropriated $640 million,[4] and as a result, some 60 RECs have been created across the nation.[5] Their goal is to provide outreach and support services to at least 100,000 priority primary care providers.

To find a REC near you, visit the CMS HIT Extension Program website (http://healthit.hhs.gov/portal/server.pt/community/healthit_hhs_gov__rec_program/1495).[6]

Other helpful resources:

- Center for Health IT at the American Academy of Family Practice[7] (www.centerforhit.org/online/chit/home.html)
- Center for Practice Improvement and Innovation at the American College of Physicians[8] (www.acponline.org/running_practice/technology/)
- Council on Clinical Information Technology of the American Academy of Pediatrics[9] (www.aapcocit.org/cocit_tasks.php; www.aap.org/ehr)
- American Congress of Obstetricians and Gynecologists[10] (www.acog.org/departments/dept_web.cfm?recno=47)

For a detailed look at the work of one REC, see the chapters by Parsons (Chapter 16) and Singh (Chapter 11) that discuss New York City's Primary Care Information Project and NYC Regional Electronic Adoption Center for Health (REACH). For more on the ambulatory EHR, see the chapter by Drs. Cole and Cheriff (Chapter 6).

Software Strategies: Best-of-Breed vs. Single Source vs. Best of Suite

One of the central debates in software selection is the choice between the best-of-breed (BoB) and single source (see Table 13-1).

The conventional wisdom argues that buying software products from a single vendor will deliver more integration. Integration means greater efficiency and cost savings in purchasing and maintaining software. Some vendors repeat what has become the mantra of single source proponents. With a single vendor, there is but "one throat to choke" (see Figure 13-1). If there are problems with any software, the CIO has but one vendor to whom he must complain.

Table 13- 1: Best-of-Breed vs. Single Source

	Pro	Con
Best-of-Breed	Best unit or departmental functionality	• Work and cost of interfacing • Many vendors to manage
Single Source	• Integrated • "One throat to choke"	• Often poor departmental functionality • Diminished negotiating cache

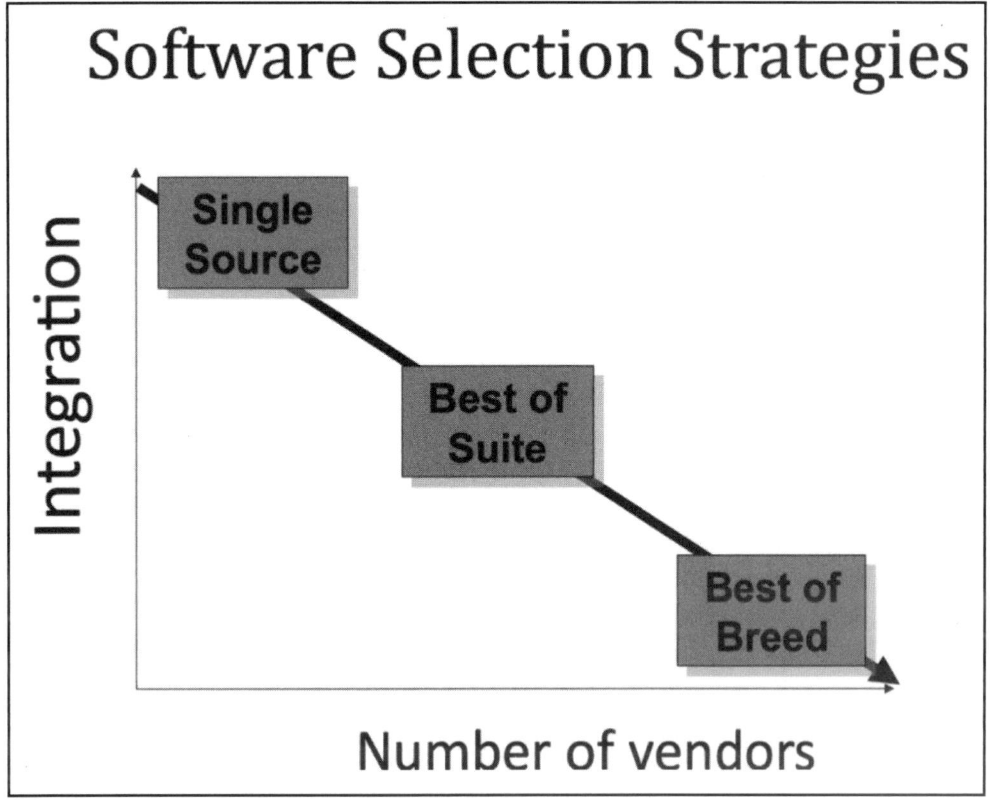

Figure 13-1: Software Selection Strategies

One of my favorite CIOs, Pete Garrison, gave a poignant rejoinder to a sales representative who made that pitch. Garrison countered, "We don't want to choke anyone's throat. We want a partner who will get us where we need to go."

Another painful reality is that the promise of integration may be either in development or illusory. No single vendor has a module for every department in a hospital. One vendor may buy a compendium of different software products but fail to integrate them. Changing a menagerie of different programs into a common database with integrated logic is an expensive and time-consuming challenge. Another vendor may be expanding its current product offerings but the newest modules may be immature.

The conventional wisdom argues that buying BoB means buying the best software. Business units or departments tend to prefer selecting the BoB software for their particular workflow, but there are at least three trade-offs. First, creating and maintaining interfaces costs money. Second, interfaces are complicated and may not function as desired, e.g., one-way only but not two-way (bi-directional). Finally, multiple vendor relationships have to be managed. Rather than one throat to choke, there are many. When an interface has issues, multiple vendors may engage in finger-pointing, and bewildering delays or downtime may occur.

A third option to BoB and single source is best-of-suite (BoS), also known as "best-of-cluster." The rationale of the BoS approach is that only a core group of software applications must be closely integrated. Applications that fall outside of the cluster need a lesser degree of integration. At the bare minimum, the cluster would include computerized practitioner order entry (CPOE), clinical decision support system (CDSS) and the pharmacy system.

The more expansive definition might include all the elements of the electronic medical record (EMR). Garets and Davis suggest the EMR environment comprises:[11]

- Clinical Data Repository (CDR)
- Controlled Medical Vocabulary (CMV)
- Clinical Decision Support System (CDSS)
- Clinical Documentation
- Computerized Practitioner Order Entry (CPOE)
- Pharmacy Management
- Electronic Medication Administration Record (eMAR)
- Workflow

CURRENT STATE: HOSPITAL SOFTWARE STRATEGIES

To better understand which of the software strategies may be better associated with a full EHR implementation, Ford et al. analyzed the 2007 survey of the American Hospital Association (AHA), as shown in Table 13-2. A total of 1,814 hospitals responded to the health IT subset of questions. A multivariate analysis controlling for profit/tax status, system affiliation, Joint Commission accreditation, and teaching status found that hospitals pursuing a BoS were 34.1 percent more likely than those pursuing a single-vendor health IT strategy to have fully implemented an EHR system. Moreover, hospitals pursuing a BoS strategy were 44.2 percent more likely than hospitals pursing BoB strategy to have fully implemented an EHR system, but this trend was only significant at the $p<0.10$ level.[12]

Why does a hospital have one software strategy rather than another? Another study using AHA data suggests an answer.

Using data from the 2007 AHA survey and the 2008 HIMSS Analytics Database, Burke et al. analyzed the software strategy of 3,343 hospitals.[13] The study found that 61 percent of the hospitals indicated a single vendor, 29 percent indicated a BoS, and 10 percent suggested a BoB strategy (see Table 13-3).

Table 13-2: EHR Strategy by Self-Reported Implementation Status[12]

Implementation Status	Best of Breed	Best of Suite	Single Vendor	Total
In Progress				
Count	166	461	793	1,420
Expected	163.6	494.7	761.7	—
Fully Implemented				
Count	43	171	180	394
Expected	45.4	137.3	211.3	—
Total[2]	209 (11.5%)	632 (34.8%)	973 (53.6%)	1,814 (100%)

[1] Pearson chi-square = 16.684; $p < .001$.

[2] Percentages are calculated using the cell count divided by the row total.

Table 13-3: Organizational Characteristics of Hospitals (n=3,343)[13]

Hospital Characteristic	Frequency (%)
Hospital bed size: Small (<99 beds) Medium (100-299 beds) Large (300+ beds)	 1,251 (37.4%) 1,401 (41.9%) 691 (20.7%)
System Affiliation vs. Stand Alone	1,966 (58.8%) 1,377 (41.2%)
For-profit status vs. Not-for-profit	507 (15.2%) 2,835 (84.8%)
Teaching hospital vs. Non-teaching facility	244 (7.3%) 3,099 (92.7%)
JCAHO Accreditation vs. Non-accredited hospital	2,449 (73.3%) 894 (26.7%)
HIT Management Strategy Best of Breed Single Vendor Best of Suite	 343 (10.3%) 2,023 (60.5%) 977 (29.2%)
Total	3,343 (100%)

Note: Number may not add up to 100% due to rounding.

Single-vendor strategies were most common among hospitals that were small, stand-alone, for-profit, non-teaching and/or non-Joint Commission-accredited. Smaller hospitals may have fewer IT staff and, in that case, managing a single vendor contract may be easier (see Tables 13-4 and 13-5).

Best of breed strategies were most common among system-affiliated and Joint Commission-accredited hospitals. Best-of-suite IT strategies were most common

Table 13-4: Hospital Characteristics and Health IT Management Strategies[13]

	HIT Management Strategy			
	Single Vendor Strategy	Best of Breed Strategy	Best of Suite Strategy	P-value
Bed size				
Small (1-99 beds)	921 (74%)	103 (8%)	227 (18%)	
Medium (100-299 beds)	817 (58%)	140 (10%)	444 (32%)	<0.01
Large (300+ beds)	285 (41%)	100 (15%)	306 (44%)	
System				
System-affiliate	977 (71%)	109 (8%)	291 (21%)	<0.01
Stand-alone	1,046 (53%)	234 (12%)	686 (35%)	
Tax status				
Not for profit	1,711 (60%)	306 (11%)	818 (29%)	0.05
For profit	311 (61%)	37 (7%)	156 (31%)	
Teaching Hospital				
Yes	71 (29%)	45 (18%)	128 (53%)	<0.01
No	1,952 (63%)	298 (10%)	849 (24%)	
JCAHO Accredited				
Yes	1,317 (54%)	279 (11%)	853 (35%)	<0.01
No	706 (79%)	64 (7%)	124 (14%)	

Note: Number may not add up to 100% due to rounding.
P-values calculated using the Chi-square statistic

Table 13-5: The Multivariate Relationship Between Hospital Characteristics and IT Strategy Pursued[13]

	Dependent Variables: Type of IT Management Strategy Pursued		
	Single Vendor Strategy	Best of Breed Strategy	Best of Suite Strategy
	Odds Ratio (95% C.I.)	Odds Ratio (95% C.I.)	Odds Ratio (95% C.I.)
Independent variables			
Bed size1	0.99 (0.98 – 0.99)	1.00 (1.00 – 1.00)	1.001** (1.001 – 1.002)
System			
Stand Alone	2.00** (1.72 – 2.33)	1.00	1.00
System affiliated	1.00	1.61** (1.25 – 2.06)	1.77** (1.49 – 2.09)
Tax-status			
Not for profit	1.00	1.82** (1.25 – 2.63)	1.00
For-profit status	1.41** (1.14 – 1.74)	1.00	0.87 (0.70 – 1.09)
Teaching hospital			
No	2.08** (1.49 – 2.94)	1.00	1.00
Yes	1.00	1.52 (0.99 – 2.33)	1.62** (1.18 – 2.22)
JCAHO Accreditation			
No	2.22** (1.85 – 2.78)	1.00	1.00
Yes	1.00	1.42* (1.04 – 1.93)	2.41** (1.93 – 3.03)

1Bed size was measured continuously in multivariate analyses
Note: Each odds ratio is adjusted for all independent variables included in that table. Only positive relationships are highlighted for significance.
*p<0.05 **p<0.01

among very large, system affiliated, teaching and Joint Commission-accredited hospitals. Both the BoB and BoS strategies require more and better experienced IT resources and the capacity to manage multiple vendor contracts.

The study's authors conclude: "The decision to pursue a specific health IT management strategy is very complex and often involves the interplay and valuation of hard and soft factors, which ultimately results in a migration path that is unique for a given organization."

No doubt every hospital wants to deploy the best technology to give the best patient care and excel beyond meaningful use. Yet, the resources are limited, and HITECH's funding comes after the hospital has made its investment, not before. As one industry watcher comments, "In that world, it's not about ripping and replacing, but patching, leveraging and surviving."[14]

THE EMERGENCY DEPARTMENT: LET'S TALK…

"The niche systems are designed specifically for (and often by) ED physicians, and their intended users sometimes advocate passionately for them. But more and more hospitals have their eye on an enterprise electronic health record, complete with clinical decision support, where a piece of data entered in any department is immediately and automatically available to all others. An interface to a separate ED system rarely behaves with equal seamlessness, and may not be enough to achieve the benefits promised by an EHR."

— *Elizabeth Gardner*[15]

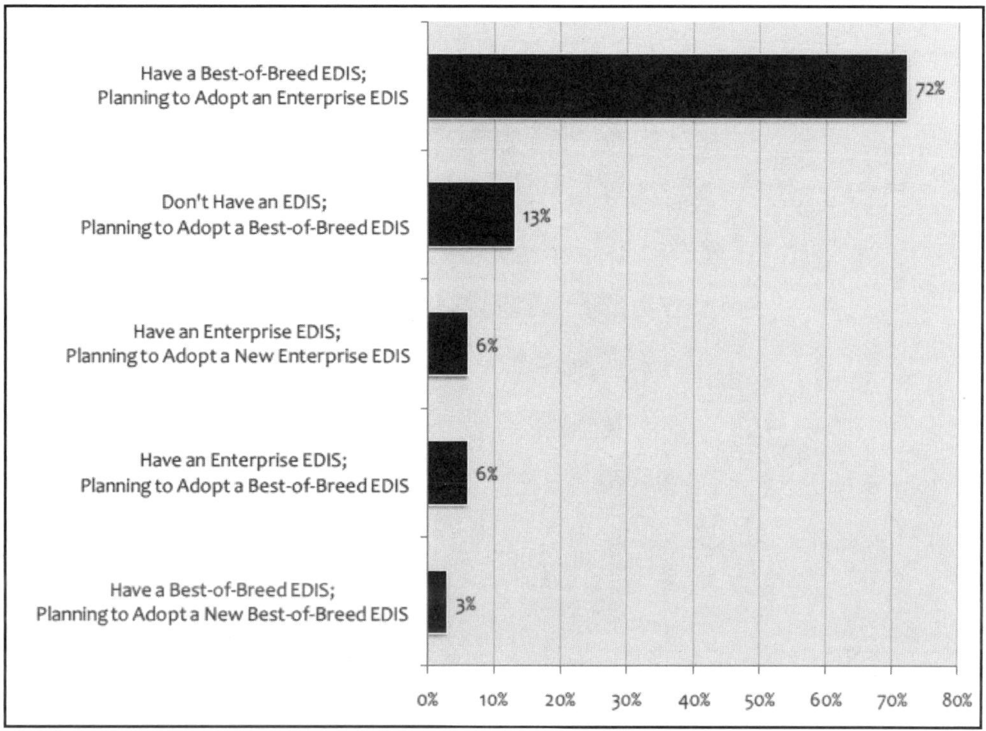

Figure 13-2: EDIS Replacement Approach (n=32) Planned EDIS Strategy (among respondents in this study who are actively purchasing or replacing their EDIS)[17]

Warning: This is an issue that makes for many passionate conversations among clinicians and managers inside and outside of hospital emergency departments (EDs). HITECH has only turned up the heat.

Whether the stage 1 core measure is CPOE, demographics, problem list, active medication list, active allergy list, vital signs, smoking status or providing patients an electronic copy of their health information or discharge instructions, the measure pertains to the eligible hospital or critical access hospital's inpatient and ED.[16]

A KLAS Research survey showed that of the 32 respondents replacing their EDIS, 72 percent were leaving a BoB EDIS solution in favor of an enterprise offering (see Figure 13-2).[17]

A couple of physician quotes provide the clinical rationale for integrated inpatient and ED systems:

> "If I'm ordering a contrast agent for a CT scan, I need to know whether the patient has any kidney damage. An isolated system cannot grab that creatinine measurement from three months ago and tell me as I put in the order."
>
> —*Reid Conant, MD*
> *CMIO of Tri-City Medical Center*
> *Oceanside, California*[15]

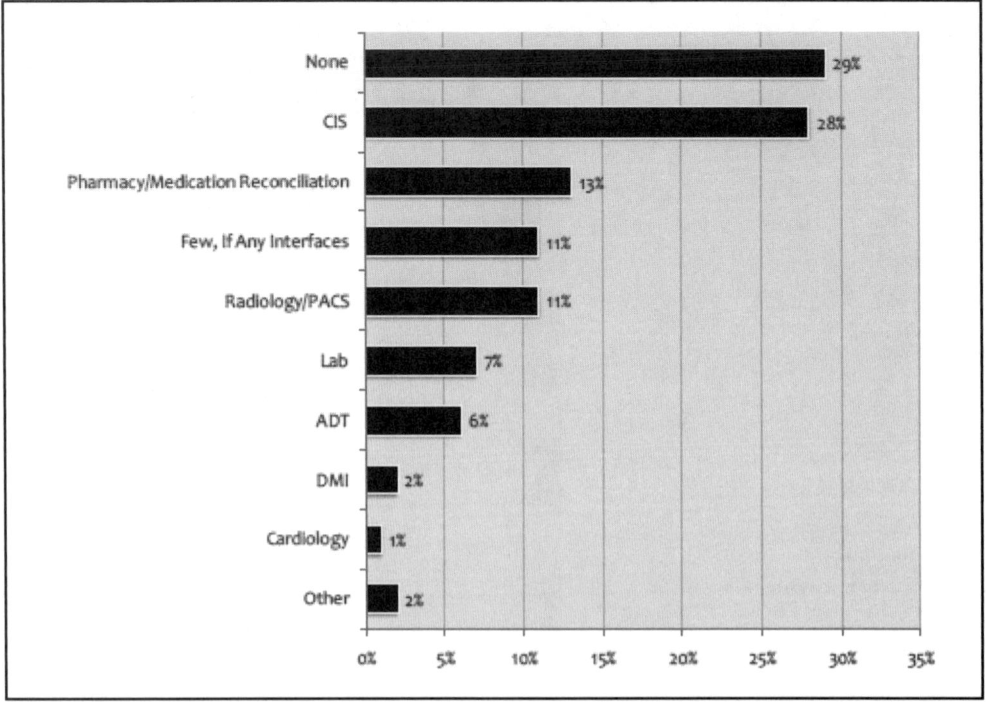

Figure 13-3: With Which Hospital Systems Are You Having Difficulty Sharing Information? (n=211)[17]

Note: the "Other" category includes ambulatory, niche systems, and medication cabinets.

> "Everybody liked it [best of breed ED system], but when we began doing CPOE and moved off paper, we found we could not make it completely safe to ensure that a patient never missed a dose or never got two doses because the medication records were on different systems. You might say, 'Oh, just interface them,' but engineers can spend four years trying to make that happen. Keeping formularies and supplier lists in parallel becomes almost impossible."
>
> —*Michael Shabot, MD*
> *CMO of Memorial Hermann Health System*[18]

Respondents to the above-referenced KLAS survey on ED systems faced interface challenges (see Figure 13-3). Some respondents who switched from niche ED systems to integrated ED systems complained that their new system was less "user-friendly" and less adapted to the ED workflow.

For those already committed to an ED system, different challenges pertain to both the integrated and niche ED systems:

- Integrated ED system: Improves both the usability and workflow of their ED module.
- Niche ED system: All EHR modules must be CMS-certified. Select an ED system that is CMS-certified and create functional interfaces between the inpatient and ED system to achieve meaningful use.

BUYING SOFTWARE IS A JOURNEY

Other than buying CMS-certified EHR software to achieve meaningful use, why does anyone ever have to buy new software? What's wrong with the old software? Why do we need software at all? These are common questions that all of us have heard before. No doubt these are questions we may have actually asked ourselves on occasion.

Why, indeed? A new project may require a purchase of software. The current version of a particular software product may sunset. A vendor sells a new software product and refuses to support the older version. Generations of software have changed from mainframe to client server or from character to Windows-driven platforms. A similar shift was seen for some products that evolved from client-server owned and maintained by the client to software as a service (SaaS) owned and maintained by a software vendor.

If a software vendor is purchased or goes out of business, their software is orphaned and left bereft of support. Even very expensive health IT may go the way of the eight-track tape player or VHS tape. Hospital or clinic mergers or other enterprise-wide initiatives may drive standardization. Standardizing software across a multihospital system can facilitate adopting best practices and lower purchase and maintenance costs for IT. Paying multiple vendors for the same software translates into multiple contracts to manage, training associated with each software product, and a Gordian knot of interfaces. Each interface can generate its own costs for maintenance and episodes of downtime.

Just as medication administration has its five rights,[19] purchasing IT does as well: the right reasons and the right process with the right people to find the right system at the right price.[20]

Sidebar 13-1: The Five Rights of Purchasing

1. The right reasons
2. The right process
3. The right people
4. The right system
5. The right price

(Adapted from Laker and Groeber.)

The right reasons should be the alpha and omega of every project. More in healthcare than elsewhere, IT must often serve both margin and mission. Should a clinical software system promote both patient safety and appropriate charge capture? The obvious answer is yes and yes. The right reasons should be translated into quantifiable and achievable goals. The right reason will have a measureable outcome. One metric that has become standard for many capital purchases is the payback period, better known as return on investment (ROI).[21]

The right process gathers the input of all major stakeholders and ensures that an evidence-based, outcome-focused selection proceeds and that the project is aligned with the strategic plan of the organization.[22] The process often includes a software selection team comprised of both managers of the business unit or organization and the relevant executive officer(s). The software selection team may be formally charged to present its project for the approval of an executive information systems or capital expenditure approval committee. The latter committee may be responsible for approving expenses that run over the projected costs or, in that most unhappy of circumstances, terminating a project if it fails to meet its milestones, projected costs or post-go-live goals. The right selection process creates the foundations for a successful installation and maintenance.

Sidebar 13-2: The Right People for a Selection Process

- Executive sponsor
- Project champion
- Project manager
- Representatives from other disciplines or business units relevant to the software application

The right people in the selection committee include an executive sponsor, a project champion, a project manager, and representatives from other disciplines or business units relevant to the software application. In addition to the formal process within the organization, the executive sponsor ensures through both formal and informal channels that the project has the buy-in of the organization's executive leadership. This buy-in includes not only the project budget but cooperation from other departments and business units to participate in the selection, the installation and successful continuation of the project. The larger the scope of the project, the more important that buy-in becomes.

The project manager may be from either the business unit or information systems. The project manager should be involved in both the selection and installation phases of the project. His/her role is to enumerate and assign each task, coordinate disparate and limited resources, identify potential or actual problems, and deliver the project on time and within budget. Project management is a body of knowledge for which formal education and certification exist.[23] But, certification is often not the most important asset a project manager brings to the table.

Heerkens suggests that the four most desired traits of a project manager are (1) thinking that is like that of a generalist, (2) a high tolerance for ambiguity, (3) a high tolerance for uncertainty, and (4) honesty and integrity.[24] Certification marks a level of competence, but experience in selecting and installing projects of similar complexity is often more reassuring.

The project champion is the person from the business unit or department who can promote and advocate others to adopt the software application, the workflow changes or the clinical transformation needed to achieve the expected project outcomes. Gladwell refers to such individuals as connectors.[25]

Rogers would categorize the ideal project champion as an early adopter: "Potential adopters look to early adopters for advice and information about an innovation. The early adopter is considered by many to be the individual to check with before adopting a new idea. This adopter category is generally sought by change agents as a local missionary for speeding the diffusion process. Because early adopters are not too far ahead of the average individual in innovativeness, they serve as a role model for many other members of a social system. Early adopters help trigger the mass when they adopt an innovation… In one sense, early adopters put their stamp of approval on a new idea by adopting it."[26]

Representatives of other relevant business units or departments should sit at the table; if their participation is important for a successful install, then they should be part of the selection process. As healthcare strives to improve quality and efficiency, collaboration and teamwork become increasingly vital. A chain is only as strong as its weakest link. Sometimes leaving just one person, one office or one department out of the selection process can compromise a successful implementation.

The right system is the one that best enables the project's goals—be it reducing no-shows for a clinic scheduling system or reducing medication errors for a closed loop medication management system.

The conventional wisdom is that a request for proposal (RFP) is the *sine qua non* for selecting the right system. In today's complex healthcare IT market, the traditional RFP is not without its problems. Laker and Groeber caution, "The classic approach is buying or building a checklist of desired features, issuing it to vendors in a request for proposal (RFP), then scoring results to see which system has the most functionality. But with today's system architectures and powerful tools, vendors can say 'yes' to nearly all questions. Most vendors' RFP responses score around 90 percent, while actual use of system functions at client sites is maybe 50 percent. Plus, sales or marketing staff answer RFPs, not the programmers and analysts who really know the product."[20]

Buying software in the 21st century can be a little like buying a new car. When hunting for a new car today, we search the Web and newsstands for rating surveys, such as *Consumer Reports*. We check the car manufacturer's website for a marketing brochure. We Google[27] online forums and blogs for opinions from consumers themselves. Whether or not they own the vehicle in question, we ask everyone we know for their opinion. We go to the car dealer to listen to that MP3-enabled nine-speaker sound system or see firsthand if the olive green looks that much cooler than the lime. During the entire journey, we share our findings with our significant other, parents, and next-door neighbor. In the end, a contract is signed and we have a new car.

Online services like KLAS[28] and MDBuyline[29] offer consumer satisfaction rankings, product specific reports, vendor specific client commentary and more. Aunt Minnie[30] is a site devoted to imaging products and their evaluation. The number one ranking in a KLAS survey or most improved ranking are coveted. Consumer ratings are an invaluable reality check for that occasional end-user who has used the existing product forever and is convinced there is nothing better.

Critics, who are more often than not vendors, lament that customer satisfaction rating services are subject to gaming. They say that vendors with the highest rankings are only better at convincing their customers to participate in the satisfaction surveys. Yet that very same tactic is open to all vendors and fails to explain why some garner better rankings than others. The vendor's website should include the number of employees, annual revenues, location of the corporate headquarters, product brochures, and contact information for sales. The product information from each vendor can be the starting point for developing the selection criteria rating tool for the selection team.

A vendor assessment or selection criteria rating tool has several tangible benefits. It represents a consensus within the selection team about what it expects the software to do. The "right reasons" should permeate the selection and implementation processes. Weighting the selection criteria can define what functionality has greater priority. The rating scale should be no more complicated than 1–3 or 1–5. Even numbered rating scales (e.g., 1–4 or 1–6) force evaluations that are more clearly positive or negative. Rating scales whose highest rating exceeds 5 or 6 do not necessarily add value. Categories of specifications should be rated rather than rating each specification itself. Selection team members find rating 10 or fewer categories practical, but 100 individual specifications impossible.

Functionality is but one section in the vendor assessment tool. Other critical sections include regulatory compliance, IT requirements, and vendor characteristics. A software product with all the latest bells and whistles is useless if its vendor's future looks dubious or if its security does not meet HITECH's heightened requirements for protecting health information.

Searching the Web for the latest news on vendors can uncover useful information. If one vendor purchases another with a competing product, one of the products will not fare well in the future. Learning of a company's reorganization, one should ask the vendor how that will affect their future and product support. Even a friendly acquisition may lead to a "hiccup" or temporary reduction in support services.

Demonstrations should be arranged and vendors rated with the vendor assessment tool. The tool can be used to ensure each vendor is asked to show the same specifications. The tool becomes indispensable if the products are complex in scope or if the number of demos includes three or more vendors over a span of days. A post-mortem or debriefing after each vendor's demo can help solidify areas of consensus and disagreement. If a product offers better support for one subset of stakeholders than another (e.g., physicians or nurses), then the team will have to decide if that tradeoff is worthwhile or if another product better serves all stakeholders. This advice is given full well knowing it is easier said than done.

Sidebar 13-3: Due Diligence—Peer-to-Peer Reference Calls

- Call current clients
- Ask about satisfaction with version of the software you're considering
- What did they like about the product? This vendor?
- What didn't they like?
- What were their 'lessons learned'?
- Would they buy this product again?
- Check client commentary in rating services, e.g., KLAS reports

After the scores from the vendor assessment tool are tallied, the finalists should be selected. Preliminary proposals and a list of current clients can be requested. "Due diligence" generally requires site visits and reference calls to existing clients. Both should be made without the vendor present. Be aware that it makes perfect sense for a vendor to refer the prospective customer to those current clients who are most happy with their product. Finding clients that have recently switched from one vendor to another is even more useful.

The right price requires a thorough review of line items in the project plan. The project plan should be part of the contract. Training is always a key issue. The "train the trainer" option lowers travel expenses, decreases time lost to training, and minimizes costs required to back-fill the staff's absence during training. A selected group of the customer's managers or super users can be trained by the vendor on site or at the vendor's corporate training facilities. The selected group of trainers can then train the remaining staff in the business unit or organization.

Subscribing to SaaS is an option many vendors now offer. Back in the day of large mainframe-based applications, the subscription model was common. The vendor would own and host the "heavy iron," the mainframe computers. The customer would pay a monthly or quarterly fee for access. Once again, courtesy of the Web, the SaaS mirrors that model and offers subscription rates. In the capital-poor environment of healthcare today, stretching the total cost of ownership over a three- to seven-year period lowers upfront capital costs.

Finally, the day arrives in a selection process when a vendor is selected. The executive sponsor and selection team present the project to the executive leadership for approval.

A successful selection process is a prelude to a successful implementation. A hasty selection can lead to missteps in implementation. The consensus required for workflow and clinical transformation is the staging platform for implementing the software and achieving the desired patient safety and business goals. Selection and planning for implementation are very much intertwined.

Sidebar 13-4: Caveat Emptor

- Vaporware
- Visionware
- Betaware
- PPOS (PowerPoint Operating System)
- Technology on the bleeding edge (newer and riskier than the cutting edge)

If you're the type who'd hesitate to buy the first model of a new car line, you should be just as risk averse with the very latest information technology. Unless your organization classifies itself in the innovator category of the adopter distribution and has the resources to devote to developing new technology, take on "the latest and the greatest" with extreme caution.

REFERENCES

1. Available at: http://www.cms.gov/EHRIncentivePrograms/. Last accessed December 2010.
2. CMIOs give meaningful use mixed reviews (Part Two in Two-Part Series). *CMIO.* July 20,1010. Available at: http://www.healthimaging.com/index.php?option=com_articles&view=article&id=23250. Last accessed August 2010.
3. CMS EHR Incentive Programs Certification. Available at: http://www.cms.gov/EHRIncentivePrograms/30_Certification.asp#TopOfPage. Last accessed August 2010.
4. Available at: http://healthit.hhs.gov/portal/server.pt/community/healthit_hhs_gov__hit_extension_centers_program/1335. Last accessed August 2010.
5. Available at: http://healthit.hhs.gov/portal/server.pt?open=512&objID=1495&mode=2&cached=true. Last accessed August 2010.
6. Available at: http://healthit.hhs.gov/portal/server.pt/community/healthit_hhs_gov_rec_program/1495. Last accessed December 2010.
7. Available at: http://www.centerforhit.org/online/chit/home.html. Last accessed December 2010.
8. Available at: http://www.acponline.org/running_practice/technology/. Last accessed December 2010.
9. Available at: http://www.aapcocit.org/cocit_tasks.php; http://www.aap.org/ehr/. Last accessed December 2010.
10. Available at: http://www.acog.org/departments/dept_web.cfm?recno=47. Last accessed December 2010.
11. Garets D, Davis M. White Paper: Electronic medical records vs. electronic health records: yes, there is a difference. HIMSS Analytics. 2006. Available at: http://www.himssanalytics.org/docs/WP_EMR_EHR.pdf. Last accessed August 2010.

12. Ford EW, Menachemi N, Huerta TR et al. Hospital IT adoption strategies associated with implementation success: Implications for achieving meaningful use. *Journal of Healthcare Management.* 2010;55,3;ABI/INFORM Global.
13. Burke et al. Best of breed strategies: Hospital characteristics associated with organizational HIT strategy. *JHIM.* Spring 2009;23:2.
14. Guerra A. Guerra On Healthcare: Application rip and replace realities. *InformationWeek.* July 29, 2010. Available at; http://www.informationweek.com/story/showArticle.jhtml?articleID=226300107. Last accessed August 2010.
15. Gardner E. Emergency situation: Best of breed, or enterprise integration? *Health Data Management Magazine.* March 1, 2010.
16. Medicare and Medicaid Programs; Electronic Health Record Incentive Program; Final Rule Available at: http://edocket.access.gpo.gov/2010/pdf/2010-17207.pdf. Last accessed August 2010.
17. Emergency Department Information Systems: Is Best of Breed Still the Best Approach? KLAS Research. December 2009.
18. Intensive care, intensive information. *Health Data Management Magazine.* May 1, 2010.
19. Neuenschwander M, Cohen MR, Vaida AJ et al. Practical guide to bar coding for patient medication safety. *Am J Health Syst Pharm.* 2003;15;60(8):768–79.
20. Laker B, Groeber V. IT purchasing strategies: Make good decisions by approaching them right. *Healthcare Informatics.* 2005;22(9):48.
21. Return on Investment: What is ROI analysis? Solution Matrix. Available at: http://www.solutionmatrix.com/return-on-investment.html. Last accessed August 2010.
22. McDowell SW. Herding cats: The challenges of EMR vendor selection. *JHIM.* 2005;17(3):63–71.
23. Project Management Institute. *A Guide to the Project Management Body of Knowledge.* (PMBOK® Guide). 3rd ed. New Town Square, Penn: Project Management Institute; 2006.
24. Heerkens G. *Project Management.* New York: McGraw-Hill; 2002.
25. Gladwell M. *The Tipping Point: How Little Things Can Make a Big Difference.* New York: Little Brown & Co.; 2000.
26. Rogers EM. *Diffusion of Innovations.* 4th ed. New York: Free Press; 2003.
27. Available at: www.google.com. Last accessed December 2010.
28. Available at: www.healthcomuting.com. Last accessed December 2010.
29. Available at: www.mdbuyline.com. Last accessed December 2010.
30. Available at: www.auntminnie.com. Last accessed December 2010.

Chapter 14

The Patient Centered Medical Home Model

Salvatore Volpe, MD, FAAP, FACP, CHCQM

INTRODUCTION

Forty-three years ago, the Council of Pediatric Practice (COPP) had a prescient opinion regarding healthcare. At that time, they were attempting to address issues regarding children with special healthcare needs (CSHCNs). The Federal Maternal and Child Health Bureau defined CSHCNs as:

> "[T]hose who have or are at increased risk for a chronic physical, developmental, behavioral, or emotional condition and who also require health and related services of a type or amount beyond that required by children generally."[1]
>
> "For children with chronic diseases or disabling conditions, the lack of a complete record and a 'medical home' is a major deterrent to adequate health supervision. Wherever the child is cared for, the question should be asked, 'Where is the child's medical home?' and any pertinent information should be transmitted to that place."[2]

Back in 1967, there were no fax machines, no secure e-mail, no EHRs with graphic user interfaces. There was, however, the realization that without the coordination of care by all the providers, the families of these children would suffer from gaps in care, redundant "care," and skyrocketing expenses. Sound familiar?

COPP made these recommendations: "The first requirement is the teaching of all medical students that a medical home and a complete central record of a child's medical care are the *sine qua non* of proper pediatric supervision. Second, the concept must spread from physicians to all agencies and people caring for children—schools, child guidance clinics, well-infant stations, surgical specialists, emergency departments, and so forth. The third step is the indoctrination of parents."[3]

While the goals were laudatory, it was not until Calvin Sia, MD, took up the gauntlet that the concept gained the exposure and funding needed to be implemented. Between

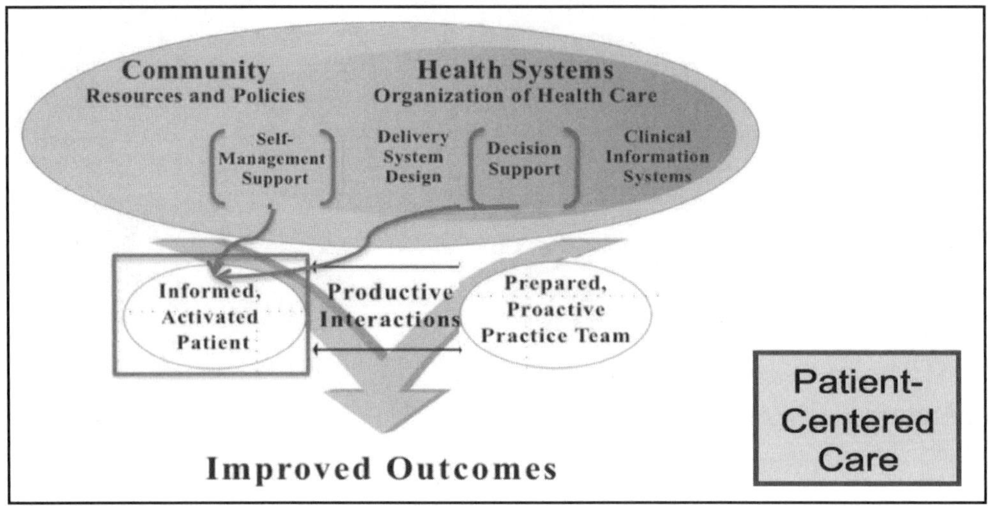

Figure 14-1: Chronic Care Model[5]
Adapted from Wagner EH. Chronic disease management: What will it take to improve care for chronic illness? *Effective Clinical Practice.* 1998;1(1):2-4.

1978 and 1979, Dr. Sia succeeded in having the term "Medical Home" incorporated in legislation passed in Hawaii. "This was the birth of the medical home concept as we know it today. It stated that a medical home would be family centered; be community based (geographically and financially accessible and available); offer continuity, comprehensive, and coordinated care; and use the resources of related services in the neighborhood."[4]

In 1998, Edward H. Wagner, MD, proposed the following model for chronic disease management based upon his work at Group Health Cooperative (see Figure 14-1).

Communities depend on healthcare delivery systems to have four key features:

1. **Self-management Support:** Patients and their families are given tools and resources to participate in management of their health.
2. **Delivery System Design:** The system to deliver healthcare has to take into account the multiple agents and facilitate communication.
3. **Decision Support:** Evidence-based clinical support tools need to be available at the point of care.
4. **Information Systems:** Information technology needs to be developed to facilitate communication between providers, patients, and the community.

In 2002, the American Academy of Pediatrics (AAP) issued the following description of the medical home:[2]

1. Provision of family-centered care through developing a trusting partnership with families, respecting their diversity, and recognizing that they are the constant in a child's life.
2. Sharing clear and unbiased information with the family about the child's medical care and management and about the specialty and community services and organizations they can access.
3. Provision of primary care, including but not restricted to acute and chronic care and preventive services, including breastfeeding promotion and management,

immunizations, growth and developmental assessments, appropriate screenings, healthcare supervision, and patient and parent counseling about health, nutrition, safety, parenting, and psychosocial issues.

4. Assurance that ambulatory and inpatient care for acute illnesses will be continuously available (24 hours a day, 7 days a week, 52 weeks a year).
5. Provision of care over an extended period of time to ensure continuity. Transitions, including those to other pediatric providers or into the adult healthcare system, should be planned and organized with the child and family.
6. Identification of the need for consultation and appropriate referral to pediatric medical subspecialists and surgical specialists. (In instances in which the child enters the medical system through a specialty clinic, identification of the need for primary pediatric consultation and referral is appropriate.)
7. Primary, pediatric medical subspecialty, and surgical specialty care providers should collaborate to establish shared management plans in partnership with the child and family and to formulate a clear articulation of each other's role.
8. Interaction with early intervention programs, schools, early childhood education and child care programs, and other public and private community agencies to be certain that the special needs of the child and family are addressed.
9. Provision of care coordination services in which the family, the physician, and other service providers work to implement a specific care plan as an organized team.
10. Maintenance of an accessible, comprehensive, central record that contains all pertinent information about the child, preserving confidentiality.

In 2007, the AAP, American Academy of Family Physicians (AAFP), American College of Physicians (ACP), and American Osteopathic Association (AOA), representing approximately 333,000 physicians, developed the following joint principles to describe the characteristics of the Patient Centered Medical Home (PCMH):

- **Personal physician** – Each patient has an ongoing relationship with a personal physician trained to provide first contact, continuous and comprehensive care.
- **Physician-directed medical practice** – The personal physician leads a team of individuals at the practice level who collectively take responsibility for the ongoing care of patients.
- **Whole-person orientation** – The personal physician is responsible for providing for all the patient's healthcare needs or taking responsibility for appropriately arranging care with other qualified professionals. This includes care for all stages of life; acute care; chronic care; preventive services; and end-of-life care.
- **Care is coordinated and/or integrated** across all elements of the complex healthcare system (e.g., subspecialty care, hospitals, home health agencies, nursing homes) and the patient's community (e.g., family, public and private community-based services). Care is facilitated by registries, information technology, health information exchange and other means to assure that patients get the indicated care when and where they need and want it in a culturally and linguistically appropriate manner.

- **Quality and safety** are hallmarks of the medical home:
  - Practices advocate for their patients to support the attainment of optimal, patient-centered outcomes that are defined by a care planning process driven by a compassionate, robust partnership between physicians, patients and the patient's family.
  - Evidence-based medicine and clinical decision-support tools guide decision making.
  - Physicians in the practice accept accountability for continuous quality improvement through voluntary engagement in performance measurement and improvement.
  - Patients actively participate in decision making, and feedback is sought to ensure patients' expectations are being met.
  - Information technology is utilized appropriately to support optimal patient care, performance measurement, patient education and enhanced communication.
  - Practices go through a voluntary recognition process by an appropriate non-governmental entity to demonstrate that they have the capabilities to provide patient centered services consistent with the medical home model.
  - Patients and families participate in quality improvement activities at the practice level.
- **Enhanced access** to care is available through systems such as open scheduling, expanded hours and new options for communication between patients, their personal physician, and practice staff.
- **Payment** appropriately recognizes the added value provided to patients who have a patient centered medical home. The payment structure should be based on the following framework:
  - It should reflect the value of physician and non–physician staff patient-centered care management work that falls outside of the face-to-face visit.
  - It should pay for services associated with coordination of care both within a given practice and between consultants, ancillary providers and community resources.
  - It should support adoption and use of health information technology for quality improvement.
  - It should support provision of enhanced communication access such as secure e-mail and telephone consultation.
  - It should recognize the value of physician work associated with remote monitoring of clinical data using technology.
  - It should allow for separate fee-for-service payments for face-to-face visits. (Payments for care management services that fall outside of the face-to-face visit, as described earlier, should not result in a reduction in the payments for face-to-face visits.)
  - It should recognize case mix differences in the patient population being treated within the practice.

- It should allow physicians to share in savings from reduced hospitalizations associated with physician-guided care management in the office setting.
- It should allow for additional payments for achieving measurable and continuous quality improvements.

STANDARDS

The National Committee for Quality Assurance (NCQA) produced a set of standards by which a practice can be recognized as having Patient Centered Medical status. Based upon a point system, a practice may be rated as having achieved Recognition Level 1, 2, or 3 (see Table 14-1). There are nine PPC® standards comprised of 30 elements. Ten of the elements are "must pass" and can result in one of three levels of recognition. Practices seeking PPC®-PCMH™ status complete a Web-based data collection tool and

Table 14-1: NCQA PPC-PCMH Content and Scoring[6]

Standard / Element	Points
PMCH 1: Enhance Access and Continuity	
A. Access During Office Hours*	4
B. After-Hours Access	4
C. Electronic Access	2
D. Continuity	2
E. Medical Home Responsibilities	2
F. Culturally and Linguistically Appropriate Services (CLAS)	2
G. Practice Team	4
PCMH 2: Identify and Manage Patient Populations	
A. Patient Information	3
B. Clinical Data	4
C. Comprehensive Health Assessment	4
D. Use Data for Population Management*	5
PCMH 3: Plan and Manage Care	
A. Implement Evidence-Based Guidelines	4
B. Identify High-Risk Patients*	3
C. Care Management	4
D. Manage Medications	3
E. Use Electronic Prescribing	3
PCMH 4: Provide Self-Care Support and Community Resources	
A. Support Self-Care Processes*	6
B. Provide Referrals to Community Resources	3
PCMH 5: Track and Coordinate Care	
A. Test Tracking and Follow-Up	6
B. Referral Tracking and Follow-Up*	6
C. Coordinate With Facilities/Care Transitions	6
PMCH 6: Measure and Improve Performance	
A. Measure Performance	4
B. Measure Patient/Family Experience	4
C. Implement Continuous Quality Improvement*	4
D. Demonstrate Continuous Quality Improvement	3
E. Report Performance	3
F. Report Data Externally	2

Note:

- 27 elements with a total of 100 possible points
- Recognition Level point requirements
  - Level 1: 35–59 points
  - Level 2: 60–84 points
  - Level 3: 85– 100 points
- * = must pass elements

provide documentation that validates responses. Level one only requires passage of 5 of the 10 elements.

As you can see, the nine "Standards" reflect the Joint Principles of PCMH.

Standard One: Access and Communication

Practices need to provide each patient with a physician who will take responsibility for his or her care. As practices attempt to fulfill this seemingly simple measure, they also need to put into place policies that will ensure that this will occur. As a physician in solo practice for over 15 years prior to making the application, I took this as a given. That notwithstanding, it was valuable to create the policies to ensure that patients had adequate access for communication, as well as office visits. Practices with more than one physician or healthcare provider need to leverage the ease of access to the patient's medical history and prior visits. This is the best way to provide continuity of care in urgent situations.

Standard Two: Patient Tracking and Registry Functions

Most practices using Practice Management and Billing software can fulfill the must-pass elements of this standard. This standard addresses the need in a Patient Centered Medical Home to address the needs of all the patients and not just the ones seen during acute illnesses. If a practice is only using a practice management system, then it can generate an ICD-9 report of diagnoses. This list can then be compared to the local health department list of the conditions with a high prevalence in one's community.

Standard Three: Care Management

The United States does not compare favorably with many other nations in the management of many chronic diseases. Studies of care within the United States show large disparities along geographic, as well as socioeconomic lines (see Figure 14-2).[7]

One way to reduce regional disparities is to increase use of evidence-based guidelines. NCQA requires documentation of evidence-based guidelines for three conditions. Most EHRs will provide evidence-based guidelines, which can be linked to diagnoses, procedures, diagnostic tests, or medications chosen during an encounter. If an EHR is not being used, consider many of the e-books and online references that are available and run on PDAs, smartphones, and computers. Use of an EHR is an opportunity to re-train one's staff from paper chart–based activities to those that will provide greater benefit to the practice. These include performing outreach to patients based upon registry reports. Sample registry reports include patients who have not had mammograms, colonoscopies, and labs based upon evidence-based criteria. Most EHRs have predefined reports which can be run with little training. Many EHRs now have relatively simple registry report tools for "custom" reports, which can be saved and used in the future. Medical assistants, who would have potentially suffered unemployment as the office became more automated, can now provide more meaningful service as they run pre-configured reports and follow outreach protocols.

Standard Four: Patient Self-Management Support

I believe that this section may be the linchpin for really changing the level of "health" in the United States. In an affluent society such as ours, the major causes of premature

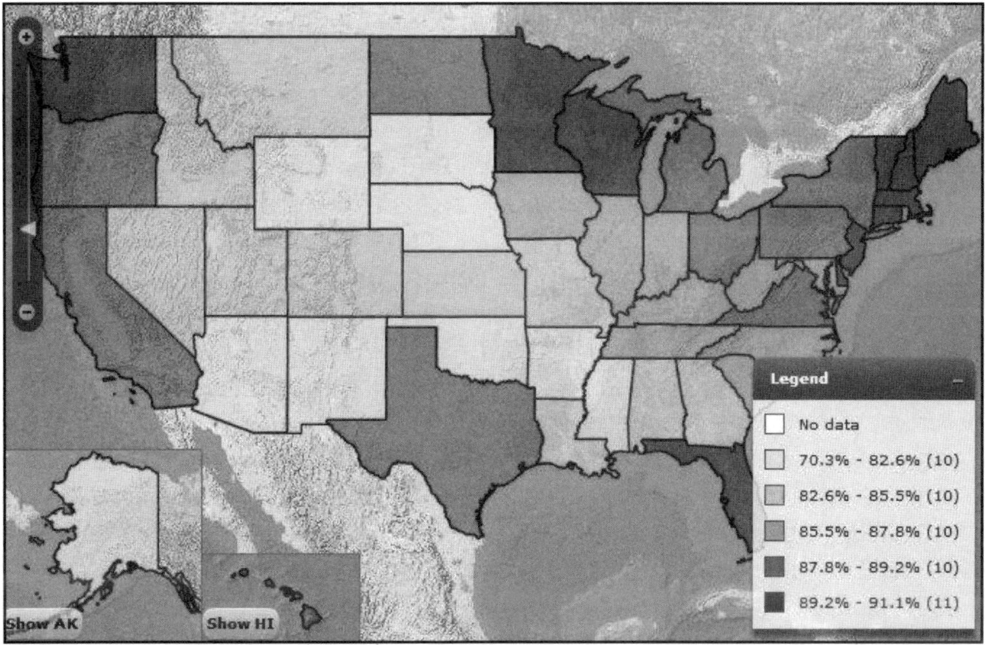

Figure 14-2: Percent of Diabetic Medicare Enrollees Receiving Appropriate Management, By Race and Type Of Screening (Race: Overall, Type Of Screening: Hemoglobin A1c Test - 2005–2006)[7]

death—type II diabetes, coronary artery disease, hypertension, smoking and obesity—are preventable. Patients and their families need to be given the information and the opportunity to improve their health.

The first step is to provide patients access to their medical records. Our practice began giving out copies of the complete office visit as soon as we implemented the EHR. Each patient becomes a proofreader of my notes. If any errors are identified, they are quickly addressed. Family members at home are encouraged to review the notes as well. These family reviewers become members of my healthcare team. In a solo practice like ours, it is a major benefit to have others identify gaps in the patient's medical history and to encourage the patient to follow through with our recommendations. Our patient portal permits the patient and designated significant others to access most of their medical record, short of the chief complaint and physical exam. We thus have family members living hundreds and even thousands of miles away, assisting with our mission.

My work as a reviewer of medical malpractice cases has made me acutely aware of the need to change the current provider/patient, provider/family, and provider/provider communication process. Most patients and their families will forgive an honest mistake in judgment if it is believed that the patient's best interests were in mind. An open/transparent record will assist in fostering this belief.

In the summer of 2010, the OpenNotes project was launched. This project involves more than 100 primary care physicians in Massachussetts, Pennyslvania, and Washington. When implemented, patients will be invited to review their records through a secure portal. As previously stated, some good ideas are formulated before their time.[8]

Ted Eytan, MD, has been a powerful spokesperson for an open record through his writings and presentations.[9]

The second step is to provide patients with access to vetted medical information. Our website includes links to the CDC,[10] Medline,[11] and other sites that provide information at the appropriate reading level, as well as in a multitude of languages.

The third step is to provide patient access to communication. This could be as simple as giving them a few extra moments to collect their thoughts to giving them access to a secure e-mail system via the patient portal and EHR.

Standard Five: Electronic Prescribing

This is not a must-pass in the current version of the criteria, but it is required at least 30 percent of the time in the current iteration of the CMS requirements for Meaningful Use of the EHR and will certainly be required by NCQA by the time this book comes to print. Electronic prescribing is probably one of the easiest means to bring Clinical Decision Support into the practice. The ability of even "free" eRX systems to check drug-age, drug-allergy, drug-drug, drug-sex interactions makes this option very valuable. The ability to do formulary checking to ensure patients get the best treatment at the best price encourages medication compliance. Until E-prescribing becomes more ubiquitous, the "magic" will not be lost on most patients. How many of you have been asked to leave an exam room to speak to a patient that was just notified of the high cost of a medication just prescribed? We have avoided such calls by addressing the issue at the point of care, often in under one minute, as we discuss the reasons for the medication chosen. You should not underestimate the marketing value of helping patients avoid waiting in lines twice: once to drop off the prescription and second to pick up the medication. E-prescribing pediatricians know how appreciative a mom with one or more sick children can be.

Standard Six: Test Tracking

One of the features that should be enabled is a bi-directional lab interface. This will permit you to submit your lab orders directly from the EHR and to receive the results directly into the EHR as structured data. Confirm that the EHR will store all lab results locally as LOINC (Logical Observation Identification Names and Codes) values. This will help ensure that results from different labs can be consolidated and queried together. Otherwise, the office would have to run separate queries for each lab company, i.e., Bio-reference, LabCorp, Quest, etc. The abnormal lab results will automatically be flagged, and normal values will be provided for reference.

One of my favorite uses of this feature is to provide patients with a table showing how their lab values have changed over time. We "imbed" this table in the progress note. This avoids the question, "Hey doc, I know my cholesterol is 168 now, but what was it six months ago?"

Structured LOINC results will also facilitate the exchange of these results with your peers and avoid the need to transcribe the results.

Standard Seven: Referral Tracking

While it is possible to track referrals for consultations, diagnostic tests, and procedures by paper, the EHR makes this somewhat daunting task more manageable. Staff that normally would have been responsible for pulling and filing paper charts can be used to contact patients about pending items and help coordinate care.

Standard Eight: Performance Reporting and Improvement

As practices prepare to meet the Meaningful Use measures, it will be important to quickly and easily assess the gaps in achieving a high level of fulfillment of various quality measures. Solo practices can benefit just as well as group practices. A simple survey of one's practice can identify easily rectifiable barriers to care, such as telephone waits on hold, time spent in the waiting room, time spent in the exam awaiting the healthcare provider and the ease of making an appointment.

These measure reports can then be transmitted to entities to coordinate enhanced reimbursement such as Bridges to Excellence[12] or to local health departments.

Standard Nine: Advanced Electronic Communications

While this standard does not currently contain any must-pass elements, I strongly recommend it for consideration. A patient portal with or without a static website will assist the practice in many ways.

As shown in Figure 14-3, the website from our own practice provides several benefits for patients.

1. A listing of the office hours
2. A listing of the services available via the patient portal: appointment requests, referral requests, medication refill requests, demographic updates
3. A list of vetted Web-based reference sites, such as the CDC and Medline
4. A list of public assistance sites
5. A list of self-help sites

Do not assume that only the Xbox/Playstation/Wii generation will be accessing your patient portal. One of my favorite experiences is of a husband and wife in their 80s. While he is hard-of-hearing, she has significant problems with her visual acuity. During office hours, I was sent his request for a follow-up specialist referral for his wife. According to the time stamps in the record, we were able to address his request in under 30 minutes without any interruption in my workflow and without the phones ringing. I was so moved by his adoption of the technology, that I sent him a thank you via the secure messaging system.

After four decades of public discourse and study, the PCMH is an idea whose time has come. The recent release of the final Meaningful Use criteria and the growing number of PCMH pilot projects[14] will accelerate PCMH adoption by providing the start-up financing needed to begin this next evolution in healthcare delivery.

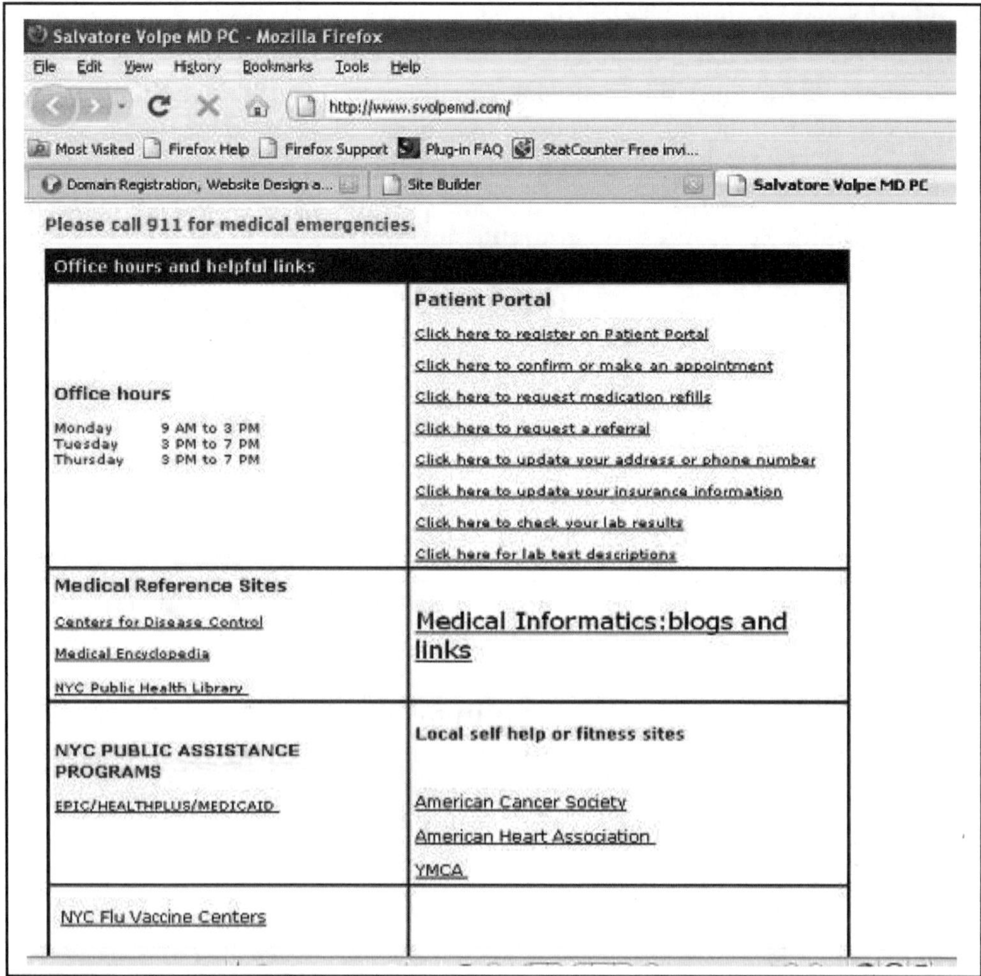

Figure 14-3: Patient Portal[13]

REFERENCES

1. McPherson M, Arango P, Fox H et al. A new definition of children with special health care needs. *Pediatrics.* 1998;102:137-40.
2. American Academy of Pediatrics, Council on Pediatric Practice. Pediatric Records and a medical home. In: *Standards of Child Care.* Evanston, IL: American Academy of Pediatrics; 1967:77–9.
3. American Academy of Pediatrics, Council on Pediatric Practice. Fragmentation of Health Care Services for Children. *News and Comment.* Supplement, April 1977.
4. *Pediatrics.* 2004;113(5):1473-78.
5. Wagner EH. Chronic disease management: What will it take to improve care for chronic illness? *Effective Clinical Practice.* 1998;1(1):2-4.
6. Available at: http://www.ncqa.org/LinkClick.aspx?fileticket=vDHh2t5aLSE%3d&tabid=631&mid=2435&forcedownload=true. Last accessed November 2010.
7. *Dartmouth Atlas of Health Care.* Available at: http://www.dartmouthatlas.org. Last accessed August 2010.

8. Shenkin BN, Warner DC. Sounding board. Giving the patient his medical record: a proposal to improve the system. *N Engl J Med.* 1973;289:688-92. [PMID: 4727972].

9. www.tedeytan.com/2010/07/25/5864. Last accessed November 2010.

10. www.cdc.gov/. Last accessed November 2010.

11. www.nlm.nih.gov/medlineplus/. Last accessed November 2010.

12. www.bridgestoexcellence.org/. Last accessed November 2010.

13. www. salvolpemd.com. Last accessed November 2010.

14. www.pcpcc.net/pcpcc-pilot-projects. Last accessed November 2010.

CHAPTER 15

Nursing Informatics: Perspectives for Healthcare Executives

Leanne M. Currie, RN, DNSc

INTRODUCTION

The purpose of this chapter is to provide healthcare executives with a view of technology in healthcare from a nursing informatics perspective. This chapter will first provide an overview of issues in nursing that are relevant to informatics, and then provide a description of the scope of nursing informatics practice and the skill set associated with different levels of informatics education.

Nursing informatics is defined as the intersection between nursing science, information science and computer science.[1,2] Staggers and Thompson (2002) provide a more descriptive definition, as follows:

> Nursing informatics is a specialty that integrates nursing science, computer science, and information science to manage and communicate data, information, and knowledge in nursing practice. Nursing informatics facilitates the integration of data, information, and knowledge to support patients, nurses, and other providers in their decision-making in all roles and settings. This support is accomplished through the use of information structures, information processes, and information technology.[3]

Healthcare executives are aware that nurses represent the largest professional group in most healthcare organizations. Indeed, there are more than three times as many nurses as physicians in the United States (2.9 million nurses[4] versus almost 800,000 physicians[5]). Nurses have been involved in system development within organizations since the first use of computers in healthcare in the 1960s.[6] However, the degree to which nurses participate in clinical information system development remains minimal. In a Web-based survey by the HIMSS Nursing Informatics Task Force, just over a third (36 percent) of respondents indicated that they have actively participated in selection or implementation of information systems at their hospital or healthcare network. Twenty-seven percent indicated that they had participated at a moderate level, but 37 percent reported that they have never participated in CIS implementation or development.[7]

The goal of involving nurses in system development is to ensure that technologies are relevant for nurses and other clinicians; however, the type of training required to be an effective contributor in computer system development has evolved. Nursing informatics leaders are excited about the opportunity for well-designed technologies to support clinical decision making for patient safety, to deploy evidence-based guidelines, to capture "what nurses do" (tasks) and to capture "how nurses think" (clinical judgment).[8] From an administrative perspective, having clinical information system data that captures nursing activities and decisions provides a strong foundation for quality improvement. In addition, from a research perspective, these data can provide a foundation for practice-based evidence, in which outcomes related to nursing activities and decisions can be examined.[8]

CURRENT ISSUES IN NURSING THAT IMPACT TECHNOLOGY ADOPTION

A very recent Institute of Medicine (IOM) report (2011) entitled *The Future of Nursing: Leading Change, Advancing Health,* highlights the complexity of healthcare work environments in which care is shifting from acute to community, the population is shifting from young to old, and organizations are shifting from a focus on individuals to a focus on systems thinking. The report accentuates the need for basic nursing competencies to include informatics (i.e., development and use of technology) and information literacy (i.e., how to access and use evidence),[9] and it further describes the need to ensure that nurses remain "up to date" in these skills throughout their careers. Several efforts are in process to facilitate keeping nurses up to date with technology; however, some of the burden will lie on healthcare organizations. For example, training in the workplace may evolve from a one-time orientation at hiring to annual training and certification, much like annual certification for infection control and fire safety.

Several efforts in the past 10 years have changed the landscape of the healthcare practice.[10-12] The IOM report *To Err is Human: Building a Safer Health System* (1999) stated that clinician practitioner order entry (CPOE) systems had the potential to drastically reduce medical errors, particularly medication errors.[11] In response to the report, integration of electronic health records (EHRs) and CPOE into hospitals and ambulatory settings has become widespread. HIMSS has developed a scale to measure level of integration of information systems, HIMSS Analytics EMR Adoption Model[SM] (EMRAM).[13] As of August 2010, EMRAM reports that 50 percent of U.S. hospitals have reached Stage 3, a level that indicates that the hospital has implemented nursing documentation including vital signs and flow sheets on at least one hospital unit. This is an increase from 35.7 percent of participating U.S. hospitals at Stage 3 in 2008. Although it is promising that the proportion of hospitals reporting use of electronic nursing documentation has increased between 2008 and 2010, electronic documentation in one hospital unit does not provide sufficient information to truly assess the level and impact of EHR integration.

A group of publications that highlighted the negative impact of information systems on patient outcomes sparked a debate in 2005 about the impact of information technology.[14-16] These reports identified several situations in which patient outcomes were negatively impacted by information systems, such as an increase in medication errors facilitated by the poor design of a CPOE system and an increase in pediatric inpatient mortality after the implementation of a CPOE system.[16,17] Proponents of well-designed information systems point out that the systems described in these reports were older systems in place in organizations that did not have robust informatics infrastructure.[18] They also noted that situations such as described often derive from poor implementation practices, including those that neglect human factors considerations.[19] For example, Reynolds, Peres and Tatham (2005) reported that rather than using a preformatted pick list, medication orders were entered using free text within a nursing communication function.[20] This type of behavior is considered a *workaround* (i.e., an alternate strategy to "get the job done"). The problem with workarounds is that they are not supported by the clinical information system and, as such, workarounds can facilitate medical errors. The effect of the medication ordering workaround described by Reynolds et al. was to bypass the clinical information system's drug-drug interaction screening, increasing the risk for medication errors.

To Err is Human also recommended the use of bar coding and electronic medication administration (eMAR) systems to reduce medication errors,[21] and, as such, these systems have increased in use. Poon et al. (2010) recently reported of a 41 percent decrease in certain medication errors on units that had bar coding compared to those without bar coding.[22] This is a promising result, and may have been related to thoughtful implementation of the bar coding system with a systematic roll out plan that was adjusted depending on complexity of medications to be delivered (e.g., oncology units were delayed until the workflow was accurately understood). However, several studies have observed problems with bar coding systems. Koppel and colleagues (2010) identified 15 types of workarounds used during bar code medication administration including nurses affixing patient labels to a piece of paper, when the label should be read from the patient's wrist.[23] Again, this type of workaround is a creative use of existing equipment which helps a nurse be more efficient, but it bypasses any potential decision support that a computer system might provide, and thus creates opportunities for errors.

An important report for and about nurses, *Keeping Patients Safe: Transforming the Work Environment of Nurses* (2004), asserts that well-designed systems can facilitate the work of the nurse and that developers must be mindful about the impact of such technologies on the work of the clinician. As with other high-risk industries such as the airline industry, information systems in healthcare that increase distractions (e.g., via interruptions) can negatively impact quality.[12] Despite these recommendations, recent literature suggests that nursing workflow is frequently not considered when systems are developed and/or implemented.[24-26] For example, Pirnejad et al. found that several usability issues were evident in a newly deployed CPOE system, including font too small to read and no method for a physician to verify that a medication had been given by the nurse.[24] Fortunately, a growing number of tools and standards are available to facilitate organizational best practices and to standardize informatics competencies.

The TIGER Initiative

An important initiative led by the nursing informatics community during the past decade is the Technology Informatics Guiding Education Reform (TIGER) initiative. The TIGER initiative was established during the *TIGER Summit*, held in 2006.[27] During this summit, nine collaborative teams were formed to address the following issues from a nursing informatics perspective: (1) Standards and Interoperability, (2) National Health Information Technology (IT) Agenda, (3) Informatics Competencies, (4) Education and Faculty Development, (5) Staff Development, (6) Usability and Clinical Application Design, (7) Virtual Demonstration Center, (8) Leadership Development, and (9) Consumer Empowerment and Personal Health Records.[27] The following provides a brief description of some relevant areas.

Informatics competencies and staff development. Three main competencies identified by TIGER include (i) basic computer competencies, (ii) information management (including use of an electronic health record), and (iii) information literacy. In 2008, the American Association of Colleges of Nursing (AACN) published the *Essentials of Baccalaureate Education* which includes essentials for all three competencies identified by TIGER.[28] Since the AACN publication, schools of nursing are increasingly including basic computer competencies in their curricula; however, for nurses not trained in these areas, the onus often falls on the employer. For those staff requiring basic informatics competencies, TIGER recommends that these can be attained by receiving training that follow criteria set up by the International Computer Driving Licence (ICDL) Foundation.[29] ICDL competencies range from basic, such as understanding how to turn on a computer and use a mouse, to advanced activities, such as performing calculations using a spreadsheet. Organizations who want to ensure staff computer competency may consider creating a method by which all staff attain their ICDL. *Information management* competencies are now part of the expectations for accreditation of baccalaureate programs; therefore, more recent graduates will have basic training. Again, however, nurses trained before these standards were in place may require on-the-job training, and nurses who are new to an organization will require orientation to the in-house system. *Information literacy* competency involves being skilled in searching for literature that may be relevant to nurses' work. The AACN criteria clearly address the expectation for baccalaureate courses to teach information literacy. Courses in evidence-based practice often teach this skill, and most nursing programs will include this in their curricula; however, for nurses who may have graduated before evidence-based practice was in the curriculum, information literacy competencies may be absent. Many organizations are providing in-house evidence-based practice efforts as part of their nursing research activities.[30] However, several barriers to effective use of library databases exist including budgetary and organizational influences such as the organizations' perception that nurses are not interested in using online information resources.[31]

Standards and interoperability. The TIGER group has worked to identify strategies to include nurses in the development of standards and interoperability. One of the main factors that has helped consolidate the voice of nursing informatics in the United States is the Alliance for Nursing Informatics (ANI) which was formed in 2005 and now boasts membership of more than 5,000 nurse informaticists.[32] Standards and interoperability efforts include identifying national policy activities that have relevance to nursing and nursing informatics, and producing joint position statements on health policy and informatics policy issues.[33]

Leadership development. The TIGER recommendations for leadership development focus on providing nurse executives with an understanding of the strengths of well-designed information systems and of having well-trained informaticists on the nursing team. The goals identified include working to bring informatics competencies to all nursing leaders, such that nurse leaders can use technology to empower nursing. Westra and Delaney (2008) conducted a Delphi study with nurse executives, nursing faculty, and nurse informaticists. They identified 92 competencies in three areas including (1) basic computer skills; (2) informatics knowledge, including management concepts, data issues, information systems concepts, staff education, and ethical and legal concepts; and (3) informatics skills, including requirements and system selection, financial, implementation and management, ethical and legal, and analysis and evaluation.

Healthcare administration masters degrees are increasingly including informatics in their curricula; however, those executives who obtain a traditional MBA may not have healthcare informatics knowledge and skills described above. A recommendation by a group of nurse executives suggested these steps: attend training, read an informatics journal, take a course, join a user group (most clinical information system vendors have user groups), join an organization such as HIMSS or ANI, and attend a conference.[34] Some suggestions for executive basic training include intensives such as a three-day pre-conference at the Summer Institute in Nursing Informatics (SINI) at University of Maryland (http://nursing.umaryland.edu/sini/index.htm), a week-long Biomedical Informatics summer course at Woods Hole, Cape Cod (http://courses.mbl.edu/mi/application.html), the American Medical Informatics online 10x10 programs (https://www.amia.org/e-learning), or an introduction to biomedical/nursing informatics course at a college/university, many of which are Web-based. Most importantly, the goal of this education would not be to fully train the executive in the field of informatics. Understanding the field will help the executive to learn gain essential knowledge and skills such that the informatics team could be effectively guided.

SCOPE AND ROLE OF THE NURSE INFORMATICIST

The role of the nurse informaticist is wide ranging and can include educator, project manager, consultant, analyst, researcher, manager, director and senior executive. In 1994, the American Nurses Association (ANA) first outlined the standards and scope of practice of the *Informatics Specialist*. Updated in 2008, the standards and scope recognizes the informatics specialist as a person with at least a master's degree in nursing or clinical informatics. Because development, implementation and management of information systems is a very complex process, there are a wide variety of titles and job descriptions given to nurse informaticists.[35,36] In general, the functional areas of informatics nursing include the following: administration, analysis, compliance and integrity management, consultation, coordination, facilitation and integration, system development, educational and professional development, policy development and advocacy, research and evaluation, and telehealth.[37]

Increasingly, organizations are seeing the need for nurse informaticists in leadership roles. Titles such as information systems clinical project leader, clinical informatics manager, director of nursing informatics, director of quality informatics, and chief nursing information officer demonstrate the level of leadership. The increase in the number of organizations defining leadership roles derives not only from organizational need, but also from a recent increase in the availability of formally trained nurse informaticists, particularly those with doctoral education. Senior nursing informatics executives will oversee wide-ranging development efforts, with a team of nurse analysts reporting to them.[35] Nursing informatics expertise at this level has the potential to promote communication with other executive leadership to ensure that an organization's objectives are realistic and that the information system is in alignment with both nurse workflow and the organization's objectives. In general, the role of the nurse informaticist will largely depend on the type of educational preparation and related work experience for the individual; however, deep knowledge of and exposure to the environment in which the system will be implemented is beneficial to those in all of the roles, and formal training can provide a solid foundation for individuals in these roles.

Skill Set of Trained Nursing Informaticists

Information systems need to support the clinical judgment and workflow of all levels of end users including patients, clinicians, administrators or researchers. The vision for information systems is for end-users to capture health related data as a byproduct of care, to verify/validate these data as needed, and to have these data available for reuse by real-time decision support systems, by administrators for quality tracking, and by researchers.[10] The data capture process should be designed to support both the patient and the knowledge worker, i.e., persons such as healthcare workers who must collect and use information to work effectively. In addition, the ideal information system must be stable, secure and perceived to be useful to patient, clinical, administrative and research stakeholders.

Toward the goal of stable, secure systems with reusable data for managing knowledge related to nursing and patient care, several key components of typical nursing informatics training include (1) information management and knowledge generation; (2) information technology, including theories, structure, development, functionality, implementation and human factors assessment; and (3) nursing practice, including models and theories of nursing and professional nursing practice (in nursing programs only), and organizational, financial and project management. For those trained on the job, skill in these areas may have been gleaned from work experience or in-house training. The importance of these components and the way in which they are relevant to nursing and organizational leadership are described in the following section.

Information Management and Knowledge Generation. Effective information management relies on the integrity and reusability of data. For data to have integrity (i.e., accurate, consistent, and well organized) and to be reusable, standardized terminologies have been developed. These terminologies are necessary to accurately reflect "what nurses do." Many healthcare executives are aware of standardized terminologies such as the International Classification of Diseases (ICD), Current Procedures and Treatments (CPT) and more recently SNOMED CT. ICD and CPT codes have been effective for billing purposes, but have limited use when used to characterize clinical practice. ICD and CPT do not capture any nursing activities, since nursing tasks and related decisions are part of a general bill rather than individual events. Toward the goal of ensuring that computerized systems accurately reflect nursing practice, several nursing terminologies have been developed. Unfortunately, these terminologies are not consistently used in clinical information systems, homegrown or vendor.

The first terminology system to be formalized in nursing was the North American Nursing Diagnosis Associations (NANDA) taxonomy, put forward by Gebbie and Lavin in 1973.[38] This taxonomy characterizes patient problems via a *nursing diagnosis*, and includes such elements as lack of education for patient or for family. Other standardized nursing terminologies that have since been developed are the Nursing Minimum Data set (NMDS), the clinical care classification system (CCC—formerly HHCC), Nursing Interventions Classifications (NIC) and Nursing Outcomes Classifications (NOC) to name a few.[39] In 2003, the international nursing informatics community approved a nursing reference terminology, which uses standardized computer representation (object-oriented) to characterize several aspects of nursing care.[40] This is important because not only was this the first healthcare terminology to attain International Standards Organization (ISO) level of standard, but it also can provide the international community with a framework to represent nursing knowledge in clinical information systems. Standards such as this are particularly important for interoperability and health information exchange (HIE)—i.e., the ability for information systems to *talk* to each other. Interoperability and HIE are critical for nursing care to be communicated to all providers across a patients' care continuum.

One of the most robust standardized terminologies used in healthcare is the Systematized Nomenclature of Medicine (SNOMED), which was developed by combining the College of American Pathologist's terminology SNOMED with the UK generated Read Codes. In 2009, SNOMED CT became SNOMED standards development organization (SDO)® during the creation of the international health terminology standards development organization (IHTSDO). All nursing terminologies have been integrated into SNOMED CT. The efforts to standardize terminologies are consistent with the Institute of Medicine (IOM) reports which advocate for standardization to improve patient safety.[41]

Information Technology. The formally trained nurse informaticist understands all aspects of information technology including development and implementation, hardware, software, security, standards and protocols, and telecommunication. One of the primary roles of the nurse informaticist is as a system analyst—a role in which the nurse is able to translate clinician needs to information technology developers and vice versa. Nurse informaticists in such roles will have skills useful at all phases of the system development life cycle (SDLC). The SDLC includes system planning phase, system analysis, system design, system implementation and testing, and system evaluation, maintenance, and support. An individual in the role of chief nurse informaticist would oversee a team that is applying the SDLC process. System planning concepts include strategic goals and priorities; vendor, product, and market analysis; resource considerations and cost-benefit analysis; and establishment of teams. The role of the nurse informaticists during this process includes administrative functions such as leading or participating in product evaluation and team formation for system implementation.

System analysis includes methods for needs assessment, feasibility assessment, process analysis (e.g., using process diagrams, decision trees, flow charts), functional specifications, request for proposal (RFP) development and system selection and contract issues. The role of the nurse informaticist for systems analysis might include formal needs assessment and requirements specification or might take on a more business perspective in RFP evaluation. System design includes understanding critical success factors within the scope of the SDLC. The role of the nurse informaticist during the system design phase may include database design, user interface design, and system quality assurance and auditing. This is different than typical hospital auditing because it refers to the quality of data from the system and is reliant on factors such as ensuring that the data are backed up, that the data can be re-used, and that the data are secure.

System implementation and testing includes functions associated with initiating a new electronic system or with managing changes within an existing system. The role of the nurse informaticist toward system implementation includes user testing, policy documentation and training. System evaluation, maintenance, and support include practices toward ensuring adequate user acceptance and perceived usefulness. The role of the nurse informaticist toward system evaluation, maintenance and support includes operational aspects that can support upgrades and enhancements; these include development of new alerts and reminders and other functions that ensure the system adequately and accurately represents the interaction between the clinician and the patients being cared for. Project management skills are critical for well-managed system implementations, and formal training in project management can facilitate a successful system implementation.

Although not typically trained in computer software programming, professional nurse informaticists understand all aspects of information technology design and implementation. Knowledge of database structure and information exchange ensures that the nurse informaticist can communicate with clinicians as well as with developers. Indeed, it is the communication role of the nurse informaticist that often provides the greatest value to an organization.

Nursing Practice. Several key factors related to nursing practice impact nursing informatics. First, in most countries, trained nurses are the most populous healthcare providers. Because of this, the role of the nurse can be widely varied. Secondly, in the acute, long-term and home care settings, nurses provide the greatest proportion of direct care to patients, which results in nurses being intermediaries between healthcare disciplines, often placing the nurse in a patient advocacy role.

Integration of the evidence to support decision making at the point of care is a primary goal of organizations that implement clinical information systems. Proponents of evidence-based practice assert that the only feasible means by which clinicians can manage the dearth of information that they are responsible to know is to have the practice recommendations fully integrated into the clinical information system.[42] Toward full integration of evidence-based practice, nurse informaticists can work with nursing practice leaders to ensure that the appropriate evidence is delivered to the appropriate individual at the appropriate time. This might involve designing alerts or reminders for clinicians at the point of care or integrating national guidelines into the clinical information system.

A great deal of work has gone into defining the decision-making process of clinicians, and recent work has focused on how decision-making processes affect patient safety.[43] As mentioned above, human factors play an important part in patient safety and the trained nurse informaticist will be able to support best practice for system design toward patient safety.

Factors related to organizational behavior, organizational change, management science and systems theory are fundamental to nursing informatics training. Nurse informaticists are aware of healthcare industry trends and regulatory requirements and, thus, can be integral in ensuring that the information technology supports such requirements.

NURSING INFORMATICS EDUCATION AND CERTIFICATION

Currently, formal training for nursing informatics involves obtaining a master's degree in nursing informatics or a post-master's certificate in nursing or healthcare informatics. This is consistent with the ANA definition of the informatics specialist which requires a master's degree. Most universities and many colleges with graduate level nursing programs offer master's level informatics programs, some of which can be completed online. As mentioned above, the role of the master's degree prepared informatics specialist can vary widely and is often contingent on organizational needs. Although some individuals without master's education are employed in health IT departments, the role of the nurse informaticist, particularly in leadership roles, will benefit from formal master's education.

A growing number of universities offer doctoral education in nursing informatics including the PhD (research doctorate) and the DNP (practice doctorate). The nurse informaticist with a research doctorate possesses applied research design, analysis and, in many cases, management skills. Nurse informaticists with doctoral education are often situated in leadership roles at healthcare organizations, leadership roles in vendor organizations or in academia. Depending on the individual's specific area of research, the nurse informaticist with a research doctorate might contribute to several of many organizational objectives. As mentioned earlier, an increasing number of organizations realize the potential of the doctorally prepared nurse informaticist in ensuring that nursing issues are addressed in relation to information technology.

Master's prepared nurse informaticists and baccalaureate prepared nurses with experience or post-baccalaureate certificates are eligible to sit for certification as an Informatics Nurse. This certification if offered by the American Nurses Credentialing Center (ANCC), the certifying arm of the ANA. The ANCC certification tests for the following elements: (1) Understanding human factors; (2) Understanding system development lifecycle; (3) Understanding critical elements of information technology; (4) Management of information and knowledge generation; (5) Professional practice, trends, and issues; and (6) Models and theories of nursing, nursing management and informatics.[44]

Many master's training programs in nursing informatics expect graduating informatics specialists to pursue the ANCC certification. A second certification available to nurse informaticists is the Certified Professional in Healthcare Information and Management Systems (CPHIMS) certification exam, offered by HIMSS.

The components of the ANCC certification are similar to the elements found in the CPHIMS certification exam; however, they differ in three main areas. First, the ANCC certification has more explicit expectations of human factors management (including ergonomics) and user interface design. Second, the ANCC certification tests for knowledge related to informatics theory, but the CPHIMS does not. And third, the HIMSS professional certification tests for management and leadership skills, but the ANCC certification does not. However, as mentioned previously, the master's degree prepared nurse informaticist will often have business administration skills, such as financial and nursing management, organizational behavior and formal leadership training.

All of these differences will be of interest to the executive because when assessing the skills of a prospective candidate, the ANCC certification does not imply management skills; however, the nurse informaticist is typically formally trained to function as a human factors expert and will be an expert in regard to nursing activities. It is important to note that neither of these certifications tests for computer programming skills; rather they test for the system analyst role, a role in which the analyst interprets end user activities and identifies an appropriate function and appearance required for an information system. In this role, the analyst would need to understand the workflow of the clinician and would also need to know the underlying process of the computerized system.

CONCLUSION

In conclusion, nursing informatics is a robust and growing field with well-defined training programs that offer significant potential for growth in organizations. Healthcare executives who are interested in ensuring the success of clinical information system development, implementation and refinement should harness the potential of nurse informaticists to ensure that the appropriate information structures, information processes and information technology are in place to support clinical decision making in all settings.

REFERENCES

1. Graves JR, Corcoran S. The Study of Nursing Informatics. *Journal of Nursing Scholarship.* 1989; 21(4):227-231.

2. Saba VK, McCormick KA. *Essentials of nursing informatics.* 4th ed. New York: McGraw-Hill Medical Pub. Division; 2006.

3. Staggers N, Thompson CB. The Evolution of Definitions for Nursing Informatics: A Critical Analysis and Revised Definition. *Journal of the American Medical Informatics Association.* May 1, 2002 2002;9(3):255-261.

4. Health Services Research Administration. *The Registered Nurse Population: Findings from the 2004 National Sample Survey of Registered Nurses* 2007.

5. Staiger DO, Auerbach DI, Buerhaus PI. Comparison of Physician Workforce Estimates and Supply Projections. *Journal of the American Medical Association.* October 21, 2009 2009;302(15):1674-1680.

6. Murphy J. Nursing Informatics: The Intersection of Nursing, Computer, and Information Sciences. *Nursing Economic$.* 2010;28(3):204-207.

7. Dykes P, Cashen M, Foster M et al. Surveying acute care providers in the U.S. to explore the impact of HIT on the role of nurses and interdisciplinary communication in acute care settings. *Journal of Healthcare Information Management.* 2006;20(2):36-44.

8. Lang NM. The promise of simultaneous transformation of practice and research with the use of clinical information systems. *Nursing Outlook.* 2008/10// 2008;56(5):232-236.

9. Institute of Medicine. *The Future of Nursing: Leading Change, Advancing Health.* Washington, DC, 2011.

10. Committee on Data Standards for Patient Safety. *Patient Safety: Achieving a new standard for care.* Washington: Institute of Medicine; 2004.

11. Committee on Quality of Health Care in America. *To Err is Human: Building a Safer Health System.* Washington, DC: Institute of Medicine; 2000.

12. Committee on the Work Environment for Nurses and Patient Safety. *Keeping Patients Safe: Transforming the Work Environment of Nurses.* Washington, DC: Institute of Medicine of the National Academies; 2004.

13. Davis M. *The State of U.S. Hospitals Relative to Achieving Meaningful Use Measurements:* HIMSS; 2010.

14. Koppel R, Metlay JP, Cohen A, et al. Role of computerized physician order entry systems in facilitating medication errors. *Journal of the American Medical Association.* Mar 9 2005;293(10):1197-1203.

15. Garg AX, Adhikari NK, McDonald H et al. Effects of computerized clinical decision support systems on practitioner performance and patient outcomes: a systematic review. *Journal of the American Medical Association.* Mar 9 2005;293(10):1223-1238.

16. Han YY, Carcillo JA, Venkataraman ST, et al. Unexpected Increased Mortality After Implementation of a Commercially Sold Computerized Physician Order Entry System. *Pediatrics.* December 1, 2005 2005;116(6):1506-1512.

17. Reynolds K, Peres A, Tatham JM. The impact on patient safety of free-text entry of nursing orders into an electronic medical record in an integrated delivery system. Paper presented at: AMIA Annual Symposium Proceedings 2005; Washington, DC.

18. Shortliffe EH. CPOE and the facilitation of medication errors. *Journal of Biomedical Informatics.* Aug 2005;38(4):257-258.

19. Bates DW. Computerized physician order entry and medication errors: finding a balance. *Journal of Biomedical Informatics.* Aug 2005;38(4):259-261.

20. Reynolds K, Peres A, Tatham J. The impact on patient safety of free-text entry af nursing orders into an electronic medical record in an integrated delivery system. Paper presented at: AMIA Annual Symposium Proceedings 2005; Bethesda, MD.

21. Gebhart F. VA facility slashes drug errors via bar-coding. *Drug Topics.* 1999;143(3):1.

22. Poon EG, Keohane CA, Yoon CS, et al. Effect of bar-code technology on the safety of medication administration. *N Engl J Med* 2010;362:1698-1707. Available at http://www.nejm.org/doi/full/10.1056/NEJMsa0907115. Accessed January 20, 2011.

23. Koppel R, Wetterneck T, Telles JL, Karsh B-T. Workarounds to barcode medication administration systems: their occurrences, causes, and threats to patient safety. *Journal of the American Medical Informatics Association.* 2008;15(4):408-423.

24. Pirnejad H, Niazkhani Z, van der Sijs H, Berg M, Bal R. Evaluation of the impact of a CPOE system on nurse-physician communication—a mixed method study. *Methods of Information in Medicine.* 2009;48(4):350-360.

25. Karsh B-T. *Clinical Practice Improvement and Redesign: How Change in Workflow Can Be Supported by Clinical Decision Support.* Rockville, Maryland: Agency for Healthcare Research and Quality, U.S. Department of Health & Human Services; 2009.

26. Karsh B-T, Weinger MB, Abbott PA, Wears RL. Health information technology: fallacies and sober realities. *Journal of the American Medical Informatics Association.* November 1, 2010 2010;17(6):617-623.

27. The TIGER Initiative. Technology Informatics Guiding Educational Reform. 2010; http://www.tigersummit.com/9_Collaboratives.html. Accessed August 30, 2010.

28. American Association of Colleges of Nursing. *The Essentials of Baccalaureate Education for Professional Nursing Practice.* Washington, DC2008.

29. European Computer Driving Licence Foundation. European Computer Driving Licence. 2010; http://www.ecdl.org/icdl/index.jsp. Accessed September 30, 2010.

30. Hart P, Eaton L, Buckner M, et al. Effectiveness of a Computer-Based Educational Program on Nurses' Knowledge, Attitude, and Skill Level Related to Evidence-Based Practice. *Worldviews on Evidence-Based Nursing.* 2008;5(2):75-84.

31. Ross J. Information Literacy for Evidence-Based Practice in Perianesthesia Nurses: Readiness for Evidence-Based Practice. *Journal of PeriAnesthesia Nursing.* 2010;25(2):64-70.

32. Greenwood K. The Alliance for Nursing Informatics: a history. *Computers, Informatics, and Nursing.* 2010;28(2):2.

33. Alliance for Nursing Informatics. Statements and Positions. 2010; http://www.allianceni.org/statements.asp.

34. Mays CH, Kelley W, Sanford K. Keeping up: the nurse executive's present and future role in information technology. *Nursing Administration Quarterly.* 2008;32(3):4.

35. Weaver CA, Delaney C, Weber P, Carr R, eds. *Nursing and Informatics for the 21st Century: An international look at practice, trends and the future.* Chicago: HIMSS; 2006.

36. Nursing Informatics Working Group. Roles in Nursing Informatics. 2004; http://www.amia.org/mbrcenter/wg/ni/roles.asp. Accessed July 21, 2006.

37. American Nurses Association. *ANA's Nursing Informatics Practice Scope and Standards of Practice.* Washington, DC: American Nurses Association; 2008.

38. Gebbie K, Lavin MA. Classifying nursing diagnoses. *American Journal of Nursing.* 1974;74(2):250-253.

39. Saba VK, McCormick KA. Essentials of nursing informatics. 4th ed. ed. New York: McGraw-Hill; 2006.

40. International Standards Organization Tc. ISO 18104:2003: *Health informatics—Integration of a reference terminology model for nursing.* 2003-12-08 2003.

41. Committee on Data Standards for Patient Safety. *Patient Safety: Achieving a New Standard for Care:* Institute of Medicine; 2003.

42. Haynes RB. Of studies, summaries, synopses, and systems: the "4S" evolution of services for finding current best evidence. *Evididence Based Nursing.* January 1, 2005 2005;8(1):4-6.

43. Patel VL, Currie LM. Clinical cognition and biomedical informatics: issues of patient safety. *International Journal of Medical Informatics.* Dec 2005;74(11-12):869-885.

44. Maag MM. Nursing students' attitudes toward technology: a national study. *Nurse Educator.* May-Jun 2006;31(3):112-118.

CHAPTER 16

Case Study: Primary Care Information Project—The Evolution to an Extension Center

Amanda Parsons, MD, MBA

PCIP BACKGROUND

Although New York City has more physicians per capita than the national average and strong investments in health IT through local and state efforts, the health system remains highly fragmented. Patients seek care in an uncoordinated, pay-per-episode environment in which primary care providers are expected to coordinate care across private practices of all sizes, community health centers and hospitals, all at different levels of health IT use. New York City faces a major primary care crisis if the burden of care cannot be better coordinated. New York City providers serve a diverse range of patients, both culturally and economically in a concentrated geographical environment. As the entry point into the healthcare system, primary care providers serve some of the wealthiest and poorest neighborhoods within one to two city blocks of each other. Despite the dramatic 60 percent increase in enrollment in New York State Medicaid programs since 2002, roughly 1.3 million people, 19 percent of the population of New York City, remain uninsured.

In 2005, the New York City Department of Health and Mental Hygiene (DOHMH) created the Primary Care Information Project (PCIP)[1] to improve public health through widespread use of health IT, with a focus on populations with the greatest health disparities. The idea, as delineated in their joint Health Affairs article,[2] and the aim of PCIP was to bring about change on three fronts: first, to design and deploy prevention-oriented medical records; second, to improve practice workflows and orient them toward population health; third, to encourage a "pay-for-prevention" based reimbursement model (see Figure 16-1).

For the first year, PCIP set about procuring a commercially available electronic health record (EHR) that would have "baked in" public health functionality such as actionable Clinical Decision Support, automated quality measurement, point-of-care alerts and

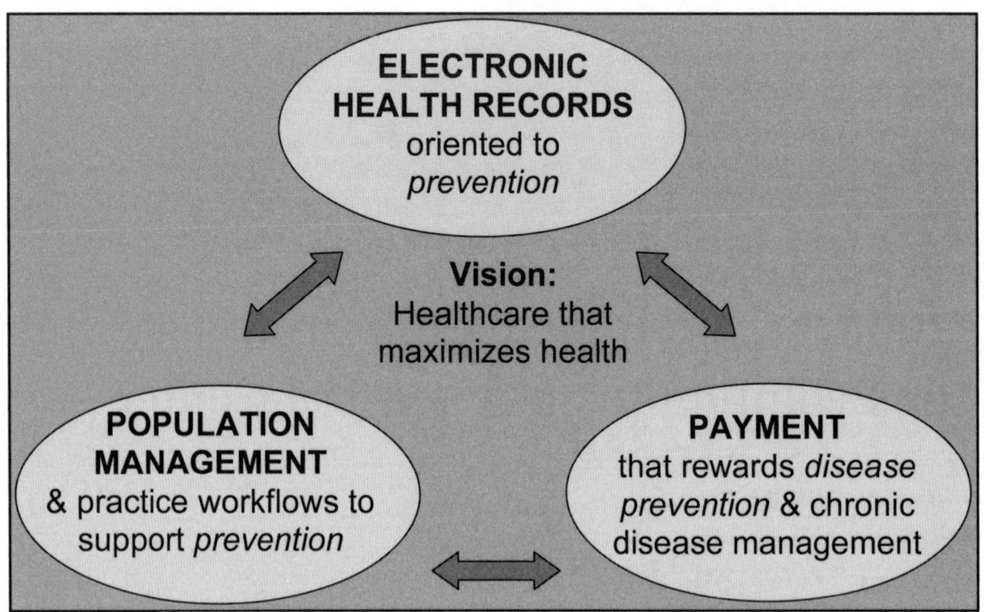

Figure 16-1: PCIP Vision

reminders, and an integrated registry function. When PCIP found that no ambulatory EHR in the market had this functionality, PCIP selected an EHR vendor that would be willing to partner with PCIP to co-develop these features. Through a series of rapid cycle development efforts, eClinicalWorks (eCW) and PCIP successfully embedded the public health features in a software build made just for New York City called the "Take Care New York" build. However, when eClinicalWorks realized the market demand and public good of these features, it mainstreamed the "Take Care New York" build into the mass retail 8.0 build, which became available to its customers nationwide.

In a little over two years from the start of the implementation process, PCIP brought more than 2,100 high-volume Medicaid primary care providers, 18 percent of the total estimated 11,887 primary-care providers (defined as MD, DO, NP, PA with prescribing privileges) practicing in New York City, live on the eClinicalWorks (see Table 16-1). Our analysis relies on the University of Albany Center for Healthcare Workforce Studies reporting of the New York State Physician Licensure Re-registration Survey adjusted for 2006–2007, supplemented by data on Nurse Practitioners and Physicians Assistants from the Medical Society of the State of New York.

Table 16-1: Breakdown of Providers Live Through PCIP Efforts

	Practices	Sites	Providers
Hospitals	5	43	810
CHCs	37	95	764
Small practices	433	457	963
Correctional Health Facility	1	1	70
Total	476	596	2,607

The city's initial investment in PCIP was intended to reach roughly 20 percent of the priority providers, with the hope that creating an early group of EHR users would help demonstrate the benefits and kick-start adoption in the city. Though city funding was not intended to meet all provider needs, PCIP was successful in identifying in-kind or matching resources, like state and private foundation grants, to supplement the services needed to help providers meaningfully use the EHR.

New York City has an overall high density of physicians, but the disproportionate concentration of providers in higher-income neighborhoods leaves many areas, including 782 census tracts (35 percent of the 2,217 tracts that constitute New York City) designated as Medically Underserved Areas by the Health Resources and Services Administration (HRSA). The NYC Health and Hospitals Corporation (HHC) and the Federally Qualified Health Centers (FQHCs), along with many small practices, target their services toward this population. Even with more than 2,100 providers live, the leadership at PCIP knew that further adoption efforts were needed to get the market past a tipping point and ensure that forces were aligned for ubiquitous EHR use. However, at the end of the New York City fiscal year 2009 (June 30, 2009), and in the midst of an economic downturn, funding for ongoing EHR implementation by PCIP from the city of New York ended. For several months, PCIP's implementation activities were funded through an array of grants and physician contributions, which was not a sustainable proposition. Therefore, when the Office of the National Coordinator of Health Information Technology (ONC) created the Regional Extension Center (REC) program, PCIP saw an opportunity to reinstate funding in support of its implementation efforts to eradicate paper charts from the primary care setting.

BECOMING A REGIONAL EXTENSION CENTER

The low levels of EHR adoption in the United States, particularly among small practices, points to significant barriers and disincentives such as high costs, a perception among providers of the biased information coming from EHR vendors, and significant practice disruption in implementing EHRs. PCIP became an expert on how to go live on an EHR by analyzing and categorically developing programs to overcome these barriers.

For providers from high-need communities who could afford the financial cost to switch from paper to EHR, PCIP offered free software through a city subsidy worth approximately $20,000 per provider. To overcome informational barriers to choosing a high-quality vendor from the hundreds on the market, PCIP ran a competitive procurement process to carefully select a vendor willing to develop a product customized for high-quality care and prevention. However, the core value that PCIP developed is a complement of technical assistance services that helps providers through every stage of planning, implementation, and quality improvement, meeting and overcoming practical and psychological barriers in provider practices at each stage. PCIP made the argument that the New York City organizations were best poised to design and deliver services by taking the lessons learned from PCIP, particularly those from small practices, and apply them to scale to over 4,500 providers.

Over the last three years, PCIP learned how to work with providers to get them to use the EHR to its full potential and described to ONC the Extension Center's need to:

1. Distill information and present it in a clear and concise way, highlighting the impact to the provider, particularly as it pertains to patient safety and enhanced reimbursement.
2. Visit the practice to observe their workflows, processes, staff capabilities, and capacity and incorporate that "practice context" into a customized solution.
3. Tailor messages to suit the specific needs of practices, recognizing that each practice will make different decisions about what they want customized, what work they want their staff members to do, what care management processes they want to improve.
4. Work across teams (e.g., EHR consulting, implementation, Quality Improvement) to share information on practices and troubleshoot their problems.
5. Connect providers to each other via phone or social networking sites to share best practices.
6. Monitor EHR vendors to help them deliver the best possible service to providers.

PCIP's long-term vision was to catalyze a fundamental reorientation of the NYC healthcare system toward prevention and health outcomes through the Meaningful Use of EHRs and EHR-derived data by physicians and health plans. It set forth a goal for NYC RECs to help 2,400 primary care providers adopt an EHR and more than 4,500 to achieve Meaningful Use in the first two years. PCIP proposed bringing providers to Meaningful Use in a way that advances the closely-tracked goals of Take Care New York,[3] the city's public health targets for 2012:

1. Ensure the majority of priority primary care providers in NYC achieve Meaningful Use of an EHR by 2012, specifically:
    a. Identify electronic medical record solutions that were best suited to the needs of primary care providers and make them available at discounted prices.
    b. Support the implementation of prevention-focused certified EHRs.
    c. Provide technical assistance to providers to support workflow redesign, privacy and security compliance, and quality improvement.
    d. Work with third-party vendors (lab companies, E-prescribing vendors) to ensure practices can electronically order medications and lab tests.
    e. Give providers visibility into their quality measures and health outcomes to drive improvements.
2. Reduce premature cardiovascular deaths by 20 percent through:
    a. The citywide implementation of Clinical Decision Support for blood pressure control.
    b. Clinical registries and training practices to enact models of care in which patients with hypertension receive timely outreach.
    c. The development and use of personal health records that allow patients to share self-measured blood pressure readings with clinicians.
    d. Multi-payer pay-for-performance driven by EHR-derived hypertension care quality measures.

3. Reduce preventable hospitalizations by 12 percent through:
   a. Care coordination through supporting practices to receive and act upon discharge summaries from hospitals and referral tracking with specialty care.
4. Reduce smoking by 29 percent through:
   a. Citywide implementation of Clinical Decision Support for smoking cessation.
   b. Electronic referrals from EHRs to smoking cessation services.
   c. Multi-payer pay-for-performance for smoking cessation.
5. Continue the decline in premature deaths in NYC and the increase in life expectancy.
   a. Supporting health information exchange and coordination of care across multiple care delivery systems (inpatient, outpatient, home health, ERs etc.).
6. Work with Extension Centers across the nation to ensure that learnings are quickly captured and disseminated.

PRODUCT AND SERVICE OFFERINGS FOR THE NYC EXTENSION CENTER

The NYC Extension Center will provide the following product and service offerings:

Education and Training for All Providers in Service Area

PCIP has four years of experience in educating providers to use health IT effectively by holding formal training classes and seminars, conducting site visits to practices to build EHR skills, and distributing written communications with best practices and tips on using the software. PCIP has multiple teams that walk providers through every stage of EHR implementation—from the point at which providers are contemplating EHRs, to troubleshooting system bugs. PCIP experience shows that providers prefer to learn in their environment, at their practice, but are willing to travel for billing, coding, and revenue enhancement classes. The PCIP Outreach team, the first to interface with providers, regularly attends local events hosted by community organizations, IPAs, and other groups to inform primary care physicians about EHRs and public health and to recruit practices.

PCIP holds open houses to disseminate general information to providers on the process of implementing an EHR. A recent open house, attended by 85 providers, offered presentations on EHR Adoption, Implementation, Meaningful Use, Quality Improvement, Patient Centered Medical Home, and Privacy & Security. In addition to holding open houses, conferences, conducting on-site training and education, and running training classes and seminars, NYC REC makes general information about EHR adoption and Meaningful Use available to all NYC clinicians through a robust communication infrastructure consisting of bimonthly newsletters, topical e-mails, a regularly updated website and On the Record, an online social network created by PCIP for EHR users in New York City. NYC REC will incorporate content developed by PCIP and the HITRC into these communications and programs.

In addition, NYC REACH will partner with vendors to develop joint communications. We believe vendors and providers will benefit from these vendor-specific presentations, in addition to all the vendor-neutral communications developed earlier, particularly when these tailored communications are focused toward providers who are already live. We have found that vendors are reluctant to reach out to their existing customer base to invite them to multi-vendor events, fearing cannibalization of customers. In addition, we have learned that presentations and conferences at which multiple vendor choices are offered are not very helpful in encouraging providers to choose an EMR that is right for them. Our early learnings in this market revealed that partnering with a vendor to discuss what the Extension Center and the vendor can do working together—highlighting the benefits of that specific partnership—is the most effective strategy to help providers select a medical record and join the extension center.

National Learning Consortium (NLC)

Over the course of implementing EHRs and practice redesign with over 1,500 providers, PCIP developed a wealth of relevant "best practices" documents including analysis of recruitment strategies, request for information (RFI) and request for proposal (RFP) templates for EHR vendor selection, formal agreements and contracts for providers enlisting in EHR technical assistance support, EHR training manuals, handbooks on documenting quality measures, curricula for billing classes, billing setup for FQHCs, quality report templates and distribution plans, and articles and updates on city, state, and federal health policy changes that affect primary care providers.

PCIP staff regularly presents key lessons learned from its implementation experience at health IT and health policy meetings hosted by a range of institutions such as the Markle Foundation, the Commonwealth Fund, NCQA, Academy Health, and AHRQ. In addition, PCIP hosted the first eCW Users' Conference in March 2009, bringing together 525 local EHR users for training, troubleshooting and networking. In 2010 this same conference, hosted jointly by eCW and PCIP, brought over 800 providers together to learn about advanced features in the EMR, Meaningful Use, Patient Centered Medical Home, Privacy & Security, and a host of other practice workflow topics. NYC REC would expand the community built through these efforts to clinicians using all EHR products. By drawing on the lessons learned in this community, the HITRC can reflect the experience of thousands of physicians who have either successfully implemented an EHR or are now in the implementation phase. To support the NLC, NYC REC will continue to create, update, and organize these materials and make them available to the national network of Extension Centers.

In June 2010, the NYC REACH launch conference event, hosted with the American College of Physicians, drew more than 300 providers, most of them not on an EHR. The seven EMR vendors, as well as the nine IT consultant firms selected through open competitive RFI processes, were invited to exhibit their EMRs and consultant services, respectively. In addition, other valuable partners such as reference lab companies, clearinghouses, Regional Health Information Organizations (RHIOs), and EMR-compatible medical device companies were also invited to participate. Presentations from local (NYC Health Commissioner Thomas Farley, MD), state (Office of Health IT Director, Rachel Block, and Medicaid Medical Director James Figge, MD) and federal (ONC, Thomas Tsang) officials helped enforce the notion that EMR-related financial incentives were real and were being offered as part of a concerted strategy to improve care, helped to dispel the common misconception among providers.

Vendor Selection and Group Purchasing

During its original vendor selection process, PCIP reviewed submissions from more than a dozen companies and selected eClincialWorks (eCW) because it successfully met both the technological and organizational capability requirements at a competitive price. PCIP worked with eCW to secure bulk discounts on the software licenses, which DOHMH then purchased and provided to practices for no direct charge.[4]

One of the first steps NYC REC took was to issue an RFI, in conjunction with the NY eHealth Collaborative (NYeC), to make a statewide selection of EHR vendors. The RFI required vendor commitment to development, quality reporting, and training in addition to compliance with privacy laws and official certification. Vendors were required provide descriptions of how their product supports Meaningful Use requirements and how they help their customers use the record. The RFI required vendors to collaborate with NYC REC through training, reporting, evaluation, HIE and assistance with quality initiatives. Response criteria were set up to narrow the eligibility of potential applicants to just those vendors that offered comprehensive solutions (e.g., documentation, CPOE, E-prescribing, quality measurement, Clinical Decision Support), as many practice-management only or modular solutions had indicated interest in applying. Vendor responses were analyzed by multi-disciplinary teams at NYC REACH and NYeHealth collaborative, as well by independent providers. Ten vendors were selected to provide a demo of their software and discuss their services and capabilities. Preference was given to vendors who offered a software as a service (SaaS) and/or application service provider (ASP) solution, as well as those product visions that were consonant with public health and quality improvement functionality. NYC REACH was one of the first RECs to undergo its selection process amidst discussions in the health IT community about the unfortunate misaligning of timing between the REC announcements and ARRA vendor certification. NYC REACH was not able to consider only those records that had ARRA certification because this process was not set to occur until early fall 2010 at the earliest. Therefore, NYC REACH used the Meaningful Use criteria from the Notice of Proposed Rulemaking as a screening criteria for each vendor.

In the end, NYC REACH selected three preferred vendors (eClinicalWorks, Greenway and MDLand) and four Tier 2 "Meaningful Use" vendors (Athena, Medlink, Eclipsys' Peak Practice and Next Gen). Discounted pricing with city-wide favored nation clauses were negotiated for all three preferred vendors, with discounts ranging from 15 to 25 percent.

Whether or not a practice works with an approved vendor or takes advantage of group purchasing, it will still be eligible to receive technical assistance to help them achieve Meaningful Use. However, the level of customization of this technical support will vary based on which EMR a practice has adopted, with more customized assistance being offered to providers who have an EMR from the preferred or Tier 2 list. When providers approach the Extension Center looking to adopt an EMR, NYC REC staff will account for practice variables such as type of practice, range of budget, and specialist connectivity and provide a practice assessment, offering unbiased advice to the provider on which vendor to select. Practices need not accept the recommendation to join the Extension Center.

Implementation and Project Management

The internal structure of PCIP mirrors the stages of the best practice EHR implementation. Four teams work closely toward getting providers live: Outreach, Implementation, IT Infrastructure, and Systems Integration. The Outreach Team contacts providers from lists obtained from the American Medical Association, state Medicaid, health plans, other healthcare conveners, or referrals to the program through word of mouth or through the PCIP website. The Outreach Team then prepares practices by working with them to identify the costs of implementing an EHR, including necessary changes to IT infrastructure and staffing. The Outreach Team conducts budget analyses and helps develop the required agreements. In PCIP's prior experience, an average of 22 calls or meetings are needed with each practice before they agree to join the program. Without this initial guidance, many practices would abandon implementation when problems arise.

Before joining the program, each practice has an IT assessment with an IT Infrastructure Coordinator to discuss equipment placement and server hosting, upgrades to the practice's network, and the importance of hiring a qualified IT consultant or staff member. PCIP requires that every practice entering the program hire an IT professional, since practices often experience implementation delays and post-go-live technical issues when the physician or other non-IT-professional tries to perform IT support on an ad hoc basis. An IT consultant RFI process was done shortly after the launch of the Extension Center to identify a pool of qualified and trusted IT consultants. Discounted services were also negotiated to ensure that providers had affordable options.

The implementation process starts with a kick-off call to determine roles and responsibilities for the practice, vendor, and PCIP; establish the billing setup and data migration plan, review optional EHR features; discuss lab interfaces, registry reporting, E-prescribing, hardware, training and a go-live plan; and review external risks and success factors. Practices also receive a Welcome Pack that includes a step-by-step explanation of what is needed from them, when it is needed, and for what purpose. The key document that keeps all parties on track is the project plan, containing important milestones and crucial go-live dates.

PCIP has found that the implementation process for small practices typically takes 22–26 weeks, which is significantly higher than the expected 12–14 weeks advertised by the EMR vendor. We believe the difference is partially accounted for by the type of provider PCIP has historically focused on (high volume Medicaid providers), as well as the robust project management support we offer. Where vendors may allow practices to defer certain tasks until post go-live if they wish, PCIP tries hard to ensure that practices go live with all the features and functionality they'll need to be successful, including bi-directional reference laboratory interfaces and interfaces to the Citywide Immunization Registry. Although EHR vendors will assist practices in implementing their product, support and oversight by a third party is essential if the practice is to be successful in using EHRs to improve health outcomes. PCIP's Implementation Team has ensured that practices understand the long-term value of investments in training, hardware, and lab and public health interfaces essential for core quality measurement.

Between the kick-off call and going live, a PCIP Implementation Specialist acts as a point of escalation for both the vendor and the practice to help move along stalled implementation processes. On-site training prepares the office staff for clinical workflow changes geared toward improving Meaningful Use. PCIP ensures that a vendor trainer returns for more intensive clinical system training for providers and mid-office staff and that the provider receives 16 CME credits for participating. After these training sessions, the practice is ready to go live on the system.

During the first month of using the EHRs, practices work with trainers to refine their use of high-level preventive functionalities: Clinical Decision Support system (CDSS), patient registries, order sets, flow sheets, and templates. The PCIP experience suggests that CDSS training is particularly crucial toward this end, and the Extension Center will focus efforts there.

NYC REC will use and expand this proven model of education, preparation, and training, which has a 99 percent success rate. This project management method works especially well with "high-need" practices, and variations on this process will be developed to address the needs of even more providers using a variety of EHR software.

Practice and Workflow Redesign

The principal objective of PCIP has always been to improve the quality of care with health IT, not merely to digitize healthcare in its current form. Workflow redesign is critical to translating the new technology into gains in efficiency and patient health outcomes at the practice level. For PCIP, the redesign process begins during the implementation stage with a detailed documentation and evaluation of current workflows to prepare for their re-formation. The Implementation Team identified the following generic workflow categories: (1) telephone encounters, (2) patient check-in and checkout, (3) document management, (4) typical visits (internal medicine, well-visit, sick visit, pediatrics, etc.), (5) labs with and without interface, (6) internal and external referrals, (7) immunizations, (8) ancillary tests (EKGs, etc.), (9) PPD, (10) prescriptions (new and refill), (11) billing, (12) new employee IT orientation, and (13) help desk.

One especially critical part of workflow redesign is developing procedures for electronic reporting within the EHR. These efforts ensure that practices can efficiently generate rich flows of information for internal analysis, regulatory compliance, and quality measurement. The ability to quantify healthcare quality, crucial to improvement, is an important result of using the system. To pull accurate, reliable quality measures, practices must be taught how to correctly document their actions and work with PCIP on any problems that arise with the reporting technology.

Workflow redesign is a sustained, iterative process, and in the months after going live, the redesign continues through the Quality Improvement services provided by PCIP and FPHNY. The Quality Improvement (QI) Specialists conduct 5 to10 on-site visits, depending on the needs of the practice, to develop workflows that improve the patient interaction. During these visits, the specialists cover both the basics of the EHR to review initial training sessions (proper documentation, administration, billing, E-prescribing, lab ordering, and troubleshooting) and demonstrate how to improve performance and results. In particular, the specialists educate the practice staff in the application of QI techniques, such as the Plan-Do-Study-Act methodology, and review the practice's quality reports to identify areas of difficulty and guide the practice toward improving key quality measures.

NYC REC will devote considerable time and resources to help practices craft procedures, beginning at the earliest stages of implementation. The Extension Center will also offer these services to providers who already have an EHR in place but need help achieving Meaningful Use. This service will include up to three on-site visits, classes, and written training materials related to each of the federal criteria. In addition, the NCQA Patient Centered Medical Home has been an important model for the PCIP QI work, and NYC REACH will encourage and support eligible practices to work toward certification, leveraging a group arrangement with NCQA that allows all participating practices to qualify automatically for Level I PCMH certification. Our aim is to provide these services, leveraging the reimbursement rates from the ONC; however, higher levels of customized services may require additional fees.

The workflow redesign process will help practices use the EHR to meet the Meaningful Use criteria and then excel beyond the minimum requirements. For example, PCIP staff recommends ways for a practice to register patients for an online patient portal as part of the workflow, and then connects them with innovative programs such as PCIP's HealtheText project, funded by Verizon, which builds on the EHR infrastructure with text message reminders for appointments and prescriptions. DOHMH also co-submitted with Google Health for a grant from the Robert Wood Johnson Foundation to enable patients at a Bronx community health center to send home-measured blood pressure readings to their physician's EHR through a personal health record. The Extension Center will continue to look for opportunities like these to encourage providers to go beyond Meaningful Use as they modernize their practice.

Functional Interoperability and Health Information Exchange

At PCIP practices, secure health exchange is facilitated through technology within the EHR, and workflow redesign is focused on the use of E-prescribing, lab interfaces, and reporting to public health registries such as the immunization registry. In addition, PCIP worked with practices to set up panel management and referral tracking processes, a crucial part of care coordination. Currently, it is difficult for providers to access comprehensive information about a patient because it is often stored in the offices of multiple stakeholders like hospitals or specialist offices, a major barrier for practices trying to follow the medical home model. PCIP works with eCW and all New York City RHIOs to refine their systems, improving the ability of providers to access longitudinal patient summaries such as the federally-recognized Continuity of Care Document (CCD).

PCIP completed significant work on one HIE initiative, the New York State Medication Management Project, which allowed a limited number of providers to access the 90-day prescription history and Medicaid eligibility status from the NY State Medicaid program. This pilot identified potential barriers of this data stream, including the need for a patient consent workflow, missing identifiers required for physician access to the system, and potential performance and issues related to speed. These lessons learned are now being incorporated into a statewide initiative. This project will also incorporate data from SureScripts, which includes prescriptions that are ordered and filled electronically, and RX Hub, the data on fill history from the leading pharmacy benefits managers. This work will allow providers to see a nearly complete prescription fill history for their patients—a critical piece of information that can prevent dangerous drug interactions, allergic reactions and can support patient compliance. It is another example of how PCIP laid the foundation for innovative technology, which the NYC Extension Center will leverage to improve care and reduce costs.

At a regional level, PCIP set a goal to enable all primary care providers to better coordinate care between individual providers through the four NYC-based RHIOs. Much of the technical-specification work for these connections is complete, and the Extension Center will be ready to move forward on the project as the NYC RHIOs develop the required technology.

PCIP has provided HIE leadership within DOHMH, successfully proposing public health surveillance and reporting projects that take advantage of data from participating practices' EHRs. These data can then be used to monitor health trends for both communicable disease and chronic conditions to guide an appropriate public health response. While the city will continue to build the capacity for exchanging health information, if funded, NYC REC will have the staff to instruct the practices on how best to integrate public health surveillance and reporting into their workflows. This will improve the accuracy and comprehensiveness of the collected data.

As a result of these efforts, NYC REC will be able to help practices meet the HIE requirements of Meaningful Use such as accessing patient information from outside sources, sharing and acting on electronic prescription information, and transmitting immunization data, lab results, and syndromic surveillance data to registries and public health agencies.

Privacy and Security Best Practices

Most security breaches are caused by lack of knowledge, confusion, and carelessness, rather than technical malfunction. The Privacy and Security Curriculum developed by PCIP addresses these hazards along with regulatory and technical issues. The Privacy and Security Team visits each practice to discuss the risks pertinent to electronic data and mitigation strategies and configure privacy and security settings within the EHR. Practice leadership receives help to formalize their security plan as a written procedures document based on a universal template. This document includes standards for regular data back-up, control and auditing of staff access to PHI, and back-up and recovery. PCIP offers guidance on appropriate hardware storage and security, encryption, back-up policies, and auditing e-records. New guidelines will be continuously researched and produced to address new regulatory requirements such as the recent Red Flag Rules[5] and new HIPAA provisions under the Recovery Act.

PCIP developed multiple layers of security safeguards to protect practices from breaches and will implement such security measures across the NYC REC:

- **Physical security:** Privacy specialists work with office leadership to ensure that computer hardware holding PHI is physically stored in secure locations with limited access.
- **Access controls:** In compliance with HIPAA, practice staff should only be able to access the information necessary to do their jobs. Privacy specialists will show the leadership how to adjust these settings within the EHR.

- **Network security, encryption:** A PCIP specialist directs practices to adopt strict security IT measures, such as an encrypted wireless router, anti-virus software and firewall, to avoid data hacking and other breaches.
- **Back-up and recovery:** Privacy specialists work with practice leadership to create a back-up plan. The NYC Extension Center will follow the existing PCIP recommendation that each practice stores back-up tapes in a secure location off site, or works with the vendor for remote storage.
- **Audits:** Practices are strongly encouraged to perform audits twice per year to make sure patient data are not used incorrectly and to check staff access levels.

The Extension Center will adopt this method and increase the number of specialized staff (as described in the budget), allowing us to offer these services to more providers working with almost any EHR system.

Local Workforce Support

Achieving citywide Meaningful Use will require work from professionals at a full range of skill levels: EHR-savvy office staff, IT specialists, EHR project managers, and software developers. The NYC Extension Center will work closely with community colleges and vocational schools to develop curricula and programs around EHRs and health IT to train a workforce for this effort and provide them with internship and job opportunities. PCIP is actively collaborating on workforce development with NYC Small Business Services, Borough of Manhattan Community College (BMCC), and SUNY Downstate. The Extension Center will also leverage PCIP's longstanding relationship with Columbia University's Department of Bioinformatics and plan to work together on curriculum design for health IT workforce training.

NYC Small Business Services (SBS) helps providers identify and hire new staff members, and NYC REC will expand on this foundation by connecting with classes for medical assistants and crafting curriculum organized around PCIP's best practices. SBS recently opened a healthcare employment center at LaGuardia Community College in Long Island City dedicated to training and placing students in the healthcare industry. Recognizing that health IT is a major growth area within New York City, SBS will prepare students for future business needs. The Extension Center will support this new endeavor by connecting qualified job seekers with future employers. In addition, Extension Center internships will offer students hands-on training.

PCIP understands the workforce needs required to meet EHR implementation objectives at practices of all sizes, The Extension Center will use this experience to help design coursework that prepares students to meet the needs of future employers, who will look for graduates with new skills: EHR super users, billing specialists, business analysts, IT consultants, health IT security experts, and clinical and office administrators with EHR skills.

NYC REC will work with both the Borough of Manhattan Community College (which has programs for medical assistants, certified nursing assistants, and EHR specialists) and SUNY Downstate (which has internships for students in the nursing, medical, and public health programs). NYC REC will support these programs through curriculum guidance, internship opportunities for students, and adjunct appointments for qualified PCIP staff.

Finally, the NYC Extension Center will continue to pursue new projects that may define innovative roles in patient care. For example, the Panel Management project introduces the concept of a shared resource, called a Prevention Outreach Specialist (POS), who visits a group of practices and utilizes the EHR registry functions to proactively manage high-risk patients. This effort will be carefully coordinated with community colleges and job placement services so that these Prevention Outreach Specialist roles can be efficiently filled by qualified applicants.

Achieving Meaningful Use

PCIP and FPHNY staff members have experience working with practices to meet a seemingly distant and lofty goal. As a public health program of a municipal health department, PCIP crafted the EHR technical assistance model to measurably improve core health outcomes: hypertension, blood pressure and diabetes control and smoking cessation. The Implementation and Quality Improvement teams have worked carefully to make the providers aware of these goals, and the Development team works with eCW to establish integrated quality measures pegged to NYC clinical priorities within each EHR, as well as automated transmission of aggregated practice and provider-level quality measures to the DOHMH Quality Reporting System. This allows QI specialists to present Quality Scorecards to providers and discuss progress toward target levels of performance to make them aware not only of the missed opportunities to improve care and save lives, but also to understand how they can qualify for various local and federal incentive programs around E-prescribing, PCMH, and other.

NYC REC, in partnership with DOHMH, will apply this model of software development, education, and feedback to ensure that providers understand what they need to do to earn Meaningful Use rewards and how close they are to this achievement. PCIP worked with eCW to integrate not only quality reporting but also EHR utilization measures to ensure the use of key public health features. NYC REC will work with vendors to include structured data fields to support the measures necessary for Meaningful Use certification and to educate providers about the documentation methods that will accurately reflect care delivered in their practice. Then QI specialists will present practices with Meaningful Use Scorecards and discuss the necessary steps for timely achievement of certification.

Monitoring progress toward Meaningful Use across the city will also position the Extension Center to detect barriers to satisfying specific measures rooted in a systemic problem in the healthcare system. For example, PCIP learned in 2008 that many small practices struggled to establish electronic interfaces with clinical laboratories. Suspecting a systemic barrier out of the control of individual providers, PCIP determined that laboratories were reluctant to establish interfaces with such small practices because of regulatory burden and constraints created by the federal Clinical Laboratory Improvement Amendments. While establishing workarounds to build interfaces with lab companies and small practices, PCIP also took up the issue at the federal level, advocating for regulatory reforms, most recently before the HIT Policy Committee Information Exchange Workgroup meeting. NYC REC will work in concert with the HITRC to resolve this and other systemic barriers that impede progress to Meaningful Use.

Since the passage of the American Recovery and Reinvestment Act of 2009, PCIP has been a resource for providers seeking more information regarding new federal Meaningful Use incentives. PCIP has met with the Centers for Medicare & Medicaid Services (CMS) New York Regional Office and follows communications from ONC closely, continually updating providers as information has emerged through bulletins, Webinars, in-person sessions, an online EHR-use social networking site, Meaningful Use update e-mails, and presentations.

NYC REC will continue to provide informed advice within the clinical community, and when CMS releases reporting requirements later this year, the Extension Center, in coordination with Regional CMS, will coordinate a communications campaign, deploying the previously described channels (one-on-one training, classes, newsletters, etc.) to instruct physicians on reporting standards and processes. As 2011 approaches, the Extension Center will incorporate technical support on the reporting process into on-site workflow redesign consulting.

CONTINUED PCIP OFFERINGS

PCIP was deliberately structured to focus on medically underserved populations, addressing the "digital divide" faced by physicians who treat these groups. Serving the profound linguistic and cultural diversity of New York City, PCIP has already worked with eCW to create educational materials in Spanish and will transfer that knowledge to other vendors. NYC REC will extend Spanish and other language development to PHRs to create patient-specific materials and improve patient engagement, with special attention paid to health literacy levels.

Reaching physicians who serve populations with specific needs, including low income, minority, non-English speaking, and the incarcerated, was a feature of PCIP's outreach strategy. The Extension Center will continue to provide free software licenses from the eCW NYC-subsidized contract to providers who serve medically underserved communities who otherwise would not be able to afford to adopt an EHR. This includes the NYC Correctional Health Services, a division of DOHMH that reaches the city's incarcerated population. Entities like this and high-volume Medicaid/Medicare providers will be eligible for this city-funded benefit.

The NYC Extension Center will continue initiatives by PCIP to establish coordination of care between primary care, behavioral health, and those providing long-term care. In coordination with the Extension Center, DOHMH will partner with the Visiting Nurse Service of New York (VNSNY), the largest home health care organization in the nation, serving over 31,000 New York City patients, to track and manage referrals from primary care providers to long-term care services. In addition, the Extension Center will partner with the DOHMH Division of Mental Hygiene and Lutheran Family Healthcare Centers to customize EHRs specific to behavioral health needs.

In order to access the Extension Center services, providers will be asked to pay a portion of the curriculum fees as a match was required from ONC for the grant. Curriculum fees are shown in Table 16-2 shown next.

The NYC Extension Center, working in close collaboration with PCIP and all their stakeholder partners, hopes to continue to serve as a national model of how public health, health IT, and a local project can develop, disseminate, and ingrain best prac-

Table 16-2: NYC REACH Pricing and Services (as of August 2010)

NYC REACH Meaningful Use Curriculum Fees	
If you are...	**Meaningful Use Curriculum Fees...**
A provider currently working with the Primary Care Information Project, and you signed your agreement less than two years ago	Free until the end of your two-year agreement with PCIP
A primary care provider (MD, DO, NP, or PA with prescriptive privileges) at a practice with fewer than 10 providers primarily focused on primary care	$600 per provider per year
Primary care providers (MD, DO, NP, or PA with prescriptive privileges) at a practice with 10 or more providers in one of the following settings: • Public Hospitals • Community Health Centers • Other settings that predominantly serve uninsured, underinsured, and medically underserved populations	$6,000 per practice per year $6,000 covers ALL physicians at a practice. Practices are defined by unique FEIN.
A specialist at a practice with fewer than 10 providers, primarily focused on primary care	$600 per provider per year
A specialist at a specialty practice *No federally subsidized services are available yet, but specialists can buy discounted services from us. We are actively looking for sources of funding to further defray the costs for specialists.* $600 Specialist Membership includes: • Access to EHR discounts • Recommended list of IT support vendors • Meaningful Use seminars and classes • Free NYC REACH events • Meaningful Use toolkits and self-assessments • NYC REACH updates and bulletins	$600 per provider Optional: (in addition to membership fee) Adoption Services (see below) $1,200 per provider *not waived* On-site Meaningful Use training $3,200 per provider
NYC REACH Adoption Services[6] **For providers using paper charts who need to purchase and install an EHR—** **available only with NYC REACH Preferred Vendors: eClinicalWorks, Greenway, MDLand** NYC REACH Adoption Service Fee is $1,200 per provider in addition to the curriculum fee. Adoption Services include • Vendor Accountability through formal agreement between NYC Health Department and Preferred EHR Vendor • Discounts on licenses for Preferred EHR Vendors • Full cost/benefit analysis for your practice • Free lab interface and integration with city immunization registry *required for Meaningful Use* • List of preferred IT support services • Personal assistance before, during, and after implementation • Option to participate in our "EHR Enabled Practices" list used by plans and patients e-mail: pcip@health.nyc.gov Phone: (212) 788-5711 Address: 161 William St., 5th Floor, New York, NY 10038	

tices in ambulatory care. Novel healthcare delivery models being considered by healthcare reform will need a way to organize and disseminate best practices, and extension centers will be well poised to do this. In addition, opportunities for extension centers to build up additional value include being able to aggregate performance information and render this information back to providers in a meaningful and actionable manner.

As PCIP as already demonstrated, such capabilities could easily form the basis of novel pay-for-performance programs that combine EMR-derived quality data with other data streams to ensure that providers are in fact being measured and rewarded based on quality of care and not just on utilization or cost data.

Regional extension centers harness the local resources and capabilities necessary to catalyze healthcare delivery system reform among the majority of the nation's ambulatory providers.

To contact the local regional extension center near you, visit the ONC website on HITECH programs.[7]

ACKNOWLEDGEMENTS

I would like to thank Thomas Cannell and Rachel Helfont who wrote significant elements of this chapter, as well as the entire staff at PCIP without whom there would not be such rich experiences to document.

REFERENCES

1. Available online at: http://www.nyc.gov/html/doh/html/pcip/pcip.shtml. Last accessed November 2010.
2. Frieden TR, Mostashari F. Health care as if health mattered. *JAMA*. 2008;299(8):950-952 Available online at: http://jama.ama-assn.org/cgi/content/full/299/8/950 Last accessed August 2010.
3. Take Care New York 2012. Available online at: http://www.nyc.gov/html/doh/downloads/pdf/tcny/tcny-2012.pdf. Last accessed November 2010.
4. The DOHMH has approximately $2 million worth of eCW license bundles (lifetime eCW software license, 10 days of eCW training, 2 years of support & maintenance) which will be allocated to the NYC REC as an in-kind contribution and distributed to practices based on need.
5. Steven Toporoff. Federal Trade Commission. The "Red Flags" Rule: What Health Care Providers Need to Know About Complying with New Requirements for Fighting Identity Theft. Available online at: http://www.ftc.gov/bcp/edu/pubs/articles/art11.shtm. Last accessed August 2010.
6. Available online at: http://www.nycreach.org/. Last accessed November 2010.
7. Available online at: http://healthit.hhs.gov/portal/server.pt?open=512&objID=1495&parentname=CommunityPage&parentid=58&mode=2&in_hi_userid=11113&cached=true. Last accessed November 2010.

CHAPTER 17

Case Study: A Small Primary Care Practice's Experience in Assessing Quality with Data Obtained from an Electronic Health Record

Deborah Johnson-Ingram; Yvette A. Ortiz, MD; Kim Benjamin Woods, MD; and Alan L. Silver, MD, MPH

Disclaimer: This material was prepared, in part, by IPRO, the Medicare Quality Improvement Organization for New York State, under contract with the Centers for Medicare & Medicaid Services (CMS), an agency of the U.S. Department of Health and Human Services. The contents do not necessarily reflect CMS policy. 9SOW-NY-THM6.3-10-05.

INTRODUCTION

The electronic health record (EHR) brings the promise of being able to collect and analyze clinical quality-of-care data. The availability of practice level statistics for various medical home/pay-for-performance efforts and electronic transfer of clinical data elements to regionally based health information exchanges (HIEs) will depend upon information obtained from EHRs. Initiatives such as CMS' EHR Incentive Program and the National Committee on Quality Assurance (NCQA) Physician Practice Connections®-Patient Centered Medical Home™ (PPC®-PCMH™) will provide form and substance to EHR-based quality data tracking. Unfortunately, current EHR products often do not produce readily usable reports.

Uptown Medical Group (UMG), a small primary care practice, is an EHR early adopter. Although the implementation was locally subsidized, UMG started using its EHR prior to any announced national or statewide programs that would provide payment to UMG for its health IT usage. Subsequent to going live, UMG became involved in several quality improvement projects.

UMG discovered that the initial quality-of-care results it obtained from its EHR based upon predefined quality metrics was variant from the staff's clinical and administrative perceptions. UMG ascertained problems in data definition, mapping, report generation, and clinician documentation that required extensive work to correct. In the near term, even small practices may require support staff to validate clinical quality data reports in order to qualify for additional reimbursement.

BACKGROUND: UPTOWN MEDICAL GROUP

UMG is an internal medicine, primary care practice located in the Morris section of the Bronx. Uptown has 1.5 full-time equivalent internal medicine physicians, Drs. Yvette Ortiz and Kim Woods, a full-time practice manager, a part-time nutrition/diabetes educator, a receptionist, a biller, and five medical assistants. The practice has an active primary care patient panel of approximately 1,800 patients. Nineteen percent of its patients are 65 years-old or older; 39 percent are male and 61 percent are female; 90 percent are Hispanic, and 10 percent are African American, Caribbean American, or other. UMG also offers multispecialty clinical access at its site for non-UMG clinicians in gastroenterology, ophthalmology, and podiatry.

UMG founder, Dr. Yvette Ortiz, always had a goal of providing high-quality, culturally competent healthcare to underserved individuals since completing her residency. In 1996, the chief executive officer (CEO) of a health plan that employed Ortiz at the time also had a vision of ensuring delivery of the best quality healthcare to its beneficiaries. Leveraging the use of technology, the CEO hired a team of people to create an EHR system. This innovative group, including Ortiz, attempted a homegrown EHR implementation. Dr. Ortiz was impressed with the potential ability to track all health maintenance issues, medication lists, allergies, and referrals. Although the project never reached fruition, Ortiz became convinced that an EHR would be an important tool in providing optimal primary care. As the years progressed, Ortiz continued to read and monitor different systems; she recognized that systems offered to small practices were either not developed enough or out of her price range.

Eleven years later, in 2007, Dr. Ortiz, now operating UMG, read a New York City Department of Health and Mental Hygiene (NYC DOHMH) bulletin in which the inception of the Primary Care Information Project (PCIP) was announced. PCIP was formed by the NYC DOHMH in 2005 to reduce healthcare disparities through a health IT adoption initiative that provides subsidized EHR licenses of eClinical Works (eCW) to physicians who serve the city's poor and uninsured population throughout the five boroughs (Brooklyn, Bronx, Manhattan, Queens, and Staten Island).[1] UMG was an ideal candidate because of its large Medicaid, underserved and uninsured population. UMG joined the PCIP Collaborative and began its implementation with the project's facilitators. It was among the first group of practices to receive eCWs licenses. UMG went live October 2007 with the eCW version 7.0 bundled package. The bundle included modules for an EHR, an integrated practice management and billing system, electronic prescription writing, lab interfacing, and medical device equipment interfacing.

BASIC SOFTWARE TRAINING VERSUS UNDERSTANDING EHR USE IN CLINICAL PRACTICE ANALYSIS

Due to its early adoption of the EHR via PCIP, UMG received two weeks of intensive general software education for all staff from both eCW and PCIP (including cross training on all aspects of EHR functionality) and an additional 2–4 weeks of post go-live shadowing from the EHR vendor, specific to individual staff work detail. With its planning, training, motivated staff, and external support, UMG felt confident they were knowledgeable about the capabilities of its application. The training was rightly focused on day-to-day clinical and office operations. There purposely was less emphasis on so-called population management and quality improvement metrics. Although this made sense in what needed to be learned first and foremost, it left the physicians and support staff without a sufficient understanding of how to use the system to measure, assess and optimally use the EHR data for quality of care. While the usage and application came equipped with a recall and registry module, the vendor did not provide a training curriculum that emphasized the value of the components. UMG did not adequately understand that the components of the EHR provide a centralized location to gather, filter, and review data. The practice was not aware of how to use the registry and recall module to perform tasks, such as sorting the data by groups of patients and then acting on clinical issues through automated processes for patient outreach. Additional training on these features would have offered a clearer directive for the clinicians and clinical support staff in the importance of documenting encounters in structured fields in order to accurately review data and support the use of adopted quality metrics.

THE QUALITY IMPROVEMENT INITIATIVES – QUANTIFYING QUALITY

UMG joined several quality improvement (QI) initiatives within months of adopting the EHR. Each program had its own specific clinical indicators that required tracking and report generation. All of the QI projects, however, were designed to promote improved patient care using valid and accepted metrics. UMG believed that in having an EHR, data could be collected and reported with very little effort from the practice. The EHR would serve as the reporting tool and mechanism for assisting in improvement. The system would facilitate more proactive practice-to-patient communication by having patient-specific cumulative data available during encounters and give UMG quantifiable information on patient-care outcomes.

The first of the three QI programs focuses on prevention. It is funded by CMS and is administered in New York by IPRO, the Medicare Quality Improvement Organization (QIO) for New York State. IPRO solicited UMG by offering *post-EHR* adoption support for three years.[2] As a participating practice, UMG would use its EHR to report patient de-identified breast cancer screening, colorectal cancer screening, and influenza and pneumococcal immunization data to IPRO and CMS. UMG agreed to provide the data quarterly for the measures listed in Table 17-1, and in return, IPRO would assist UMG by assessing its EHR capabilities and current care processes related to breast and colorectal cancer screening and immunizations. IPRO also offered guidance on improving reporting outcomes by sharing best practices.

Table 17-1: Medicare Prevention Quality Indicators

Influenza	# of adult patients appearing in the EHR who were age 65 or older as of day of the last measure period who had a flu vaccine during the most recent flu season; for example September 1, 2009 – March 31, 2010
Pneumococcal	# of adult patients appearing in the EHR who were age 65 or older as of day of the last measure period who had received at least one pneumococcal immunization during his/her lifetime
Colorectal Cancer Screening	# of adult patients appearing in the EHR who were age 51–80 or older as of day of the last measure period who had either a fecal blood test in the previous 1 year or flexible sigmoidoscopy in the previous 5 years or double contrast barium enema in the previous 5 years or colonoscopy in the previous 10 years from the last day of the measure period
Mammography Screening	# of female patients appearing in the EHR who were between the ages of 52 and 69 as of the last day of the measure period and had at least one screening mammogram in the previous 2 years

The next QI project is administered by NYC DOHMH–PCIP and funded by the Robin Hood Foundation. The Healthy Hearts (eHearts) initiative is a pilot pay-for-quality incentive project. It recognizes and rewards EHR-enabled practices for achieving high clinical performance based upon accepted metrics in cardiovascular disease.[3] Unlike some other pay-for-performance programs, eHearts enabled UMG's EHR system to directly transmit prevention-oriented quality measure reports to a remote data repository. The participating practices were provided with software that automated the retrieval of population level data needed to assess performance of the clinical measures. UMG would be paid a financial reward based upon a proportion of eligible UMG patients that fulfill the quality metrics[3] (see Table 17-2). The indicators are a set of quality measures in cardiovascular health (the "ABCS").

The measures related to the eHearts program criteria are[4]:

A – Antithrombotic therapy for patients with ischemic vascular disease (IVD) or diabetes (DM)

B – Blood pressure controlled to recommended levels in patients with hypertension

C – Cholesterol controlled to recommended levels in patients with hypercholesterolemia

S – Smoking cessation treatment or counseling for current smoker

The third program, also a pay-for-performance initiative, was funded by a local insurance company. This 18-month pilot program randomly assigned the participating practices into two groups. Group 1, the supported group, received a practice facilitator and a nurse care manager. Group 2 was a control group that received no clinical practice support but did receive access to a redesign toolkit developed by the insurer. With the goal of improved patient outcomes, Group 1 was to use the facilitator to assist and assess participating practices' capabilities in achieving NCQA PPC®-PCMH™-recognition with the adoption of EHRs and to ascertain changes in clinical performance and operational efficiency. In addition, the practices were provided with an on-site nurse care manager who performed chronic care support activities.

Table 17-2: eHearts Core Measures[4]

Measure Name	Measure Numerator	Measure Denominator
A – Antithrombotic therapy for patients with IVD or DM	# of patients who have documentation of use of aspirin or another antithrombotic	# of unique patients seen in the reporting period 18 years and older with a diagnosis of ischemic vascular disease (IVD) or age 40 years and older with a diagnosis of Diabetes Mellitus (DM)
B – Blood Pressure control in HTN w/o DM	# of patients in denominator having both a systolic blood pressure below 140 mmHg and a diastolic blood pressure below pressure below 90	# of unique patients 18–75 years of age, with IVD AND HTN without DM who were seen for a visit in the reporting period
B – Blood Pressure control in HTN (140/90)	# of patients in denominator having both a systolic blood pressure below 140 mmHg and a diastolic blood pressure below 90 mmHg, on their last blood pressure measurement within or prior to the reporting period	# of unique patients, at least 18 years of age with a diagnosis of HTN established six months or more prior to the last day of the reporting period, AND no diagnosis of IVD or diabetes, and who were seen for a visit in the reporting period
B – Blood Pressure control in IVD w/o DM	# of patients in denominator having a recorded blood pressure measurement in the past 12 months up to and including the last day of the reporting period, having both a systolic blood pressure below 140 mmHg and diastolic below 90 mmHg	# of unique patients 18–75 years of age with IVD without a diagnosis of DM
C – Cholesterol Control	# of unique patients denominator whose most recent recorded LDL level is < 100 mg/dL	# of unique patients seen in the reporting period 18–75 years of age, with a diagnosis of (IVD or DM) AND (a diagnosis of lipoid disorder] and [an LDL cholesterol level measured in the past 12 months up to and including the last day of the reporting period)
S – Smoking Cessation	# of patients in the denominator who received cessation counseling (e.g., advise to quit, referral for counseling) and/or pharmacologic therapy in reporting period	# of unique patients 18 years of age or older, seen for a visit in the reporting period, whose smoking status was current smoker at the beginning of the reporting period

UMG was randomly assigned to the control Group 2. For this program UMG agreed to perform two NCQA PPC®-PCMH™ surveys (an initial baseline assessment of the practices' medical home level and a final re-measurement post-project completion), provide patient encounter data to a patient-experience-with-care survey vendor and to submit CPT II codes that reflected clinical performance status on several Healthcare Effectiveness Data and Information Set (HEDIS®) quality measures. Both Groups 1 and 2 received increased reimbursement based upon the number of sponsoring insurance company participants, with Group 1 having the highest achievable payment potential. Both had scalable reimbursement amounts based upon a practices' capability to achieve NCQA PPC®-PCMH™ recognition level 1, 2, or 3. The health plan rewarded practices by a formula that weighed a combination of data including patient satisfaction scores, patient-encounter efficiencies and effectiveness based upon a risk-adjusted ratio of expected to actual episode-of-care costs, NCQA PPC®-PCMH™ recognition level and observed reductions in patient hospitalization.

A NEED FOR QUALITY-OF-CARE SURVEILLANCE TRAINING

UMG used its EHR to collect and/or transmit data for each project. The results were surprising. There were major gaps between what UMG assumed was captured when using the EHR and what the initial EHR-calculated performance rates were for the individual quality measures. In retrospect, if UMG fully understood what they needed to measure, they could have placed a greater emphasis on ensuring metric validity when implementing the EHR.

UMG understood the EHR as a mechanism for obtaining encounter information during a patient visit. The practice did not understand fully what it meant to use an EHR to capture clinical performance information. UMG staff had not been adequately trained in quality improvement approaches or the need to collect data in structured fields in a standardized way. The staff assumed that because all the information was in an EHR, it could be collected for any quality measure at the push of a button. If UMG had better understood the need to track groups of patients (denominators) to ascertain clinical performance (numerators), the training and workflow redesign that occurred in the beginning of the implementation would have been more suited toward capturing quality data. Instead, UMG had to restructure its workflow almost nine months post-go live.

RESULTS FROM QUALITY IMPROVEMENT INITIATIVE #1

The CMS Prevention Project was not tied to a financial incentive but did provide free consultant services which helped to identify several issues:

Clinical Quality Measure Data Results

UMG and IPRO identified opportunities for workflow redesign to fully capture and validate UMG's quality metrics. For example, the practice began to perform additional data recovery for completed colonoscopies. UMG retrieved documented results from additional system locations. Previously the completed colonoscopies were measured only if located in one EHR area—the referrals section. UMG also started to check the code mapping for the metrics. Associating results to outstanding colonoscopy orders, for example, gave it credit for the full and appropriate data that were retrievable in the system's primary care registry panel. The changes from June 2008 to July 2010 yielded mixed results. Immunization rates increased. Cancer screening rates increased from baseline but decreased from their highest rates in December 2009 (see Table 17-3).

UMG added a process to referral tracking by closing out orders and referrals simultaneously. It had previously indicated referrals as "complete" when the referral report from the outside clinical service came back. This workflow did not have a process to determine whether incomplete "orders" were in the patients' records. In the new workflow, the staff checks for the outstanding orders, links the appropriate documents, and then indicates the orders and referrals as "complete" in the EHR. Now the full cycle is closed (referral-result-review).

UMG also addressed data mapping. Colonoscopies did not map to the registry component of the EHR if the providers ordered them as a procedure and not a diagnostic image. Colonoscopies ordered as "procedures" were retrievable in a different reporting section of the EHR that was installed post-go live. This separate section tracked performance on a more narrowly defined colorectal cancer screening measure that related to the CMS quality metric. UMG would obtain different results for colonoscopy rates dependent upon which reporting tool in the EHR was accessed and which way the providers ordered them as either a diagnostic image or a procedure. The EHR vendor was made aware of this problem and advised UMG that they would work to remedy the issue. At this writing, this issue has not been addressed.

Accuracy

Addressing the need to clean the patient data base, UMG's patient demographics were migrated from a legacy practice management system. UMG did not understand that data migration occurred without removal of patients who were inactive, (i.e., moved, sought care with another provider, or expired). For UMG, this inaccuracy resulted in an exaggerated total number of patients in the EHR. When UMG initially ran queries in the EHR system to formulate denominators, adjustments were not made for the database housing patients that had aged out of the practice. Therefore UMG's adherence rates were significantly lower than they should have been. The denominators were adjusted from calculating "all patients in the EHR..." to all patients in the EHR who had visit encounters in the past two years...." Addressing this issue resulted in an increase in UMG's quality metrics (see Table 17-3). UMG estimated that there was a considerable time cost to cleaning the patient data base. The work required staff to identify "dead file" patients and remove them to avoid being captured in the registry.

Attribution

Reviewing the denominators helped identify a larger-than-expected pool of patients. Patients scheduled to see specialty providers were counted in the quality metrics algorithm because they had a visit encounter to the practice even if they were not followed by the UMG primary care physicians (see Table 17-3, baseline and Dec 2009 data).

Table 17-3: Medicare Prevention Quality Indicators

Clinical Measure	Flu Vaccine Numerator	Flu Vaccine Denominator	Flu Rate %	PPV Numerator	PPV Denominator	PPV Rate %	CRC Numerator	CRC Denominator	CRC Rate %	Mammography Numerator	Mammography Denominator	Mammography Rate %
June 2008 Baseline	99	469*	21%	26	469*	6%	159	1116*	14%	11	435*	3%
Dec. 2009	116	693*	17%	171	693*	25%	549	1552*	35%	199	625*	32%
July 2010	127	273	47%	201	273	74%	149	670	22%	98	533	18%

* Totals represent an inflated denominator due to attribution.

Patients were scheduled specialty services in the EHR under a "resource schedule," a section of the appointment system set aside for encounters such as non-billable appointments, lab visits, and, in this case, appointments to a specialist. UMG did not realize that any encounter would be counted in the quality measure assessment. The solution was for UMG to filter their registry reports to identify patients who had an encounter with the primary care providers and not *specialty* providers (see Table 17-3, July 2010 data). This was an easy fix once UMG was able to determine the problem.

The specialists were placed in the EHR as referring providers. They are not licensed eCW users. UMG uses the "resource schedule" element of the EHR to accept appointments for the specialists and document patient arrival at the practice. Otherwise the specialists keep their own paper charts for the visit and bill separately from UMG. The specialists do not enter any data into the EHR. UMG staff gets these specialist results as paper and treat this information no differently than any other external referral source.

RESULTS FROM QUALITY IMPROVEMENT INITIATIVE #2

UMG received a final report detailing the number of patients meeting goals and calculated incentive payment in July 2010. The report reflected data on patients that had visit encounters from April 1, 2009, to March 31, 2010. Participating practices were not required to meet a minimum threshold for payment.[5] According to eHearts, UMG had a total of 182 patients who met the aspirin prohylaxis measure, 243 patients who met the blood pressure control measure, 693 who met the cholesterol measure, and 75 who met the smoking measure. UMG did not receive patient-specific data, i.e., patient lists, in keeping with the quality initiative design.

Throughout the 12-month initiative, UMG received progress reports indicating its current status on patients meeting the measure. The reports helped practices, to a limited degree, identify their progress in assessing whether all eligible patients were assigned appropriately for each of the quality metrics. A facility not capturing clinical quality measures could put corrective actions in place and review the data quarterly to see if improvement activities yielded measurable success. This proved difficult for UMG, since it was unable to match its patient-specific data with numeric values reflected from the eHearts repository. At best, UMG could hope to match numerators.

UMG believed that it had a much higher adherence rate than what the eHearts report reflected for the four measures. Attempts to replicate the denominator and numerators were unsuccessful, since the practice extracted different totals when querying the registry system (see Table 17-4). UMG sought clarification on how the denominators were identified. They did not know if the eHearts software extracted patient diagnosis codes entered in the patient assessment, or from the problem list, or both. Since the progress reports did not identify patients explicitly, as per the program parameters, UMG had to recreate the report queries to validate data and identify patients who would benefit from having outstanding quality measures addressed.

PCIP was aware of these difficulties and did advise practices of the need to be very careful in entering data. "PCIP has been working with primary care providers to increase the delivery of preventive services with a specific focus on patients with cardiovascular risks. Tracking patient health with the electronic health record can be automated, but it requires patient information to be entered and updated in specific areas of the record.

Table 17-4: UMG Internal Review from EMR Registry*

Quality Measure	UMG Internal Numerator	eHearts Year 1 Report Numerator	UMG Internal Denominator	eHearts Year 1 Report Denominator
Aspirin	253	182	355	Not available
Blood Pressure (3 measures combined)	74	243	794	Not available
Cholesterol	715	693	774	Not available
Smoking	75	75	176	Not available

* Number of patients who had office visits between April 1, 2009, and March 31, 2010

The clinical decision support system (CDSS) is a tool that can assist providers with documentation."[6] Providers were also reminded that documenting where it counts was imperative and that providers should record all diagnoses in their problem lists.

UMG concluded that adherence, on behalf of the providers, required using specialized condition-specific data collection forms (Smart Forms) and that not using these forms yielded a lower-than-expected number of patients meeting the smoking cessation criteria. PCIP stated providers needed to enter data in very specific ways to count in the quality calculation algorithm, such as using the Smart Form with all patients to document their smoking status; that a patient's blood pressure, height, and weight needed to be entered in the vitals section and that tests would have to be ordered through the laboratory section for assessing a patient's hemoglobin A1c (glycosylated hemoglobin) or cholesterol.[5]

Providers do not always use EHRs as intended[7] and UMG was no exception. There was marked variation in how the clinicians and support staff interpreted EHR use and data entry. This variation likely reduced the number of patients who met quality indicator goals. Despite EHR design to facilitate structured entry of specific data elements,[8] providers at UMG, like most clinicians, will develop shortcuts to using the EHR based upon the time constraints of the clinical encounter, the biases of how they conceptually view the data (e.g., is a colonoscopy a referral or a lab test or a procedure) and the layout of the EHR. Quality metric monitoring needs to be an iterative process.

RESULTS FROM QUALITY IMPROVEMENT INITIATIVE #3

The local insurance initiative submitted a feedback report reflecting UMG's status on meeting the requirements for incentive payment. UMG was successful in completing the NCQA PPC®-PCMH™ survey for both the pilot project's baseline and final measure periods and ultimately achieved level-3 recognition. They also exceeded the additional necessary components of successfully entering CPT II quality measure codes to identify patient blood pressure values and submitting patient names (post-encounter) to the patient experience survey vendor.

The NCQA PPC®-PCMH™ survey requires practices to submit a range of measurable components in order to ascertain whether a facility meets its medical home standard. The lengthy survey process, coupled with UMG's exposure to other QI programs, helped them plan a course of action that led to success for this initiative. The medical home submission encourages and permits facilities to define clinical quality measures on chronic conditions that affect their patient population and to structure self-administered reviews on their performance.

A major component of UMG's process of meeting the initiative's goals was the development of an updated practice policy and procedure manual. The policies supported a well-defined structure and workflow. The manual was a written process on steps ranging from patient/staff communication, to prescription refills, to a contingency plan if the EHR is down.

Since UMG had the ability to develop its own components and measures for the PPC®-PCMH™ survey, it was able to provide quality clinical data with higher accuracy. Having the EHR and developing skill at assessing and validating data across groups and/or clinical conditions benefitted UMG even though it did not get support from a facilitator or care manager. Not having the data automatically exported, as in QI program #2, gave UMG the opportunity to remove and or expose outliers during its self-administered data review process. Although UMG believes this approach has greater internal validity, it recognizes that without outside metric formulation or review, the external validity of its measures likely is limited.[9] As NCQA and CMS move toward incorporating quality metric performance in their programs, this will become more problematic as it was in the first and second quality initiatives presented earlier.

SUMMARY

The automation of clinical encounters does not by itself equate to improved healthcare outcomes. There is an extra step that providers will have to be willing to take, since assessing quality care by any measure will be an expanding component of physician reimbursement. Clinicians will have to educate themselves on their own performance in order to maximize any future financial health IT adoption incentives, such as Meaningful Use. Alternately they will have to hire staff that can validate clinical data and ensure that data capture reflects clinical performance. The implementation of an EHR does not give practices all the answers, but it certainly provides a more efficient tool when attempting to aggregate patient population data. UMG did not know the "what" and "hows" of measurement at go-live, but the QI programs gave them a crash course on getting key issues addressed. Addressing issues such as workflow, attribution, mapping, and eligibility provided UMG with a head start for what the future of medicine likely will become.

UMG learned that a practice can take all of the right steps when implementing an EHR but omitting QI needs from the process can result in a potential future financial loss. A fuller or more robust and continued education on the structure of the EHR from the vendor or others, such as insurance companies or external quality performance contractors, is needed to educate providers and their staff on the nuances of quality data measures and improvement. However, this effort will cost money and time—two important things that most small primary care providers cannot spare.

The Office of the National Coordinator for Health Information Technology has launched a variety of programs to support EHR implementation and appropriate use.[10]

These include the HIT Regional Extension Center Program (REC) and several curriculum development efforts to improve training of professionals to support the use of health IT. Ultimately these should supplement existing efforts, such as the IPRO QIO work in this paper's Quality Improvement Initiative 1 and the PCIP work in Quality Improvement Initiative 2. Based upon the staging of the CMS EHR implementation program and the requirements of the REC program, the major REC focus at least for the next 1–2 years will be implementation and not quality improvement.[11] At this writing, it is not clear whether the next QIO contract cycle (August 2011–July 2014) will include targeted quality improvement assistance efforts focused on practices that have implemented EHRs. Clinicians will need to include quality improvement training and support in their EHR implementation work plan and be sure that learning starts early on how to use health IT to change clinical practice capability.

The authors' experience supports early incorporation of quality improvement activities. The assistance and ongoing feedback UMG received from two of their QI programs yielded success in the third. UMG's future goals are to leverage sustainability for their efforts and continue to provide effective and efficient evidence-based quality care to their community.

REFERENCES

1. NYC DOHM eHearts FAQs (2010). Available at: http://home2.nyc.gov/html/doh/downloads/pdf/pcip/pcip-ehearts-faq.pdf. Last accessed November 2010.
2. CMS 9th Scope of Work Prevention Background (2010). Available at: http://www.ipro.org/index/9sow-prevention-about. Last accessed August 2010.
3. NYC DOHMH Healthy Hearts Rewards (2010). Available at: http://www.nyc.gov/html/doh/html/pcip/ehearts.shtml. Last accessed August 2010.
4. NYC DOHMH Sample Quality Measure Report (2010). Available at: http://home2.nyc.gov/html/doh/downloads/pdf/pcip/pcip-qualityreport.pdf. Last accessed August 2010.
5. NYC DOHMH CDSS Increases Documented Preventive Services. Available at: IPRO_Chart_Review_Prelim_Results[1].pdf (2010). Last accessed November 2010.
6. NYC eHearts Rewards (2010). Available at: http://www.nyc.gov/html/doh/html/pcip/ehearts.shtml. Last accessed September 2010.
7. Miller RH, Sim I. Physicians' use of electronic medical records: barriers and solutions. *Health Aff* (Millwood). 2004;23:116-126.
8. Roth CP, Lim Y, Pevnick M. The challenge of measuring quality of care from the electronic health record 2009;391.
9. Cook TD, Campbell DT. *Quasi-Experimentation Design & Analysis Issues for Field Settings.* Boston: Houghton Mifflin Co. 1979; Chapter 3.
10. HITECH Programs. Available at: http://healthit.hhs.gov/portal/server.pt/community/healthit_hhs_gov__hitech_programs/1487. Last accessed September 2010.
11. Connecting America for Better Health EHR Incentive Program. Available at http://www.cms.gov/EHRIncentivePrograms/. Last accessed September 2010.

CHAPTER 18

Case Study:
Citizens Memorial Healthcare

Denni McColm, MBA

WHO WE ARE

Citizens Memorial Healthcare (CMH) is a rural healthcare network based in Bolivar, Missouri. CMH operates healthcare services across the continuum of care. The network serves a rural community and service area that includes five rural counties with a population of 100,000. CMH operates an acute care hospital licensed for 76 beds. The hospital holds a sole community provider designation from the Centers for Medicare & Medicaid Services (CMS). CMH provides emergency medical services through an emergency department (ED) with trauma level III designation. CMH also offers ambulance services for two counties and hosts air ambulance services on the CMH campus.

In addition to acute and emergency services, CMH offers ambulatory care, rural health clinics, specialty physician clinics, home care, long-term care, residential care, independent living apartments, rehabilitation services and oncology. Services are offered directly and through partnerships and affiliations. CMH is a registered name representing two corporate entities. One is a Missouri public hospital district, officially Citizens Memorial Hospital District. The other is a 501(c)3 nonprofit corporation known as Citizens Memorial Health Care Foundation. The community recognizes Citizens Memorial Healthcare as both entities.

Annually, CMH provides inpatient care for 4,500 patients, including 500 babies delivered at the CMH BirthPlace; 20,000 ED visits; 3,600 ambulance runs; and more than 120,000 rural health clinic and specialty physician clinic visits. CMH maintains a census of 500 residents in five long-term care facilities.

CMH employs 1,550 people across the five-county service area. The hospital and clinics are accredited by The Joint Commission.

WHERE WE WERE: STAGE OF ELECTRONIC MEDICAL RECORD (EMR) ADOPTION

The Citizens Memorial Hospital District was formed in 1979 by a vote of the population in the hospital district. The hospital district includes all but one township in Polk County, Missouri. Following the formation of the hospital district, general obligation bonds were approved and issued. Citizens Memorial Hospital opened in September 1982.

Upon opening, CMH began using a hospital software package for admissions and billing from IBM, known as HFMS. It operated on an IBM mainframe system. Soon after the hospital opened, IBM discontinued the product and support. CMH hired a programmer to continue support. The same programmer supported multiple hospitals in the region using the same product. CMH continued to use this product, supported and expanded by local programmers, until 2002. CMH purchased a lab information system, a pharmacy information system, and a physician practice management system prior to 1999. All systems were running on an AS400 by the year 2000. All systems were modified and prepared for Y2K, and the transition to the new century was successful.

CMH had adapted and was making full use of the systems in place. The lab information system was used hospital-wide to facilitate order entry and communication to ancillary departments. The scheduling module of the physician practice management system was also used for outpatient radiology scheduling. Interfaces pushed charges from the lab and pharmacy systems to the billing system. With only lab and pharmacy systems in place, CMH was at Stage 0 on the HIMSS Analytics EMR Adoption Model[SM] (EMRAM).[1]

WHY WE ADOPTED THE EHR: MISSION, GOALS

In 1999, CMH conducted strategic planning, looking forward over a five-year planning period. Strategic planning had been conducted every two to three years over the life of the hospital. During 1999, it was recognized that the hospital and related foundation had grown to include a full continuum of healthcare services—cradle to the grave—hospital, home care, long-term care, and physician clinics. One strategy adopted that year was to re-brand the organization and drop the multiple names and logos that had accumulated over the years for various service lines and buildings. The decision was made to rebrand under the Citizens Memorial Healthcare name and logo for all services and to promote to the community that CMH could provide "seamless care across the continuum."

It was a great idea, if it had been true. CMH did have services across the continuum of care. The problem was that they were not seamless. Services were not seamless from the point of view of patients or healthcare providers. For patients, it was most evident by the fact that CMH asked for demographic and medical history information over and over as they moved from one CMH service to another. More importantly, CMH healthcare providers did not have access to the lab results, radiology reports, and physician and nursing notes they needed to provide care. Paper medical records were kept in 33 different locations, including clinics, the hospital, home care, long-term care, and storage facilities. It was impractical, if not impossible, to pull a patient's complete medical record together. And, even if a provider could get all of that paper together, how would they trend it, filter it, or make it useful?

As a result of this analysis, CMH set out to solve the problem. On a smaller scale, this is the same problem that faces our nation—pertinent patient information is not available when and where it is needed to facilitate care.

CMH contracted with VHA Consulting to provide help in deciding how to approach the issue. A multidisciplinary team was formed. Project Manager, Wayne Stuckey, with VHA Consulting, led the team through a year-long series of steps to assure that information systems (IS) efforts would support organization strategies.

The IS Assessment and Planning Process was conducted by a team that eventually became the CMH IS Steering Committee. The time line for the process was:

- Information Technology & Systems Assessment, April 2000
- Information Systems Strategic Planning, January 2001
- Vendor Selection & Contract, December 2001
- Information Systems Implementation Planning, January 2002

INFORMATION TECHNOLOGY & SYSTEMS ASSESSMENT

An IT and systems assessment was conducted in April 2000. The assessment included a complete inventory of existing information systems and resources in use at CMH and a demonstration of those systems by end users.

As a result of that assessment, the team identified these "Top IT Issues:"

- Disparate systems and databases
- No common patient identification
- Lack of continuity of patient care information across the delivery system
- Lack of clinical documentation systems
- Operational inefficiency
- No availability of medical record in electronic format
- No decision support capability
- Minimal IT standards
- Insufficient IS resources

The team reached the following conclusions and made these recommendations:

- Establish an IS Steering Committee and IT Strategy
- Review organization strategic objectives and align IT strategies to support those initiatives
- Develop an integrated information system to serve hospital, clinics, long-term care, and home care
- Replace existing information system within realistic time frame and resource constraints
- Expand IS resources (staff and budget)

These guiding principles were adopted for application prioritization and software and technology acquisition:

- The IS strategic direction is guided by the long-term vision and strategic plan for the organization.
- Common system solutions will be implemented for like functions across departments where the system can meet 70–80 percent of individual depart-

ment requirements. This will provide operational integration across the continuum of care.

- Investments in new systems and technologies must demonstrate a positive ROI based on business and clinical benefits.
- Existing investments in systems will be preserved and expanded wherever appropriate.
- Priority will be given to those systems that best support overall organizational needs.
- To achieve integration, CMH will look to a single core vendor whenever possible but will select other vendors for niche systems in which benefits outweigh the lack of integration.
- Improvement in provider productivity, as well as reducing the "hassle" factor for physicians will be considered key requirements for system selection.
- System acquisition will be driven by weighted criteria including functionality, ease of use, technology and support requirements.
- CMH will adopt systems and technologies that are on the upward curve of their system lifecycle, will be an early adopter of proven technologies, and will avoid alpha/beta relationships and custom development particularly for mission-critical functions.
- System acquisition will follow a formal process including needs assessment, requirements definition, and vendor due diligence.
- Information Services will develop the infrastructure to support known upcoming strategic projects with capability for quick incremental growth.

The pros and cons of integration versus best-of-breed (BoB) strategies in system acquisition were discussed and debated by the IS Steering Committee. The Committee very deliberately chose and continues to support an integration strategy for CMH. This strategy has proven successful and is one reason CMH has been able to rapidly implement the EMR and CPOE across care settings.

The selection process at CMH was employee driven. Teams of employees were involved in each step. When the decision was made to pursue a new system that included the EMR and MEDITECH was selected, there was strong consensus around the plan throughout the organization. That consensus has been a key to CMH's success in implementation. In fact, one of the biggest challenges in the implementation was keeping up with the demand. Departments and employees were so excited about the new system that they all wanted to be first to implement.

STEPS IN THE SELECTION AND CONTRACT PROCESS

Project teams made up of end users were convened. The teams, which numbered 39, were challenged to identify functional requirements for a new system, develop demonstration scenarios, participate in and evaluate demonstrations, conduct reference checks, participate in site visits, and recommend a vendor(s) of choice. The teams were asked to think big by asking themselves "In my wildest dreams, what would information systems do for me in my job and department?"

A time line was established for the RFP process, with a goal of completing contracts by December 2001.

The RFP included more than 200 pages of functional requirements identified by the project teams. Vendor analysis was done by scoring each vendor against those functional requirements. The top three vendors were invited to present product demonstrations. Evaluation surveys were completed by more than 100 project team members attending each vendor demonstration.

Reference checking was done. A second demonstration for physicians and board members was done to ensure that they were "on board." A corporate visit was made to the MEDITECH headquarters. Five site visits were conducted, including one specifically for physicians and clinics, one specifically for home care services, and one specifically for long-term care facilities.

MEDITECH was chosen as the recommended vendor based on their proven technology, which is utilized in over 2,000 healthcare organizations. MEDITECH has a 36-year history in the industry lending to confidence in their stability. The MEDITECH Client/Server platform was selected in order to maintain flexibility and ease the transition for end users accustomed to using Windows products at home.

A detailed budget was prepared for Project Infocare, the name by which the project came to be known.

HOW WE IMPLEMENTED THE INPATIENT EHR AND OTHER RELATED TECHNOLOGY

Implementation planning was conducted in a two-day session in January 2002, using Franklin Covey's 4 Roles of Leadership model.[2] The planning was conducted off-site to minimize interruptions. A facilitator skilled in Franklin Covey processes was utilized. The Implementation Director and Implementation Specialist from the major vendor (MEDITECH) participated along with the IS Steering Committee (ISSC) (see Table 18-1).

Vision

The vision for the project was articulated as:

- Enable a patient to enter anywhere into our continuum of care and have a personal identity that is maintained across that continuum.
- Physicians and other caregivers will have access to all of that patient's information within the healthcare system.
- Providers will be able to document efficiently within the software system, which will free them to spend more time with patients.
- The investment of time, talent, and money will enable CMH to be a technologically advanced healthcare organization poised to grow and offer new services to our patients and the community at large.

Objectives

These specific objectives and strategies were embraced during planning:

- **Patient Information:** Patients will be asked to supply information only once. CMH will store, protect, and make that information accessible (only as needed) without redundancy.

Table 18-1: Summarizing the Planning Effort

Information Systems Implementation Planning **4 Roles Planning Highlights**	
Pathfinding These key stakeholders were identified: • Patients & community • Physicians & other caregivers • System end users & employees • Administrative decision makers & boards of directors The Project Infocare vision statement was enthusiastically developed and embraced.	**Aligning** Understanding the importance of aligning to achieve the vision, the team agreed to use these techniques and practices in the implementation: • Understand and become experts on the system before training • Train in the basics of computer operations, so end users will not feel intimidated by the new technology • Begin with current users and gain support • Phase in functions and applications in order to ensure sufficient resources for support during training, implementation, and post-live • Build a foundation upon which an EMR can be developed • Seek process improvements in each step to enhance workflow for end users • Identify problem people and make a positive effort to engage them in the process • Market the project to end users throughout the continuum of care
Modeling The role of the ISSC was determined to be to • Allocate resources • Remove obstacles • Establish parameters • Serve as cheerleaders • Implement system to maximize functionality • Serve as communication liaisons	**Empowering** The planning team identified the need to form Implementation Teams for the many applications to be implemented. Key qualities to seek in Implementation Team Leaders were decided on and included knowledge of department or function, trusted/respected, works well with other departments, interest/enthusiasm, communicator/listener, organized/can meet deadlines, and motivated. An Implementation Kick-Off event was planned to include the CMH CEO with all team members. A meeting was scheduled to introduce the project and responsibilities to the chosen Implementation Team Leaders. A chart was developed to show the organizational relationships of the Implementation Teams, IS Staff, and Administration.

- **Patient Billing:** Patient-friendly billing processes, forms, and practices will be adopted.
- **Access:** Patients will be able to schedule appointments for all services from all CMH locations.
- **Care Documentation:** Documentation will be captured at the point of care. Charges to patient accounts will be created automatically as care providers document in the system.
- **Information for Providers:** Direct care providers will have access to easy-to-use, reliable, timely, accurate, and complete information that is available from any location.
- **Performance Improvement:** CMH will employ the new system tools to enhance patient care, improve delivery and safety of care, and support decisions with access to knowledge bases.
- **Data Collection and Storage:** Information will be stored digitally in a retrievable format. Paper documents will be phased out. Queryable data elements will be selected over scanned images.

- **Organization-wide Perspective:** Project Infocare will serve CMH and the healthcare providers that make up the continuum of care. This continuum consists of many integrated units all serving the same patients across care settings. In making decisions and establishing processes, CMH will consider the effect on the whole continuum.
- **Implementation of Project:** Project Infocare has been conducted in phases. For each phase, the system was configured, testing was conducted, end users were trained, and a parallel run was performed before the implementation date.

Implementation Phases

Implementation of Project Infocare began in March 2002 with a kick-off event including 150 participants from teams ready to begin implementation. The CMH CEO presented the importance of the project. He expressed confidence in the success of the implementation and the positive impact it would have on patient care, quality, and service.

The financial applications were placed in operation in October 2002. This first step included General Ledger, Payroll/Personnel, Accounts Payable, and Materials Management.

Core clinical applications were placed in operation in December 2002. These applications replaced disparate systems with integrated solutions and created the shell of the EMR to begin "collecting" data immediately. The applications were Medical Records, Abstracting, Admissions/Registration, Billing/Accounts Receivable, Lab, Pharmacy, Imaging, Community-wide Scheduling, EMR, Order Entry, Operating Room Management, and an Executive Support System.

Home Care Services software was placed in operation in January 2003, including the use of in-home documentation utilizing portable devices. Nurses and therapists carry handheld devices and download daily information via a telephone link. Home care visits are available in the EMR.

Physician Clinic Practice Management was placed in operation in June 2003 in 16 CMH Physician Clinics. The system replaced a separate system with one that is integrated and established the foundation for ambulatory clinical records within the EMR. Even at this time, each visit in the CMH physician clinics created a visit in the EMR that included diagnosis and demographic information, lab results, and transcribed reports.

Long-Term Care Billing was placed in operation in June 2003 in five long-term care facilities. This system replaced a separate product with one that integrates to the EMR.

The Nursing and ancillary application was placed in operation in November 2003 in the hospital including online documentation of care plans, assessments, vital signs, and medication administration on all hospital inpatient units.

CPOE was fully functional in the hospital, scanning was implemented for any remaining paper items in the medical record, and CMH was paperless in the hospital for current records by December 2003.

Full CPOE implementation was the completion of an intense effort over a period of months that included training, communication, building, rebuilding, designing, redesigning, follow up, and support for physicians. CPOE and utilization of the online EMR were phased in as follows:

- **Phase I:** Electronic signature on transcribed documents and viewing transcribed reports and lab results online. Printing of the documents was discontinued.
- **Phase II:** Ordering procedures (lab, radiology, nursing services, ancillary services) online.
- **Phase III:** Ordering medications online and viewing miscellaneous scanned documents associated to a record. Paper charts were eliminated.

Picture archiving and communication systems (PACS; digital radiology) became operational at CMH in January 2004. Digital images are available throughout the network on any workstation. Diagnostic-quality monitors are available in the emergency department, imaging department, medical/surgical, physician resource room, and ICU. Images are available in physician clinics and by remote access.

The first long-term care facility implemented nursing and ancillary documentation and CPOE in February 2004. This implementation at a 111-bed facility was incredibly successful. All nursing and ancillary staff at the facility complete documentation and the online medication administration record in real-time, using wireless devices on carts, portable devices, or hardwired computers. Physicians admitting to the facility enter and review orders and care documentation online.

CMH implemented an interface with LabCorp Referral Lab in April 2004, so that lab results from this source are captured as data elements and are available for trending.

Remote access to the EMR was made available to physicians via Citrix in July 2004.

Also in July 2004, CMH implemented Patient Friendly Registration processes to further enhance the registration process. Processes include an Express Registration card that is issued to patients. The card includes a bar coded patient identifier to facilitate quick and accurate patient identification. New processes also include "quick links" to common routines, the ability to view previous insurance cards, the ability to print consents with preprinted patient information, scripting and standardization of registration processes.

In February 2005, CMH launched HealthStream online learning system. In addition to the education required by regulation and accreditation bodies, CMH sees the need to provide ongoing education on the new computer system. Any upgrade to the system requires the re-education of hundreds of employees who work in geographically dispersed locations on varied shifts. New nursing personnel can now take most of their orientation training online.

In March 2005, CMH's first Physician Clinic implemented clinical documentation with the Electronic Ambulatory Record and began phasing out paper charts. Also in March 2005, CMH began implementing the ED module, which includes a patient tracker, nursing documentation, discharge instructions, patient triage, physician order entry, and documentation.

In 2006, CMH added bar code verification to medication administration, which was already being done using an electronic medication administration record.

In-home tele-management for home care patients was added in 2007. The system allows patients to take vital signs at home. Those are transmitted to the CMH EMR system via telephone lines where nurses and physicians can view and use them in providing care.

CMH introduced speech recognition in 2008, as well as expanded the use of PACS to include mammography.

In 2009, CMH began an effort to more actively engage patients in their own care through a patient portal and through training methods that encourage physicians and nurses to share the computer screen and EMR with patients. In this same year, CMH integrated portable vital signs monitors and glucometers into the EMR at the point of care. E-prescribing was introduced for ambulatory patients.

In early 2010, CMH implemented the final piece to qualify for Stage 7 on the HIMSS Analytics EMR Adoption Model^{SM} (EMRAM). That was interoperability. The interoperability is a standards-based, bi-directional exchange with the GoogleHealth PHR. Patients can request a link between their GoogleHealth PHR and the CMH EMR system. Lab results, medications, allergies, and procedures are all transmitted from the CMH EMR to the patient's GoogleHealth record. When patients are admitted to CMH, their PHR information can be retrieved into the CMH EMR for use by physicians.

LESSONS LEARNED

- **Agree on the why.** For CMH there was a clear strategic initiative to provide seamless care across the continuum for patients. That vision was agreed upon and expressed in a vision statement. That vision statement kept people focused on why we were making the change to EMRs.
- **Adopt an approach.** CMH specifically committed to an integration strategy, as opposed to a BoB approach. The CMH IS Steering Committee was clear that priority would be given to systems that meet overall organizational needs and not just departmental preferences. This commitment to an approach helps guide decisions.
- **Secure resources.** The CMH IS Steering Committee spent considerable effort identifying the full cost of the project to assure that Administration and the Board were fully aware of the commitment. They did not downplay the size of the budget but rather made an effort to assure that the needed resources were understood and appropriated. This strategy has proven successful. During the implementation of the new system, the team did not need to expend energy in securing resources, which allowed all efforts to be focused on implementation excellence.
- **Evaluate the alternatives.** CMH took time to re-demonstrate existing systems and to look to the market to determine the best fit for a long-term investment. This evaluation gave users confidence that the best possible decision had been made going forward.
- **Be all inclusive.** CMH included anyone and everyone who would participate in defining requirements, evaluating vendors and participating in site visits and reference calls. At the end of the evaluation, a consensus was clear and the broad input made a difference and helped gain commitment throughout the implementation.

- **Document the official "go ahead."** CMH documented the board and medical staff meeting in detail when the decision was made to forge ahead with the EMR system. Later, during the implementation when it became challenging for physicians to change their workflow, the minutes of that meeting served to remind everyone that they were a party to the decision and committed to the project.
- **Plan the implementation.** Making the decision to implement an EMR system and selecting a vendor are exhausting, but they are only the beginning. It is important to stop at some point(s) along the way and plan the implementation. Almost any planning model will suffice. CMH used Stephen R. Covey's 4 roles model to pinpoint pathfinding, aligning, modeling, and empowering decisions. The planning was specific and targeted and helped define expectations for implementers and users.
- **Articulate the objectives.** More specific than the vision are objectives, such as "patients will be asked to supply information only once." These objectives help guide decision makers and give users a clear understanding of the reasons behind decisions.
- **Talk. Talk. Talk.** Use both outbound communication and marketing but also listening posts. CMH used multiple methods to gather information from users on their perceptions, needs, and issues. In particular, active solicitation of issues and concerns among the medical staff proved to be a helpful strategy. Instead of waiting for issues to be brought forth, CMH staff continually asked physicians what could be improved during the implementation and followed up on every issue or concern identified. Even if the answer is "no, we can't make the system do that," closing the loop was important to the physician users.
- **Cater to the physicians.** CMH established a room known as the physician resource room. It is a small, former office near the hospital's medical/surgical floor. The room houses nine computers with large screens, telephones, and speech microphones for speech recognition. An IS staff member was in the physician resource room continually during the implementation of physician order entry. Seven years later, an IS staff person or super user staffs the room on weekdays from 6:00 a.m. to 9:00 a.m. during physician hospital rounds. This gives the physicians easy access to help in ordering and documenting care provided.
- **Make it personal.** Physician training was conducted one-on-one. In preparation for that training, each physician's most common orders were identified from the system and pre-populated as favorites. This personalization gave physicians a head start in using the system and demonstrated how it can be customized for their style of practice.
- **Involve pharmacy.** There is a difference in the way pharmacists and physicians approach medications. Pharmacists must consider the inventory of medications in the pharmacy. Is the 30 mg of a medication going to be given as one 30-mg pill, half of a 60-mg pill, or two 15-mg pills? The physician does not care. The physician just wants his or her patient to receive 30 mg. Bridging this gap so that physicians can order easily and that order will link to the appropri-

ate inventory in the pharmacy makes life better for both parties. Also, pre-populating the common and safe dosages are available to physicians also helps.

- **Use a phased approach.** In the end, CPOE is simply eliminating the middle man. Instead of the physician writing an order and someone else entering that order into the EMR, the physician does it directly. Instead of an abrupt off-on for CPOE, CMH trained the physicians and encouraged them to use CPOE "part-time" for a few weeks, pending the official go-live date. This allowed physicians to enter a few orders without as much pressure and to become used to the system. When the official go-live date arrived, it was barely noticed and went smoothly.
- **Go paperless.** Unless a hospital eliminates the paper chart completely, they will have dual workflow. CMH finished the transformation by completely eliminating the paper chart. Anything that does need to be scanned (for example, an advance healthcare directive) is scanned at the point of origin, or where it is first known to be available. This eliminates the entire process of creating, moving, scanning, and disposing of the paper after the patient is discharged. In addition, it assures that all of the information about the patient is accessible during the admission when it is most important to care decisions.
- **Expect it to be hard.** Physicians and other users may go through what feels like the Kubler-Ross stages of grief: denial, anger, bargaining, depression, and acceptance. CMH staff members kept administration appraised, and administration provided support and encouragement to all users to "keep going."
- **Continued support.** Implementing an EMR system is not ever really finished. The support needs for current and new physicians continue indefinitely. CMH staffs the physician resource room every weekday, provides training for enhancements and upgrades, as well as for new physicians. CMH continues to encourage open communications and follow-up on issues and concerns.

Subject matter experts with technical aptitudes make the best support team. The team members from various professions and departments who are most enthusiastic and who learn the system the best make the best support people. They already have a good understanding of workflow and patient care flow to which they can apply the technology. For CMH, the best physician support person is a former coordinator of ward secretaries. She knows physicians, she is trusted by physicians, and she knows exactly what should happen when an order is placed.

Extend and enhance through super users. Super users are invaluable in staying connected to end users in every area. CMH has more than 50 super users throughout the organization. These special individuals act as liaisons, assist with testing and training, and provide enhancement ideas. CMH super users are paid a stipend for their work, and they can float to a budgeted super user budget pool in the IS department when performing testing and training, in addition to his or her normal job.

- **Train for patient-friendly use.** CMH had assumed that users would naturally utilize the EMR during patient encounters and share the screen with patients to show trends. Only a few CMH users readily adapted to this model. CMH later began an effort to train users and give them the script and confidence to engage patients using the EMR. In retrospect, this would have been helpful to have included in initial training.

- **Plan for quality reporting early.** Quality reporting from an EMR system is assumed to be easy. It is not. Although many of the data fields needed for quality reporting are normally found in an EMR system, many—particularly quality measure exclusions—are still found in narrative reports. Early planning and building of data capture fields would be helpful in getting to fully electronic quality reporting.

CONCLUSION

CMH has achieved many specific positive results from the implementation of the EMR system. Those include a reduction in transcription costs, a reduction in clerical staffing, an increase in charge capture, improved clinical documentation, a reduction in re-admission and emergency department usage rates for home care patients, increased productivity, and improvements in quality metrics.

REFERENCES

1. HIMSS Analytics EMR Adoption Model.[SM] Available at: www.himssanalytics.org/hc_providers/emr_adoption.asp. Last accessed September 2010.
2. Available at: www.franklincoveycoaching.com/leadership. Last accessed September 2010.

CHAPTER 19

Case Study: Sentara Healthcare

Bertram S. Reese

INTRODUCTION

In 2010, Sentara Healthcare achieved Stage 7, the highest level of the HIMSS Analytics EMR Adoption Model^{SM} (EMRAM). HIMSS Analytics developed the EMR Adoption Model in 2005 as a methodology for evaluating the progress and impact of electronic medical record (EMR) systems for hospitals.

HIMSS Analytics Stage 7 Hospital Standards:

- Deliver patient care without the use of paper charts.
- Are able to share patient information by sending secure standardized summary record transactions to other care providers.
- Use their vast database of clinical information to drive improved care delivery performance, patient safety clinical decision support, and outcomes using business intelligence solutions.
- Are the best practice example of how to implement sophisticated EMR environments that fully engage their clinicians.

The HIMSS Analytics validation process confirms that a hospital has reached Stage 7, which includes a site visit conducted by a HIMSS Analytics executive and independent chief information officer (CIO) to ensure an unbiased evaluation. The validation team visits representative hospitals that have the same EMR applications and clinical utilization of the hospitals under consideration.

This case study strives to share the challenges, successes, and considerations Sentara Healthcare experienced in its journey to Stage 7 recognition. The format and structure is aligned with frequently asked questions of potential Stage 7 candidates.

Sentara Healthcare

Sentara Healthcare is a not-for-profit, integrated healthcare system in southeastern Virginia and northeastern North Carolina. Sentara includes eight hospitals, health plans with 415,000 covered lives, and a 400 physician medical group (SMG). Sentara is the only health system to be listed in *Modern Healthcare's* Top 10 for 12 years. In 2009,

U.S. News and World Report ranked Sentara Norfolk General Hospital in the Top 50 Hospitals for cardiology and heart surgery, kidney diseases, diabetes and endocrine disorders, and geriatric care; Sentara Leigh Hospital for orthopedics. Also in 2009, the National Committee for Quality Assurance awarded Optima Health Plan, Sentara Health Plan, and Optima Health Plan's HMO Medicaid the highest accreditation. *Modern Healthcare* also honored Dave Bernd with the 2010 CEO-IT award.

THE EMR PROJECT

EMR implementation requires sound strategy, strong leadership, and collaborative governance over the life of the project. Sentara planned, implemented, and proactively managed the EMR project (called Sentara eCare Health Network—a.k.a. "eCare") over a five-year period. Today, eCare is a comprehensive EMR system that integrates non-teaching hospitals, physician offices, diagnostic sites and pharmacies, allowing ubiquitous electronic documentation and communication in real time. By way of the "MyChart" patient portal, patients can review test results, renew prescriptions, schedule appointments, and find information.

Goals and Objectives

eCare was the cornerstone to Sentara's strategic imperatives. In January 2005, Sentara executed a deliberate effort to instill collaborative EMR leadership. Sentara solicited input from its 18,000 employees and the local community in the planning, implementation, and optimization phases of eCare execution. Based on a year-long campaign, the Strategic Management Committee announced the results:

- **Vision:** Be the healthcare provider of choice in the communities we serve
- **Mission:** We Improve Health Every Day
- **Goals:** Be the regional best and aspire to national top 10 percent. Transform care delivery. Pursue growth. Add value to the communities we serve.
- **Objectives:** Improve quality outcomes, patient safety, and embrace transparency.

The EMR Journey

In February 2005, Sentara's CIO took a group of IT leaders, physicians, and process redesign experts to the HIMSS annual meeting. The weekend before the annual meeting started, this group of 15 professionals met with six national EMR vendors. The purpose of these meetings was to hear the status, progress, and prognosis of the EMR industry to determine whether it was time to pursue an EMR strategy. The unanimous consensus at the end of the sessions was that it was time, as there was sufficient evidence that an EMR would provide significant improvements to quality, safety, and cost savings.

Upon returning, the CIO assembled a cross-functional committee to develop the strategy and a business case—called the eCare group. The eCare group split up assignments and conducted more in-depth research. The IT leaders in this group pursued the technology perspective to include site visits, on-site vendor demonstrations to a large group of operational leaders, phone calls to early adopters, and document searches for best practices. The process redesign experts pursued the business case benefits (qualitative and quantitative) for why Sentara would want to pursue this expensive and high-risk undertaking. They conducted document research, contacted best practices identified by the research and by whom the semi-finalist vendors had identified as doing the best job of implementing their EMR and tracking benefits.

Based on the original round of research, the eCare group made a presentation to Sentara executives about the potential of a system-wide integrated EMR. This presentation, titled "Imagine If," presented a compelling argument as to why the time was right to invest in an EMR and identified the major processes at which benefits are expected. Executives supported the strategy and encouraged operational leaders of the most impacted processes to work with the group to help build the business case and evaluate the alternative EMR products.

The process owners became actively involved and spent considerable time reading research literature, talking with best practice organizations and attending demonstrations, and making site visits. Over a period of several months, they became comfortable with estimates of return on investment (ROI) and value of the investment (VOI) benefits. Eventually, they committed to achieve a specific level of return once the EMR was fully functional. Their estimates became the basis for the business case presented to the board of directors. Meanwhile, the IT leaders conducted extensive research into the various vendors and eventually narrowed the potential vendors to three finalists. They invited the finalists to do "scripted demonstrations" of the actual software, not PowerPoint slides. There were more than 700 attendees at a multiple-day demonstration. Attendees were asked to rate the vendors against specific criteria.

Seeking Board Approval

In June 2005, the CIO presented the eCare concept to the board of directors. His presentation included the reason for committing to an EMR, the total cost of ownership, the estimated ROI and VOI, and the implementation milestones. It also included how Sentara would track early adopters to identify problems before moving ahead. The overarching message was that the entire leadership team, not just IT, believed in the vision and was committed to transforming care, not just "installing an EMR." The phrase *"eCare is bigger than Epic"* became a cornerstone for the project and remains a core principle to this day. The EMR project fund was the largest expenditure ever requested by Sentara's leadership. For the first time, the IT project forecast included costs for process redesign and implementation training.

After the board approved the eCare project, negotiations began in earnest with the vendor selected as providing the best continuum product and greatest level of potential benefits (Epic). The IT leaders began organizing their Design, Build, and Validation (DBV) team requirements. They identified the number of recruiting and worked diligently to recruit and train team members. Most of those selected were from operations. The CIO's belief was that it was easier to teach a clinician how to design an IT software system than to teach an IT professional the clinical processes that they would be changing.

Having signed a contract with Epic in September 2005, efforts to organize the project accelerated. Meanwhile, the CIO challenged the process redesign team to train members of the eCare team on Lean Six Sigma principles. In November 2005, a three-day "foundations" class was conducted, and more than 80 eCare members were trained in a common set of redesign tools and processes. This was followed by a three-month "surge" during which more than 200 leaders, facilitators, staff members, and eCare members participated in very aggressive process redesign work. All the while, the eCare team was getting trained, certified and participating in the process redesign efforts.

eCare Goals and Objectives

In June 2005, the Sentara leadership introduced the eCare concept to the board of directors as "...the Gateway to Clinical Excellence." At that time, the CEO challenged the organization to imagine an EMR system that could forever enhance care delivery and the community's well-being. Throughout the life of the project, the board enthusiastically supported the eCare concept and diligently challenged the eCare team with questions of accountability: What is eCare's effect on quality and patient safety? What is eCare's influence on the physician practices? How does eCare impact staff morale? Is the project on-time, on-budget, and on-target to achieve the strategic imperatives? With the strategic EMR goals in place, the eCare team was able to develop a sound project plan with specific performance metrics and milestones.

Beginning in 2006, the eCare vision was refined over a period of months with input throughout the organization. The CIO was adamant that everyone understand that eCare was an operations-owned project—not an IT project. The eCare goals were to (a) revolutionize inpatient and ambulatory care delivery, (b) develop physician/system integration initiatives, and (c) adopt the Institute of Medicine's "Six Aims of Care"—Safety, Patient Centered, Efficient, Effective, Equitable, and Timely.

Leadership and Governance

Sentara approached the eCare transformation from an organizational development perspective. Believing that success depends on user engagement, the project teams represented all stakeholders, including physicians. As shown in Figure 19-1 (eCare Project Management Office Organization Chart), several stakeholder groups oversaw the design, build, and testing of the eCare functions and features. The Executive Design Committee (EDC) was responsible for the EMR design and implementation decisions. The EDC was comprised of senior leaders from the hospitals and physician practices preparing for EMR adoption. After EMR implementation at their home site, operational EDC members transitioned to the ongoing Executive Optimization Committee.

The Physician Advisory Group (PAG) provided key physician leadership. PAG was comprised of over 25 community physician leaders from the major inpatient and ambulatory specialties. PAG was instrumental in vendor selection, software design, and eCare implementation. Much like super users, PAG members volunteered to share their experiences and make recommendations. Compensated for their time, PAG continues to focus on eCare optimization. Each hospital and physician practice had a medical director who provided leadership and consulted with the medical staff during implementation. The hospital Physician IT Steering Committee and the Medical Staff Officers Council provided implementation oversight and direction. A Community Collaborative of independent practices provided consultation on community issues.

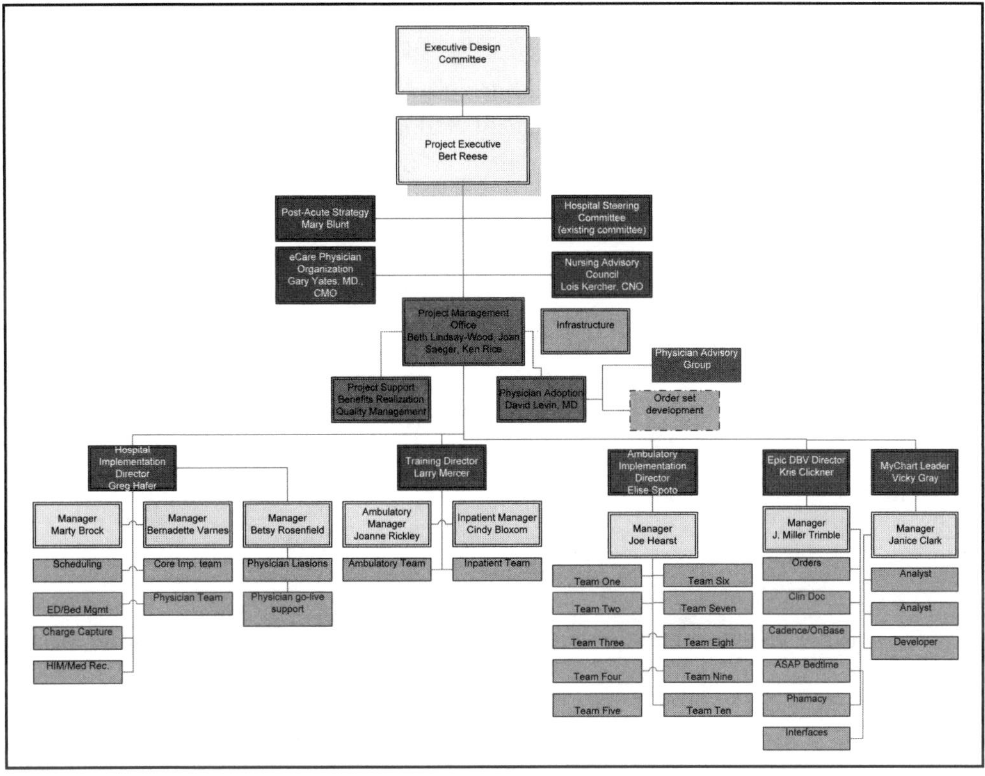

Figure 19-1: eCare Project Management Office Organization Chart (2006–2009)*

** The Core Hospital Implementation team includes Inpatient core processes, Cardiac, Pharmacy, Critical Care, Inpatient Ancillaries, ED Orders/Documentation, Inpatient Support Services, and O/P Therapies/Procedures.*

Stakeholder Involvement

Gaining consensus among key clinical and business stakeholders is critical to EMR adoption. Sentara engaged all disciplines in determining the EMR requirements, vendor selection, implementation, and eCare optimization. Collectively, the stakeholders created "a day in the life of a patient" workflow scenarios. The scenarios covered the major patient flows from admission to discharge, from physician's office to lab. Each EMR vendor was required to present his or her proposal strictly on the Sentara-created scenarios. Key stakeholders across the organization viewed videotapes of the vendors' proposals. By the time the eCare business case was developed, 3,000 caregivers and 1,000 physicians had viewed the proposals.

Needs Identification and System Acquisition

Prior to eCare, Sentara had disparate "best-of-breed" (BoB) legacy IT systems. In 2005, after implementing a picture archiving and communications system (PACS) and eICU system, the CEO challenged the organization to provide seamless electronic information conveyance across the system. Following painstaking EMR research and Total Cost of Ownership analysis, the board decided that despite the inherent risks, transformation of care demanded a greater commitment to IT. The CEO set a clear and purposeful vision for determining the EMR needs and system acquisition strategy. Understanding the risks of predicting the future of technology, the CEO was passionate about finding the right IT platform at the right cost. Under the specific chief financial officer's (CFO) guidance, the Process Improvement and Business Intelligence departments conducted a rigorous needs assessment and cost-benefit evaluation. As a result, 18 key workflow processes were identified that could be enhanced through an integrated EMR system. In 2005, following a CPOE retreat, the board of directors authorized $237 million dollars for the eCare program, which remains the largest and most complex project the board had ever approved.

Marketing and Communications

Sentara marketed the eCare vision, goals, objectives, and progress extensively. Marketing activities included advanced demos, widely distributed tent cards, posters, and gifts. Marketing analysts also conducted multiple MyChart community focus group sessions. An exclusive eCare employee portal provided daily updates. Each hospital identified celebratory themes for its EMR implementation and celebration.

Project Risk Management

To identify the risks of implementing the EMR, Sentara conducted site visits to several early adopter health systems, attended state and national conferences, solicited guidance from reputable consultants, conducted extensive literature review, and vetted multiple vendors. Based on a predefined Project Charter and Implementation Plan, the eCare Project Management Office (PMO) conducted weekly meetings to monitor the project plans, budgets, and user impact analysis. Internal auditors to the PMO provided the final approval on each hospital go-live. The PMO identified several potential high-risk processes as briefed at regular intervals by the application DBV teams.

Implementation Planning

With strong board and medical staff support, the eCare leadership decided to pursue a Big Bang (all departments, all applications) implementation to provide a single-view access for integrated results retrieval across all environments of care. A Big Bang implementation avoids the risks associated with delivery of patient care in "two worlds—paper and electronic documentation.

The eCare features include CPOE, access to protocols, decision support tools, and clinical documentation built on architecture to facilitate patient record integration. eCare software applications include Epic's inpatient and physician practice EMR, pharmacy, health information management, emergency department, oncology, bed flow management, and scheduling. Supplemental applications include bar coding, faxing, and patient health record.

A phased hospital implementation approach (shown in Figure 19-2) was used with the philosophy of "build once, roll many." This approach followed the design principle to customize the Sentara Healthcare system, then standardize across Sentara hospitals.

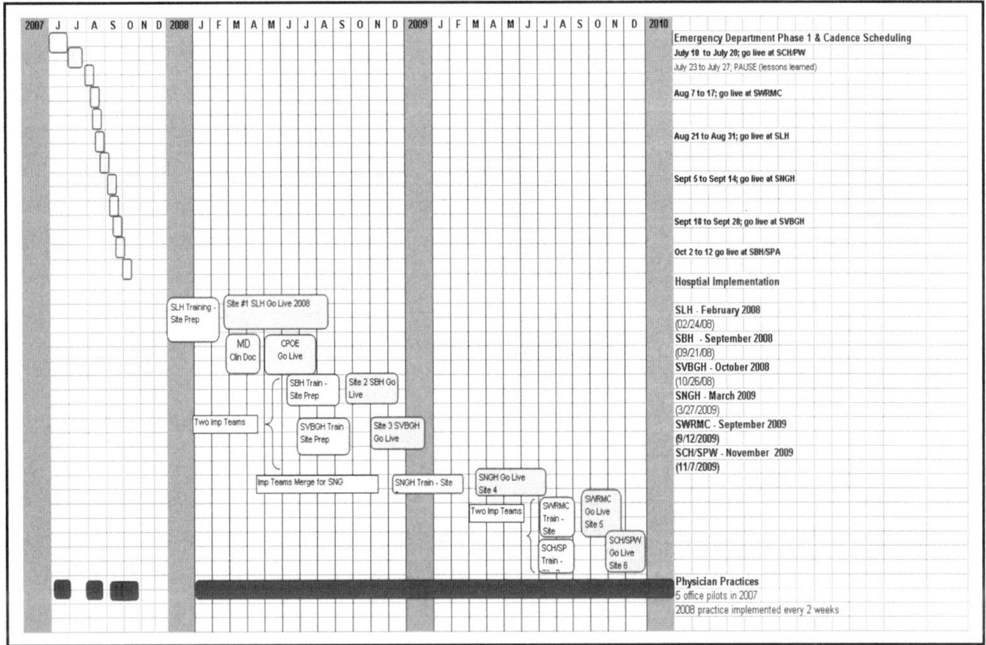

Figure 19-2: eCare Plan B Implementation Schedule (2007–2010)

The following dates list the major milestones:

- June 2005 .... Sentara Board approved EMR funding
- September 2005 .... Signed contract with the EMR vendor (Epic)
- November 2005................ Conducted Six Sigma initiatives
- May 2006 .... Conducted design, build, and validate
- August 2007...................... Implemented five pilot physician practices
  Implemented centralized scheduling and limited functionally in all emergency departments
- February 2008 .... Implemented pilot hospital
- November 2009................ Implemented last of six hospitals
- December 2010................ Implemented last of Sentara physician practice

The physician practice pilot phase lasted six months. Afterwards, one practice was implemented every two weeks through 2010. The original hospital Plan A was to roll one hospital at a time on the Epic release Spring '05. However, Sentara decided to delay the pilot hospital by three months to install the new Epic release Spring '07, which included significant clinical enhancements. Moreover, Plan B accelerated the rollout plan to minimize the monthly $3 to $4 million dollar burn rate. As shown in Figure 19-2, the pilot hospital implementation included an extended support time frame to allow a delayed CPOE ramp-up. CPOE started at go-live for the remaining five hospitals. Future eCare phases include hospital and physician practices billing and registration, as well as home health and long-term care. Two Sentara hospitals are not fully on eCare because they were acquired after the eCare project was approved.

Implementation Staffing

To instill operational ownership, Sentara recruited the eCare team from operations, when possible. Moreover, the preferred strategy was to train IT skills to clinical professionals rather than train clinical workflows to IT professionals. At the peak of accelerated Plan B implementation activity, the eCare team consisted of 190 full-time employees—73 more than the original Plan A. The implementation staff was the same as the planning phase staff. To minimize disruptions to patient care during the implementation, the hospitals backfilled their staff with agency and nurse pool personnel. A cadre of "black shirts" supported the hospital and practice physicians at the elbow.

EMR Applications Implemented

Six Sentara hospitals have implemented the *Spring '07* version of EpicCare Inpatient (including CPOE, clinical documentation, and results review); Cadence (Scheduling); ASAP (Emergency Department); BedTime, Epic RX, Medication and Positive Patient Identification Barcode Scanning, Onbase Scanning, Beacon (oncology), CPM (nurse care planning), Zynx (standard order sets) and Clarity (reporting). Sentara Medical Group (SMG) physician practices implemented Epic Ambulatory, Cadence and MyChart (private health record). The Epic EMR is interfaced to the following applications: Cerner Lab, Cerner Radiology, Pyxis (medication dispensing cabinets), Tracemaster (EKG), Chartscript (dictation/transcription), HBOC (registration and billing), ePrescribing (ambulatory only), Picis (surgery application), bedside monitoring and device integration (ICU, ED, and procedural areas) and Visicu (eICU—flowsheet documentation and medications).

Implementation Training and Support

The eCare project included the implementation team, training team, and DBV teams along with super users (1:5 staffing ratio). The implementation training strategy was based on vendor guidance and principles of adult learning. End users were required to complete classroom training and pass a proficiency test to gain sign-in eligibility. The training content was limited to "just enough and just in time." EMR demonstrations, job shadowing, and role-specific workflow-guided practices maximized user competency. Hospital employees were assigned by application type. The physician practice training sessions were grouped as administration, nursing, and physician. The 12-hour hospital physician program was targeted on a need-to-know basis: 4 hours of view-only, 4 hours of documentation, and 4 hours of order entry training. Allowing managers to enroll their staff via the Learning Management System and providing Continuing Medical Education credits were helpful in gaining broad participation. Course attendance and proficiency test results were the key measures of training effectiveness, as well as the no-show and room occupancy rates, and the trainer-to-trainee ratio. During the weeks of hospital go-live, trainers augmented the implementation team's 24-hour support on the units, while the DBV teams operated the command center help desk phones.

Ongoing Management

eCare leadership continues to track and report results on a quarterly basis. In 2008, Sentara installed a three-person optimization team at each hospital to (1) enhance physician adoption, (2) assure the business case, and (3) achieve additional benefits. The optimization teams report to the Executive Optimization Committee (EOC) to monitor progress, resolve issues, and remove barriers. The EOC also reviews potential projects and prioritizes resources.

Remaining Paper Medical Record

Paper portions of the medical record maintained during or after the patient encounter include the consent forms, driver's license, and insurance verification. Starting at go-live, all documents are scanned into the record within 24 hours.

Ongoing Planning

Winning the HIMSS Analytics Stage 7 Award was a stirring recognition of success. Sentara's chief operating officer (COO) and CIO presented the HIMSS Analytics Stage 7 plaques to each hospital to express their pride and gratitude for operations' commitment and results. Based on eCare success and organizational enthusiasm, Sentara has committed $12 million dollars each year to further IT enhancements, clinical improvements, and informatics development.

Ongoing User Support

eCare Application User Groups manage enhancement requests. The Executive Optimization Committee approves all enhancements. The 24/7 general and physician help desks provide ongoing support. Each hospital VP for Medical Affairs determines the procedures for dealing with infrequent physician users. Infrequent physician users can dictate and/or scan written documents into the electronic record.

Ongoing User Training

Human resources orients new hires, using the same curriculum and content used during the initial go-live. As time passes, training will rely more on computer-based training and less on instructor-led training. eCare Optimization teams and department super users provide training for new enhancements and upgrades.

Leadership Lessons Learned

In all areas of EMR implementation, the lessons learned are innumerable. Below is a high-level listing:

- Develop and gain commitment to a compelling EMR vision.
- Manage benefit expectations, as initial costs will outweigh benefits for years.
- Map benefits to processes and hold process owners accountable.
- Embed the benefits in performance goals and budgets.
- Operational leadership support is vital.
- Optimization ensures benefit realization, but operations has to own it.
- Implement supporting systems to the EMR ahead of time (scanning/scheduling).

FUNCTIONALITY

Computerized Practitioner Order Entry

The PAG led the CPOE design. The order entry process was automated via the CPOE application, including inpatient and physician office practices orders. As a system, Sentara has an 87 percent CPOE rate, 9 percent verbal orders rate, and 3 percent written orders rate for inpatients. CPOE adoption rates started above the 80 percent threshold at the first four hospital implementations. The last two hospital implementations started out at greater than 90 percent CPOE.

CPOE significantly reduced turnaround time for order processing and patient care delivery. The average time for administration of a NOW medication dose after order creation was reduced from 90 minutes to 30 minutes or less. Order sets are standard across the system and are evidence-based. Using Sentara customized Zynx and existing paper order sets, CPOE eliminated the ambiguity of written orders. Clinical decision support tools, such as medication alerts, have reduced the need for nurses and pharmacists to validate orders through callbacks.

Streamlined Processes and Documentation

Online documentation has streamlined clinical care processes. Nurse care-plan content now drives clinical best practices among all inpatient disciplines. Since the beginning of the eCare project, an interdisciplinary clinical care team from all hospitals has evaluated several approaches for care plan content. They decided to utilize CPMRC® (CPM Resource Center) evidence-based clinical content for the interdisciplinary care planning and clinical documentation. CPMRC is an international consortium of more than 100 clinical settings that provides evidence-based content with ongoing review and revision of clinical standards. CPMRC methodology has initiated the transition to a truly integrated patient record that reflects care provided from all disciplines. Today, the medical record reflects the patient's story of care, rather than the discipline's interactions with the patient. Moreover, the CPMRC team continues to champion improvements to clinical workflows.

Medication Administration Bar Code Scanning

Point-of-care bar coding radically redesigned medication administration. Nurses scan the patient, the medication, and themselves to ensure closed-loop medication administration. This workflow facilitates communication and cooperation among nursing, pharmacy, and information technology staffs. Sentara continually measures compliance with patient bar code scanning and medication administration and analyzes the reasons for near misses and failed scans.

Sentara has a 96 percent compliance rate for patient and medication scans. There were 12,459 (1.53% of all medications administered) potential medication administration errors prevented in March 2010 because of the medication bar code scanning process. The nursing staff has accepted bar code medication administration scanning as a significant safety improvement. It has brought their documentation process to the bedside where they can focus more on the patient. Bar code administration scanning has improved safety, timeliness, and has revolutionized the way nurses administer medications.

Changes to Patient Flow

Sentara redesigned the care management processes to enable real-time communications of patient status, bed need, and bed availability. A "pull" process allows staff to direct the patient to the appropriate bed on a given unit without a central staff intervention. Length of stay (LOS) is visible to caregivers on the patient banner, increasing awareness of actual versus expected LOS. Using EPIC, e-Discharge, and other software applications, Medical Care Management pushes data on patients awaiting placement to long-term care facilities, which facilitates better handoffs and information transfer. The redesign of the workflows brought representatives together from many inpatient disciplines. Their efforts resulted in a 16,000 patient day LOS reduction and a reduced turnaround time for bed availability from ED to inpatient of 90 minutes.

Changes to Medical Records and Coding Processes

A commitment to real-time documentation and scanning capability have transformed EMR and coding processes. Paper generated from diagnostic equipment not interfaced to the EMR is scanned real time to assure that it is available to caregivers. No paper charts remain in medical records departments. Medical records realized a $3 million dollar reduction due to the paperless environment. There has been a $1.4 million dollar reduction in transcription costs and malpractice premiums. Claims denials have decreased by $500,000 annually. Medical records departments now require minimal hospital space.

Comprehensive Data Capture

eCare captures and retains data from all critical systems that contain electronic clinical information. The EMR receives and stores cardiology, vascular, and pulmonary studies; laboratory results; surgical summaries; and radiographic interpretations and images. Interfaced information, such as a handwritten order, is scanned into the patient's record via the document management system. All data elements are retrievable on an episodic, longitudinal and cross-episode basis. However, some degree of handwritten orders will likely remain.

Point-of-care Testing Devices

Sentara makes extensive use of point-of-care testing devices. Point-of-care testing devices can perform up to 24 discreet tests. Two-thirds of those test results are sent electronically into the EMR via Sentara's enterprise laboratory system. Care providers enter the remaining point-of-care test results into the record as discreet results. eCare does not accept point-of-care testing performed by individual patients (e.g. home glucose testing). Where appropriate, patient-collected data logs are scanned into the record or referred to in the progress notes. Moreover, Sentara customized Zynx and existing paper standard orders and documentation templates to ensure efficient data entry in a format that conveys data across all venues of care. Automation provides checks and reminders for data entered incorrectly. For example, alerts fire for incorrect medication dosage if the value is improperly entered or if a flow sheet cell exceeds or falls below threshold for the patient's age.

Dictation

Physicians are not required to type notes such as the history & physical and discharge summary. They have the option of dictating these and procedure notes for transcription. Once transcribed, notes are filed in the EMR with prompts for electronic signature. The use of voice recognition technology has been successful in the Sentara physician practice setting and has helped to reduce transcription costs. Sentara also continues to use scribes at its Williamsburg Hospital Emergency Department, where pre-med students are readily available.

Non-physician clinical staff can enter verbal and handwritten orders. Verbal orders are co-signed electronically by physicians. Handwritten orders are scanned into the patient's record. Pharmacists compare the scanned handwritten medication orders to the orders entered into the system during the verification process to ensure transcription accuracy.

Bedside Monitor Device Integration (BMDI)

Sentara has employed the use of BMDI technology to make flow sheet documentation of bedside monitor and ventilator data more efficient for its nursing staff. BMDI is deployed in the critical care units, emergency departments, obstetrics, and endoscopy suites. As the EMR receives data, nurses are prompted to review the data for appropriateness before filing them on the flow sheet.

E-prescribing

E-prescribing provides the ability for the physician practice prescriber to check the patient's medication history within the EMR provided by the claims processors. While the information is limited by whether the patient's payer participates with Surescripts/RxHub system, it can give the prescriber information about patient compliance. The increased ability to track and act on a more complete medication history, as well as the medication bar code scanning process, has provided significant improvements in ensuring a safe medication management system. Similarly, a medication reconciliation tool provides prescribers in the hospital environments a display of medications the patient was taking at home, including prescriptions created in the physician practice or ED. This list allows the prescriber to continue the medications in the inpatient environment or to hold them for a decision on whether to continue them at discharge. The list can be reviewed, along with the active inpatient medications, at the time of transfer to each level of care. Using the medication reconciliation tool, inpatient medications can be converted to outpatient prescriptions or discontinued at discharge.

Information Availability

The cross-continuum EMR and CPOE process ensures that a complete picture of the patient's medication history and profile is available at each level of care. The EMR also allows unprecedented access to patients' charts across all venues of care except home health and long-term care environments. Non-Sentara providers who send patients to a Sentara facility for care or testing have access to the Sentara EMR for retrieval of clinical data. Consolidation of clinical data into a single source offers care providers clinical data that have never been available electronically. The key to accomplishing this integration was the implementation of an Enterprise Master Patient Index prior to the EMR implementation. These successes have led Sentara to investigate further integration opportunities with home health and long-term care, and non-Sentara EMRs.

Tailored Decision Support

To accommodate the variety of user types and disciplines afforded access to the EMR, Sentara created unique user templates to facilitate workflows. The Sentara EMR uses workflow components called "navigators." The navigators guide the end user through the most efficient process for specific workflows (e.g. admission, transfer, discharge, clinic visits, etc). In addition to providing efficient processes for data entry and retrieval, the navigator helps ensure standardization of workflows and consistent data capture. Customized data retrieval templates show combinations of clinical data appropriate for specific providers and venues of care. Streamlined "View Only" templates are available for providers with limited data retrieval needs.

Decision Support

Sentara has a long history of developing and customizing algorithms for clinical decision support specifically related to medication therapy. The focus of these efforts has been to reduce the number of unnecessary alerts while increasing the number of appropriate alerts. Inpatient physicians see medication alerts for drug-drug interactions, drug-allergy, maximum dose, and pregnancy/lactation. Recent data analysis demonstrated that 23 percent of the time, the physician providers took action when these alerts appeared during order entry. The success Sentara has achieved in this area is due to customization of the vendor-supplied external alerts logic within the EMR application.

The EMR also provides formulary substitute alerts. These alerts direct the prescriber to the appropriate choice of medication based on pharmacy and therapeutics committee decisions. Sentara has taken a cautious approach to the implementation of alerts and reminders to avoid compromising adoption. Many medication alerts are utilized (e.g. duplicate therapy, drug versus laboratory results, drug versus disease state, etc.) by pharmacists to ensure safety while not overburdening physicians with alerts. Other disciplines have taken advantage of the alerts and reminders. For example, alerts are in place for nursing staff to help ensure compliance with immunization protocols. Nurses and clinicians can use custom columns on their patient lists to display specific values when thresholds are exceeded. This functionality affords a quick and high-level overview of specific conditions over a large population of patients.

Practice Standardization

Clinical decision support tools that take on a more passive role in the EMR include order sets, care plans, patient education templates, navigators, patient-level customized views of clinical data, and cascading flowsheets. These tools help to standardize care based on best practice and provide information relative to the patient's conditions at the point-of-care. Requests for decision support functionality typically come from user groups and quality-related committees. A new clinical decision support committee was formed to provide a more formal governance structure for the development and management of clinical decision support.

Provider Communications

eCare has revolutionized communication conveyance among caregivers. The Sentara EMR system has an internal messaging system that is at the core of communication between providers and patients. The internal messaging system manages the processing of unsigned documents, provides reminders to physicians regarding chart deficiencies, and sends information about abnormal laboratory results. Nurses can notify pharmacy to replenish medications. It allows direct communication between physicians and nurses in the practice setting and facilitates communications between patients and physicians via the patient portal and direct communication among providers.

Knowledge Access

The method for providing context-sensitive information to the providers has changed because of the EMR. Medications have associated hyperlinks which, when selected, will refer the provider to a drug database containing information specific to the medication selected. Work is ongoing toward bringing disease-specific references to ICD-9 diagnoses displayed in various sections of the medical record. Links to clinical evidence and protocols are provided within specific order sets. The use of interdisciplinary care plans facilitates communication among care providers within a common space in the patient record.

Data Sharing

EMR implementation has opened many possibilities in the area of data sharing. Sentara sends data to state and national registries, such as the Essence Health Report project, the CDC Biosense database, and the Virginia Department of Health. Care providers and medical records staff can route patient summary data to the next provider(s) of care via facsimile server from within the EMR when the patient is to be seen by a provider not on EMR. The patient portal is proving to be an important mechanism for patient-physician communication. The portal allows patients to view physician-specified test results; request and view office appointments, request prescription refills, access disease and medication reference materials, and communicate via internal messaging with their physician. By May 2010, there were more than 24,000 MyChart users. Future functionality will likely allow patients to enter medical and family history data for assimilation into the record by the care providers.

Secondary Uses of eCare Data

The Sentara EMR integrates with the external hospital and practice management registration and billing system. Patient charges originated in the EMR flow via HL7 interface to the hospital and practice management systems. A significant portion of charges generated in the EMR is the by-product of clinical documentation. This ensures greater accuracy between patients' bills and the clinical documentation. Moreover, the EMR has led to significant clinical and quality report development. Sentara improved its quality measures since the EMR implementation as a result of the ability to monitor compliance and make appropriate interventions. Real-time reports are used to identify patients who may need interventions to assure quality and safety compliance. Staff and leadership use historical reporting to analyze and report management, quality, and safety data to internal and external stakeholder groups. As a non-teaching health system, Sentara is modestly involved in clinical trials and research initiatives.

TECHNOLOGY

Scope and Design of eCare System

The eCare platform supports 3,000 end users employing a mix of Windows and UNIX server technologies. At the heart of the multi-tier server architecture lays the primary and failover UNIX database servers. These servers are equivalently architected Hewlett Packard (HP) Titanium Superdomes containing 12 Titanium 1.5 GHz processors, 32 GB of physical memory and run HP-UX version 11iv2. These servers deploy an Intersystems Cache database shared among all eCare applications. In the event of hardware failure on the primary database server, failover to the second database server can occur within 10 minutes. The average Central Processing Unit utilization on the database server during peak load is 25 percent. Ten HP Titanium RX26600 servers handle the application-processing layer, each containing four processors, 16 GB physical memory and running HP-UX 11iv2 for their operating system. Utilizing Intersystems Enterprise Cache Protocol, application processing is separated from the backend database process, which provides the ability to scale the platform by adding application servers.

Figure 19-3 provides a diagram of the eCare network configuration. As illustrated, production data are replicated to three other HP Titanium Superdomes UNIX servers. One server acts as a read-write copy of the database and is used in the event of a catastrophic failure on the primary storage hardware. The second server is used as a reporting server, which provides the ability to query production data in near real time. This offloads reporting requests from the production database. The third server provides a read-only copy of the database. During system maintenance, eCare users have read-only access to the production data. Replication between the production database and the three shadows occurs by utilizing the shadow functionality within the Intersystems Cache database. Latency between production and the shadow servers averages around 15 seconds during peak utilization. All servers hosting critical functionality are architected in a redundant fashion. No single server component or complete server failure will cause system unavailability.

Storage

An HP XP12000 with 3 terabytes of usable Raid 10 disk space and 36 GBs cache memory provides storage for the production database server.

Desktop

Epic is deployed to 11,000 desktops utilizing Citrix 4.5 running on x86 OS platform. The Citrix farm includes 70 dedicated servers for the eCare environment. Using Citrix servers allows quick additional capacity without software loads on individual desktops. Sentara uses flowcharts (workstations on wheels) and wall units but not tablets or iPads.

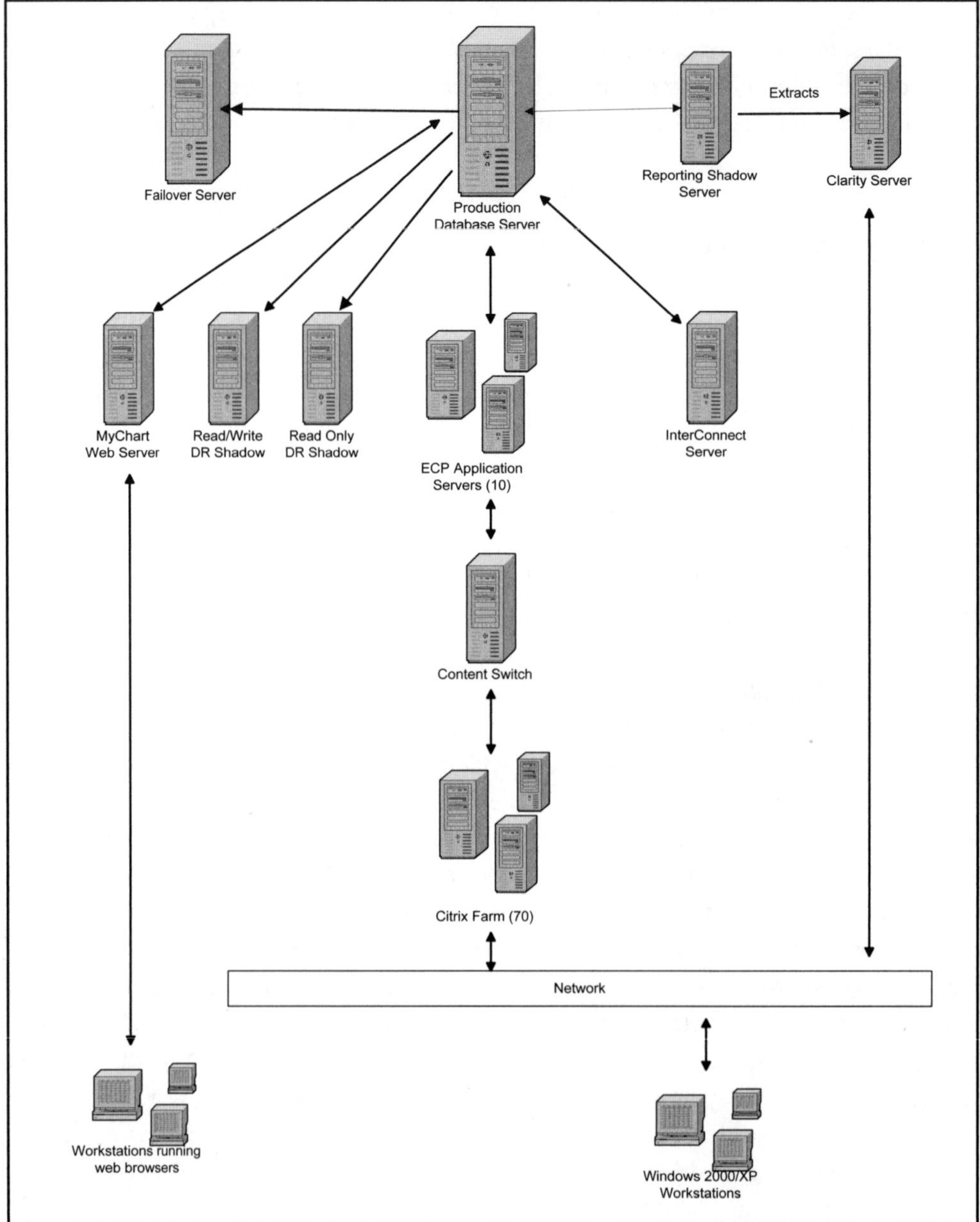

Figure 19-3: Physical Layer Network Configuration for eCare Health Network

Remote Access

Remote access to the EMR environment for physicians is provided using the Citrix solution via a Web portal. MyChart provides a patient portal to the EMR. Patients have access to portions of their medical record by their primary care provider. MyChart is hosted on a pair of load-balanced HP Windows servers. As of May 2009, more than 25,000 patients have MyChart access. Additional practices are added monthly.

Interfaces and Integration

The EMR system shares a single database that integrates clinical and financial data from all SMGs, hospitals, labs. New functionality will soon allow other Epic and non-Epic sites to share patients' clinical data in real time. eCare has replaced many of the legacy systems within the Sentara enterprise, yet some ancillary systems and medical devices remain; for example, Cerner Lab, PACS radiology and Picis Surgery.

Interoperability

eCare is integrated with most clinical systems within the Sentara enterprise and shares information with other agencies. The *Care Everywhere* application from Epic allows Sentara to share clinical data with any other Epic hospital, whereas *Care Elsewhere* supports sharing clinical information with non-Epic EMR systems. Sentara shares ED data with the Centers for Disease Control and Prevention (CDC) in an effort to assist in detecting and monitoring outbreaks. Sentara also extends our EMR to community physician practices. Sentara participates in the statewide health information exchange testing.

Scalability

By using Citrix, Sentara can deliver a fully functional application client through their local area network and via the Web, providing a consistent presentation of the Epic application. As the need to access the application grows, additional servers support the increasing load. As updates are needed, they are patched to the servers at the data center, which patches the client whenever the user launches the application. When the user load is low, the servers can be pulled out of the mix, updated, and then put back into service to reduce user downtime.

Data Warehouse

Sentara is moving its enterprise informatics strategy to a consolidated enterprise warehouse model. Sentara's strategy brings clinical, financial, operational, human resources and materials data together. This allows a broad array of analysis and predictive modeling. The clinical repository stores information from our primary EMR. Benchmark information from industry vendors is incorporated, allowing for external comparisons. Clinical information will be extracted from other ancillary systems in future phases. Sentara's technology architecture is primarily the Microsoft Business Intelligence solutions.

Sentara uses MS/SQL server as the primary database, MS/SSIS as the ETL layer, and MS/Analytical Services as the OLAP layer. Cross-continuum of care analysis is being incorporated into the informatics strategy that allows analysis from the physician's office, hospital setting, home care, long-term care and health plan. The analysis will focus on population and disease management and provide information on appropriate care delivery, such as preventable readmissions.

Network Facts

- 333 Communication Closets
- 2,369 Networking Devices
- 5,024 Wireless Devices

- 29,979 Customer Devices
- 33,588 Voice Devices
- 290 miles of fiber between hospitals

Security and Data Integrity

To protect privacy and confidentiality, Sentara implemented a role-based security model for the EMR. Each user type is built to include only the security functions necessary to perform their job duties. The training curriculum is tailored to this role-based model to ensure employee competency. The eCare security team performs quarterly audits and reviews all active users to validate that they have the appropriate security for their job role. Sentara's EMR technical services team runs daily integrity checks on the production database.

Confidentiality

Sentara requires employees and non-employees to sign a statement of confidentiality and complete integrity training on an annual basis. The confidentiality agreement states that the employee will only view patient data specific to the patient care requirements. A privacy hotline is in place to report suspected security breaches or inappropriate use of the system. During the breach investigation, the eCare security team can run Clarity audit reports on the patient record, perform a full chart audit, and forward to the Privacy Officer for review. If a breach occurs, the appropriate disciplinary action is taken, up to and including termination.

System Integrity and Disaster Recovery

Sentara uses multiple technologies to protect system integrity and provide disaster recovery. Some options are hot stand-by systems, fault tolerant systems, or clustered systems. Sentara contracts with SunGard for disaster recovery services.

Data Model

eCare has a centralized database that documents both the ambulatory and hospital-based patient care. eCare employs Smart Tools that allows for standardization of terminologies and maintaining data definitions. Smart Tools contains preconfigured text that can be used to standardize documentation, such as notes, within the system. SmartTools include SmartLinks, SmartLists, SmartPhrases, and SmartTexts.

Standards

When possible, patient data are entered or interfaced into the eCare database. The data are entered directly or are electronically interfaced using an HL7 feed from other third-party systems. Interfaced data include lab results, imaging results, medical device data, transcriptions, pharmacy, and scanned documents. Interfaced data allow eCare to provide a complete clinical display to care providers from a single platform.

Response Time

Response time on the eCare system is monitored at several levels. Robotic probes measure Citrix initiation and login response time. The probes identify exceptions and send daily management reports. A Response Time Tracker monitors specific workflows in

Epic Hyperspace, and both Sentara and Epic review response times. Epic Instrumentation is installed on the workstation to address specific response time to user complaints and to track exceptions and pinpoint causes.

Continuity Planning

eCare has built-in mechanisms to account for system or network outage. In the event that the entire system is unavailable, a separate Disaster Recovery Shadow server keeps the system functional. In the event of a wide area network outage, eCare has Business Continuity Access (BCA) Web servers at each hospital that contain patient lists and schedules that are updated throughout every day. In the event of a local area network outage at a facility, eCare has BCA workstations in every department and every ambulatory site. These BCA workstations also contain patient lists and schedules that are updated throughout every day.

Analysis and Reporting

eCare applications offer great flexibility to design, program, and distribute operational and analytical information. eCare provides innumerable reports, queries, and graphs for real-time display and printing, such as revenue cycles, clinical outcomes, etc. Moreover, eCare allows the capture, storage, and extraction of discrete data into another database for analytics and information conveyance. eCare supports over 500 reports and more than 50 work queues. Concurrent reports allow real-time LOS analysis, usage patterns, chronic disease management, bar code compliance, CPOE statistics, and Joint Commission reporting. Retrospective reports include physician utilization, medical utilization, and procedure volume.

VALUE

Total Cost of Ownership

Information technology, aided by Decision Support and Finance, developed the Total Cost of Ownership (TCO) 10-year forecast. The TCO was based on extensive research into the best practices for implementing an EMR across the continuum of care (hospitals, ambulatory sites, and physician practices). A TCO was calculated for the three top vendors, as were the benefits, so that the comparative business cases could be properly evaluated. To ensure the TCO was realistic, a consulting firm with EMR experience was hired to conduct a thorough assessment and to validate the assumptions and estimates.

The TCO was vetted by the directors of finance from all divisions, as well as by an extensive number of operational and senior leaders. Process owners presented the benefits to their counterparts to further refine and validate the estimates and expand the "ownership" of the benefits commitment. Draft TCO and benefits were presented to the CEO Work Group and the chairman of the board in separate meetings to obtain guidance and commitment. These "premeetings" resulted in guidance to obtain additional benefits commitments from process owners, as the initial estimates were too conservative. The TCO over 10 years showed the magnitude of the effort. Below is the final TCO and benefits estimate:

Capital .... $ 67 M
Operating expenses .... $ 170 M
Hardware maintenance .... $ 15 M
Software maintenance .... $ 50 M
Disaster recovery .... $ 3 M
Work redesign .... $ 36 M
Training .... $ 16 M
Implementation .... $ 22 M
Ongoing support .... $ 22 M
Other non-salary support .... $ 6 M
Total Cost of Ownership over 10 years .... $ 237 M

The benefits (ROI, VOI) agreed to by process owners, Sentara executives, and IT leaders in June 2005 were:

Hospitals Total .... $30.0 M
Reduced nursing overtime & improve retention .... $ 5.2 M
Reduced IT maintenance .... 4.2 M
Reduced medical records/transcription .... 4.1 M
Increased outpatient services .... 3.2 M
Reduced length-of-stay .... 3.1 M
Improved Rx process/reduced adverse drug events .... 2.9 M
Reduced paper/storage .... 2.4 M
Other improvements .... 4.9 M
Home Health Total .... $2.7 M
Sentara Health Plan Total .... $2.8 M*
Sentara Healthcare Total .... $35.5 M†

Values of investment (VOI) expectations presented to the board were:

- Provide one patient chart with real-time information.
- Provide accessible charts anytime, anywhere to all providers.
- Improve communication among nurses, primary care physicians, specialists, etc.
- Streamline medication process in hospitals, physician offices, and home health.
- Reduce illegible orders and wasted time due to handwriting issues.
- Improve physicians' ability to round for others from office/home.
- Enhance recruiting and retention of physicians and staff.
- Increase ease of scheduling in office, patient's homes, anywhere.
- Eliminate duplicate tests, which cause delays and unnecessary work.
- Provide evidence-based medicine alerts and reminders.
- Streamline care management and discharge processes.
- Optimize staff time by minimizing time spent retrieving patient information.
- Improve reporting capability to help with research, pay for performance, etc.
- Enhance patient education and disease management programs.
- Bottom line: The EMR will improve health and save lives.

---

* 62% of Sentara Health Plan benefits will be passed on to employers.

† Excludes $2.7 M in Sentara Medical Group (SMG) benefits which will accrue to SMG physicians.

Process Redesign Efforts

The CIO tasked the redesign professionals to work with operations and the eCare team to analyze and redesign core processes to ensure the transformation of care. There were more than 200 individuals assigned to 18 process redesign teams. The selected processes were those that had the most significant financial or qualitative potential.

1. Arrival Management (registration, ambulatory testing, order entry)
2. Bed Management
3. Case Management
4. Charge Capture
5. Claims Processing
6. Clinical Communications
7. Disease Management
8. Emergency Department
9. Home Health
10. Medical Records
11. Meds Management
12. Monitoring/Recording
13. Order Sets
14. Patient Care Transformation
15. Patient/Member Satisfaction (MyChart)
16. Physician Practice
17. Physician Processes
18. Scheduling

These 18 redesign teams of Sentara salaried employees committed several hours a week for three months to a Lean Six Sigma effort. The teams analyzed current processes, measured performance, identified opportunities, and designed the ideal processes. The redesigned processes were then sorted into four categories; (1) changes that would be achieved by Epic, (2) those for which Sentara needed to do something to exploit Epic, (3) those in which the changes had nothing to do with Epic, and (4) changes for future consideration. The compensated Physician Advisory Group of 25 members reviewed the results for validity.

In April 2006, the redesigned processes were reviewed over a two-day period with more than 100 Sentara executives, eCare team members, operational and IT leaders, and Epic managers. The eCare DBV efforts commenced after the process redesigns were completed and the team members had been to training at Epic. The DBV teams included many of the process redesign members to ensure that the system was built so benefits would be realized. In several cases, the teams learned through the build phase that many benefits would not be realized just by installing the EMR.

DBV, PAG, and Implementation

Design/Build/Validate efforts lasted nearly two years. The efforts were heavily influenced by the process redesign work, best practice research into workflow processes, and by a commitment to transform performance. The DBV team relied extensively on the PAG to ensure the processes and the EMR were designed with providers' perspectives in mind. While the DBV and PAG efforts continued, implementation and training teams were formed to work with operations on plans that would enable a smooth transition to a paperless world.

After the first go-live, subsequent hospital staff was able to shadow experienced EMR users. Being able to ask questions of those who had successfully made the journey helped them have a more meaningful transition experience.

Optimization

The CIO placed optimization teams into the divisions before, during, and after go-live to help operations do the following priority tasks:

- Stabilize facility and increase physician adoption.
- Achieve eCare business case.
- Leverage eCare to achieve additional benefits.
- Find divisions and systemwide non-eCare opportunities.

The optimization teams, made up of eCare experts and process improvement professionals, adhered to the concepts:

- Measure ("what gets measured, gets improved")
- Budget-expected benefits
- Align goals
- Hold process owners, operations, and optimization accountable

The ongoing optimization teams report to the Executive Optimization Committee (EOC). The EOC sets priorities, monitors progress, and resolves issues related to the EMR project. The Optimization Project Management Office reviews potential projects, prioritizes resources, and shares best practice ideas.

Benefits Tracking

In keeping with the notion that eCare is bigger than Epic, the Executive Design Committee (EDC) decided to use 2006 as the baseline year. In 2007, expected benefits were embedded in the 2008 goals for key executives and in divisional and departmental budgets. Moreover, a scorecard, as shown in Table 19-1, was established and baseline performance measured.

After the first hospital went live, daily meetings were held to review various performance metrics to identify potential problems before they became entrenched. More than 40 measures were utilized around financial performance, throughput times, and volume metrics. After three weeks, reporting was reduced to every other day and even-

Table 19-1: Scorecard

eCare Benefits in Addition to Business Case
2009 Q4 Benefits Achieved

		Hospital						
#	Benefit	SLH	SBH	SVBGH	SNGH	SWRMC	SCH	Total
1	Reduce IP Labs	$196,993	-$50,813	$114,770	$196,577	-$36,038	$39,499	$460,987
2	ED Registration Staff	$22,940	$43,710	$18,290	$20,770	$15,810	$43,710	$165,230
3	Order Entry/ AA Staff	$311,201	$125,552	$405,246	$676,556	$184,718	$331,009	$2,034,282
4	Endoscopy Staff	-$19,000	$0	-$20,500	-$19,500	$0	$0	-$59,000
5	Rehab Transcriptionist Staff	$31,000	$31,000	$31,000	$0	$0	$0	$93,000
6	Leapfrog EMR Benefits							$177,611
	Total Additional eCare Benefits	$543,134	$149,449	$548,805	$874,403	$164,489	$414,219	$2,872,110

tually phased out as a monthly ROI scorecard began to be populated and process performance was measured.

Perhaps the most important metric tracked was bar coding performance. Medications bar coding was simultaneously implemented with Epic EMR and Onbase document scanning. CPOE was phased in over several months at the first hospital and initiated at go-live at the subsequent hospitals. However, the document scanning process had major performance issues with nursing and pharmacy processes.

A major lesson learned is that the process redesign experts must work with the systemwide process owners, as well as the individual department heads. This worked well with all departments except medical records/scanning, surgery, and endoscopy, in which the magnitude of the changes exceeded our ability to get the departments prepared for go-live. Through post go-live process redesign efforts, performance improved, and future hospitals benefitted from lessons learned at the first hospital.

Documenting eCare Value

In 2009, the financial ROI and the qualitative value of investment benefits far exceeded projections based on an expected slow rate of adoption of best practices. The following is a summary list of realized benefits.

Streamlined Care Processes and Enhanced Medication Alerts

- 88,500 potential medication errors were avoided due to bar coding scanning alerts.
- 7 of 10 EDs improved their triage performance; 4 of 10 EDs improved their admit time performance, and all hospitals improved their patient throughput times.
- The median percentage for all 14 patient flow metrics improved; over half of them by greater than 25 percent.
- Percentage of patients with angioplasty within 90 minutes of arrival increased from 78 percent in Q1 2009 to 90 percent in Q1 2010.
- Percentage of outpatient surgery patients who had antibiotics started within 60 minutes of incision increased from 84 percent in Q1 2009 to 92 percent in Q1 2010.

Ordering Process

- CPOE reduced medication order entry to administration time from 59 minutes to 4 minutes.
- CPOE and medication bar coding decreased time from order written to medication administered (NOW orders) from 132 minutes to 38 minutes.
- Elimination of duplicate orders reduced inpatient lab tests by 5.5 percent.

Medical Records

- SMG transcription, medical records, and malpractice premiums reduced by $1.4 million dollars.
- Hospital medical records savings of $3.9 million due to paperless environment.

Efficiency Benefits

- 190 FTEs redirected to more value-added activities.
- $9.4 million in savings as a result of reduction in nursing overtime and purchased labor.
- Increased outpatient revenue $4.4 million dollars due to being "easier to do business with."

Length-of-Stay Improvements

- $9.4 million in LOS savings as a result of streamlined care processes.
- Sentara Health Plan realized $2.2 million as a result of reduction in severity-adjusted LOS.

Turnaround Times

- The time from bed assignment to admit an ED patient has decreased 90 minutes.
- Central scheduling average speed to answer was reduced from 71 to 10 seconds, and the abandonment rate was reduced from 9 to 3 percent.

Quality Improvements

- Readmission ratios reduced at each hospital from 23 to 18 percent.
- Compliance with influenza immunizations enabled Sentara to identify the epidemic had passed and to notify the state health department of its findings.
- SMG implemented Physician Quality Reporting Initiatives in primary and specialty practices.
- Sentara's CMS core measures percentages of green metrics doubled from 36 percent (Q1 2009) to 72 percent (Q1 2010).

Miscellaneous

- 87 percent CPOE for six hospitals.
- 25,000 registered MyChart users have access to portions of their chart and electronic communications with their physician offices.
- Risk Management Claims reduced $250,000 per year.
- Denials reduced with annual savings of $700,000.
- Enhanced communications with and among physicians and their ability to round from office or home improved the timeliness of care decisions.
- Expectation of being 100 percent compliant with Stage One Meaningful Use requirements.

Sentara Medical Group EMR Benefits

- Automated Referral Process – Sentara can now track physician-to-physician referrals, which improves patient safety by eliminating overdue referral messages.
- Automated Central Authorizations – The Referral Management System automatically conducts the MRI and CT authorizations upon physician order entry.
- My Action Plan – Primary care providers provide this automatically generated health maintenance document to patients at check-in. The plan enables

patients to take ownership of the accuracy of their medical information and motivates them to ensure that preventative care items are addressed.
- Optima Health Plan Integration – This allows Disease Management caseworkers to view the patient's record and document their interactions. Also, HEDIS claims-based data can be validated without pulling charts.
- Template Development – Sentara is piloting standardized templates to achieve two goals; (1) guide physicians to use nationally accepted protocols for managing specific diagnoses, and (2) ensure that physicians select the appropriate billing code for the amount and type of documentation.
- Quality Intelligence – Sentara is now producing disease registries and exception reports for diabetes and heart/stroke quality indicators. This has led to the implementation of best practices, and qualifies SMG for NCQA (National Committee for Quality Assurance) recognition.

User Satisfaction

End-user satisfaction with the EMR is an evolving process that requires ongoing measurement and evaluation. Sentara adopted several formal avenues for physician and staff feedback. We triangulate our survey findings based on paper and automated survey tools, conduct open-ended interviews with key stakeholders, and solicit randomly-selected caregivers for their informal feedback. Sentara utilized the Epic post assessment methodology and an in-house tool. End users were evaluated at one, four, and eight months post go-live. Overall, the results of both formal avenues of assessment demonstrated "good" end-user satisfaction. The Epic assessment reflected a 7 out of 10 level satisfaction. (One represented "extreme dissatisfaction" and 10 represented "extreme satisfaction.") The Sentara assessment demonstrated "good" end-user satisfaction with results of four or higher on a 5-point Likert scale.

The survey results were shared throughout the organization and used to prioritize optimization activities. Many workflow and software changes were also initiated. For example, the clinical staff identified that the "effective hand-off tool" should be streamlined to allow for easier communication between caregivers. The physician staff identified areas of improvement within ordering and documentation processes. Through user interaction with medical staff and interdisciplinary teams, the PAG improved order-set content, streamlined documentation tools, and worked collaboratively with the Epic user community. Key changes were made to the educational program including additional computer based training and interactive learning sessions such as skills day and department-based education. Training was also enhanced from a generalist approach to be more user-role specific. This resulted in improved user satisfaction and performance.

WHAT'S NEXT?

In the journey to achieving HIMSS Analytics Stage 7, Sentara did not encounter any significant negative EMR experiences. With six hospitals and over 100 physician practices implemented, eCare is a resounding success. Moreover, eCare provides a solid platform to launch advanced strategic programs in the pursuit of improving patient safety, quality clinical outcomes, and affordable patient care delivery.

CHAPTER 20

Case Study: NorthShore University HealthSystem

Thomas W. Smith

WHO WE ARE

NorthShore University HealthSystem (NorthShore) is headquartered in Evanston, Illinois. It is a comprehensive, fully integrated healthcare delivery system that serves the greater North Shore and northern Illinois communities. NorthShore includes four hospitals located, at most, 15 miles apart. The system has more than 2,000 affiliated physicians, including a multi-specialty group practice, with over 75 office locations as part of its employed Medical Group of 650 physicians. Further, NorthShore is committed to excellence in its academic mission and supports teaching and research as the principal teaching affiliate of the University of Chicago's Pritzker School of Medicine. The NorthShore University HealthSystem Research Institute has more than $100 million in grants and focuses on clinical and translational research, including leadership in outcomes research and clinical trials.

NorthShore has annual revenues of $1.6 billion and a staff of more than 8,000. The integrated health system has significant capabilities in a wide spectrum of clinical programs, including cancer, heart, orthopedics, high-risk maternity, and pediatrics. NorthShore is a national leader in the implementation of innovative technologies, including the electronic medical record (EMR). In 2003, NorthShore was among the first in the country to successfully launch a systemwide EMR with demonstrable benefits in quality, safety, efficiency, and service to patients. NorthShore University HealthSystem has been recognized by multiple national organizations for this notable achievement, including having received the 2004 Davies Award. NorthShore has worked hard to share its EMR experience and has hosted over 100 site visits, including more than 10 from international organizations. NorthShore was formerly known as Evanston Northwestern Healthcare, a name that was changed in 2008 to reflect its change in teaching affiliation. In 2009, HIMSS Analytics selected NorthShore as one of the first two organizations for its EMR Adoption Model℠ (EMRAM) Stage 7 Award.

IMPACT OF ADVANCED CLINICAL SYSTEMS FOR PHYSICIANS, NURSES AND PATIENTS

NorthShore University HealthSystem is the first integrated healthcare system to put a totally EMR system into an acute care setting at the same time as it was implemented in the physician office setting. The EMR install built upon a series of successful installs of major ancillary systems, including a large distributed picture archiving and communications system (PACS). The significance of this state-of-the-art EMR system—in use by 100 percent of all physicians, nurses, and other medical professionals at NorthShore University HealthSystem—is that all patient-related documentation and orders are now paperless throughout the organization. All practitioners work from a single, integrated source of clinical information that is secure, current, legible, organized, and instantly accessible in all NorthShore University HealthSystem locations and anywhere Internet access is available. The EMR includes links to images in the respective ancillary system, such as Cardiology or Radiology by a hyperlink at the bottom of the specialists' interpretative report. This link allows the clinician access without an additional patient search or another sign-on.

Each year NorthShore has more than 60,000 admissions, 1,200,000 office visits, and 125,000 emergency department (ED) visits. All of this data are added to the same clinical and administrative database. The patient portal (NorthShore*Connect*) has more than 125,000 users. NorthShore is a highly centralized, integrated health system, with one set of information systems applications supporting all of its processes across the system. In addition, NorthShore has one professional staff across its four hospitals.

WHERE WE CAME FROM

The history of computer systems at Evanston, or NorthShore, started in the early 1970s with mainframe billing and payroll systems. By the mid-1970s, there was also a minicomputer laboratory system in place. Some small cardiology systems were in place by the mid-1980s.

It was not until the late 1980s that the first local area network (LAN) and a small number of personal computers (PCs) were installed in the finance department. In 1990, there were 250 dumb terminals connected to the mainframe systems covering the then two hospitals and fewer than 20 PCs in place for financial analysis at the corporate office building. The connectivity between the data center and the second hospital was only a single 56k data line.

The number of PCs and LAN drops quickly grew, and by the mid-1990s, the organization had several clinical systems that were connected through the LAN for registration and billing purposes. Reporting of results at this time was still on paper. At this point, a clinical clerk order entry and results reporting system was installed on the mainframe. This system interfaced with the previously stand-alone minicomputer systems. Results could be accessed for the major departments from the mainframe system (CliniPac) through mostly dumb terminals on the floors. The paper chart was still the main source of information for the physicians. Fewer than than 20 percent of our active physicians would have signed on to a computer in any given year at this time.

By the mid-1990s, the trend was away from the mainframe and the development of particularly clinical systems on minicomputer platforms. These machines could connect to a LAN; and therefore, soon the organization became wired throughout by connecting by hard wire the various systems and access to some of them directly from the floor. A plan was established to follow a Best-of-Breed (BoB) with a major vendor who had purchased many individual companies and was integrating these systems into a "complete medical record." This plan was followed until 2001 with mixed results.

In 1998, a new chairman of Radiology was selected and, with him, planning for a PACS system was started. This resulted in a radiology information system (RIS) and a PACS system being both selected and installed in 1999. In 2000, a post discharge chart-imaging product was implemented. This required all physicians to complete their charts online. At this time then, all physicians had—and used (even if for a limited purpose)—a computer sign-on.

The success of these two systems was significant to the decision to proceed with an EMR in 2001. Both projects were successful. The LAN had good uptime percentages, and it was not a huge step to consider removing charts if we had successfully removed all patient films. We also installed a SONET Ring between our major buildings (our third hospital had joined us in 2000) to provide the necessary bandwidth and reliability for the radiology image transfers. This decision and subsequent implementation also served us well when we decided to proceed with the EMR.

In 2001, we decided to implement an enterprise-wide EMR that would cover both the then three hospitals and the approximately 50 office practices for our employed medical group. The plan was to extend the EMR by offering it to the independent physicians (through the Stark provisions) once the employed offices were all installed. Our previous success in the area of PACS and the chart imaging system, as well as the SONET, were part of the background that allowed us the confidence to proceed. In 2001, there were no other integrated health systems that we knew of that had a centralized patient database that covered both hospitals and offices. At this point, the major sites of success were self-developed systems at major academic centers. There were several successful installs of office billing systems and a limited number of office EMRs in place for large physician groups often attached to a major university or a teaching hospital. We were not aware of any organizations that had installed commercial systems that covered both offices and hospitals.

WHY WE ADOPTED THE EMR

In 1999 and 2000, the Institute of Medicine (IOM) issued two reports: "To Err is Human" and "Crossing the Quality Chasm." The research in these reports that evidenced medical errors that resulted in unnecessary deaths were difficult to ignore. The natural question to ask, then, was how we could stop these errors and improve care for our patients.

Many of the medical errors in the IOM reports could be prevented by an effective computer system. For example, handwriting errors in placing medication orders could be eliminated by CPOE. The ability to check on allergies and other medications when placing a medication order could also be made part of the CPOE process.

The beginning of the internal discussions focused on two points:

1. An EMR that will improve some of the IOM issues is the "right thing to do."
2. Can we select and implement such a system, given that no one else had done this across both our hospitals and physician offices with a commercial system?

We decided to proceed with two main objectives:

1. Improve patient safety through the tools of an EMR
2. Establish a longitudinal, patient-centric database, covering both hospitals and offices

In 2001, the current long-range plan for NorthShore included the goal of becoming the best integrated healthcare system in the region. NorthShore senior management agreed that a successful EMR implementation would greatly aid this goal.

NorthShore has a history of tightly centralizing all administrative systems and departments. The concept of being able to apply this centralization and, more importantly, consistency across all clinical settings was viewed as a very important goal; it was a goal that was worth the obvious risks involved in deciding to pursue a joint hospital and office clinical system that would replace all paper charts and develop a longitudinal patient-centric database.

During informal discussions between administrative and physician leadership and board members, the board members were strong supporters of the concept. Many of them were used to a comparable system in their businesses, which often used products such as SAP to oversee large parts of their operations.

In March 2001, we made the decision to select such a system. This decision was driven by the commitment to reduce or eliminate the sources of medical error identified by the IOM reports. It was possible to take on a high-risk decision due to the long-term tenure of the CEO/COO/CIO and other key management and physician staff and the trust that had developed over time. For example, the key physician had practiced his whole career at NorthShore and was then president of the professional staff. His role and the confidence the professional staff had in his judgment were critical to the project.

The CEO made gaining approval of this implementation project a personal objective. He ensured the project was clearly led by users—both administrative and clinical. Once the project was approved by the board, the incentive system was used to support the project. In a normal year there might be 100 or more individual goals spread among 200 individuals that would be used to calculate success and payments of incentives. For the years 2002 through 2004, there was only one goal for any participant in the incentive system—install the Epic inpatient and ambulatory EMRs on-time and on-budget. This focus created a great deal of support and led to quicker decision making and great support for the project as a whole.

The county surrounding the NorthShore service area (Cook County, Illinois) is one of the hardest areas in which to acquire malpractice insurance coverage in the United States. NorthShore has for years carried a $20 million (and now $25 million) deductible, with only claims over that level covered by an umbrella plan secured out of the country. We had a great incentive to improve patient safety and improve processes to reduce patient harm. These cases often were clearly ones that could have been stopped or greatly reduced by the implementation of an EMR. This was also reinforced by the

IOM reports. This connection was not lost on our board members when they were asked to approve the additional capital dollars for the EMR project.

While we were starting with the hospitals and the employed medical group, it was always our intention to reach out to the independent offices through the Stark provisions. This started in 2004 and allowed a method to tie in the offices that generate over 50 percent of the hospital admissions that come from our independents. This allowed our focus of patient data and improved patient care to be increased by adding the sites which would bring in the most patient data. Today we have over 1,200,000 office visits added to the database each year.

A Steering Committee was established with the two project directors, the top seven management positions, and two physicians. The project directors, the CIO, and the senior vice president of the Medical Group had both been at NorthShore for several years and had worked on several projects together in the past. The Steering Committee established project objectives and goals to insure that the system was implemented across the health system in a consistent manner. The goal was set to use the EMR as a tool to further integrate the care of patients across the hospital floors, outpatient departments, EDs, operating rooms, and the physician offices. Goals for improvements in specific areas such as medication errors were set along with improvements in administrative processes.

We chose between two final vendor options. One had several hospitals that had installed their inpatient EMR but had no office installs. The second vendor (Epic) had many successful full EMR installs in large physician groups but no hospital installs. Epic was selected for several reasons, but their past success with physicians in the office settings was significant. We knew that the physicians were going to endure the biggest changes in their day-to-day activities, and we wanted a vendor experienced in meeting their needs.

NorthShore established an aggressive timetable for the implementation, believing that rapid implementation created the greatest potential to reduce the number of patient care errors and improve the quality of care. The sooner all healthcare providers were on the system, the sooner an individual provider would benefit from sharing the patient's EMR with another provider. As such, the organization chose a no-pilot, all-at-once approach to provide an integrated system as quickly as possible. Leadership believed that results within a hospital would not be realized until the implementation and integration from patient admission through discharge was completed within that hospital. The goal was to get to one set of information as quickly as possible and to reduce the risks inherent with requiring users to go to dual systems—paper and electronic.

At the start of the project, NorthShore made an important logistical decision for the inpatient roll-out. The clinical applications—ED, clinical documentation, CPOE, and pharmacy—would all go-live on the same day for a given hospital. In the ambulatory roll-out, the physician offices would go-live with scheduling, billing, ordering, clinical documentation, and CPOE on the day of go-live.

However, as described in detail next, NorthShore revised that strategy and implemented the system in two major phases for hospitals: (1) documentation, and then (2) order entry. For the physician offices: (1) administrative functions, and then (2) clinical. The hospital selected for the first implementation was Glenbrook Hospital because it was the smallest and most flexible in terms of culture.

EMR IMPLEMENTATION

Planning and Governance

Planning for the implementation ran on two parallel tracks. Track A was the hardware and technical track, which focused on selecting hardware for mobile devices in the clinical areas, installing our first wireless network, and setting up the central computer room hardware.

Track B focused on redesigning workflows and then building and installing the software to support these new workflows. Early on, the Steering Committee knew that to succeed, most if not all workflow processes would need to be examined and redesigned. Existing processes were too inconsistent and convoluted to have an electronic system dropped on top of them. Project management assigned a team leader to each of the seven operational areas involved, as well as a technical team led by the chief technology officer and a training team led by the chief learning officer. In selecting team leaders, project management selected those individuals with clinical experience, process redesign and performance improvement experience, and who had the trust of the operations staff. This team would be responsible for the detailed planning and preparation for the implementation.

Preparation

To implement a consistent set of processes for managing clinical information, NorthShore first had to develop a consistent set of processes. The Steering Committee and team leaders knew that while quality of care was believed to be excellent, variability in the delivery of that care was significant from facility to facility, floor to floor, shift to shift, and clinician to clinician.

Throughout the implementation process, NorthShore worked with the vendor, Epic Systems, to make enhancements to the applications to meet NorthShore's needs. Through this collaboration, Epic Systems interpreted the knowledge and skills of NorthShore clinicians to build a system with the flexibility to function for the variety of processes within an acute care setting. As we were the first hospitals to use Epic's software for CPOE, etc., Epic recognized these changes as needed for a system that would function in an acute care setting and built them into its applications.

To prepare for what was to be the project step that was going to involve the users the most, team leaders and key physician leaders participated in a training class on the capabilities of the new software. With this understanding, team leaders began to redesign workflows throughout the three hospitals. For three months, they led more than 150 end users through a complete analysis of the patients and information flow throughout their areas and the organization. This analysis touched every major workflow and revealed redundancies, workarounds, and hand-offs that significantly slowed the flow of patients and information and created numerous opportunities for error. With this insight into current processes, team leaders then worked intensively with end users to redesign the flow of information and create integrated workflows. The result was 500 high-level workflows that provide for consistency in managing clinical infor-

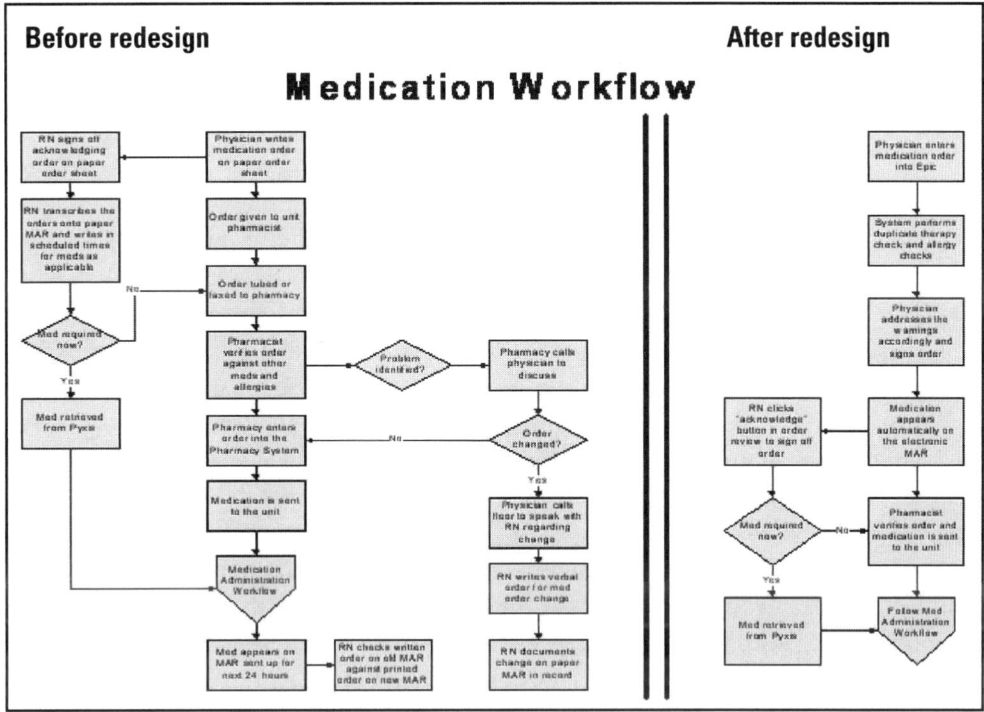

Figure 20-1: Sample Workflow Process: Medication Administration

mation across the organization. These 500 eventually were expanded into 2,000 detailed workflows, as we continue to believe that users relate better to workflows then master files or even screen layouts.

The high-level workflows laid the foundation for the simultaneous development of:

- Deeper, more detailed department and unit workflows (see Figure 20-1)
- Policies and procedures to support the new workflows
- Training materials
- System planning and build
- Communications for change management

As teams proceeded with the redesign of deeper workflows, they simultaneously gathered all paper documentation tools and order sets. Working with clinicians, the teams also analyzed and classified the data elements that were collected and reviewed. This enabled a complete redesign of the clinical information gathering by units. They then worked with IS to build the forms for documentation in the Epic system, so that users would enter data into the system only once. From there, it could be shared, retrieved, and reused by any clinician in the care and outcomes management of the patient across the continuum of care.

Simultaneously, physicians began standardizing physician documentation and order sets. They built templates to enable electronic documentation by physicians and established standards for order entry build. An indication of the success of these templates is the fact that many physicians quickly discontinued the practice of dictating notes and results and now enter them directly into the EMR. Similarly, the standard order sets developed for physicians practicing the same specialty provide a consistent quality of care. The physicians developed more than 1,000 order sets, which are widely used across the organization.

For the then 68 office practice sites, the ambulatory team developed a basic set of workflows to serve as a model for all sites. The standardized workflows assured that each office performed critical workflows in the same efficient manner, while allowing for the unique set of physicians, specialties, personnel mix, and physical characteristics at each location and practice. Organization-wide registration conventions ensured that equivalent information was collected and entered into the system in the identical way from largest site to smallest outlying office. This helped to establish basic routines from co-pay collection and payment posting to scheduling patients or taking phone messages from patients. Skeleton processes were formulated to standardize clinical workflow, while leaving ample room for individualized patient care.

Process and Staffing

The more technical application components of the implementation process began in summer 2002, following completion of the initial workflow analyses. It required conversion of the legacy patient demographics database from Medipac and the conversion of the clinical data repository (HNS). Cadence scheduling then replaced the organization's legacy Patient Appointment Scheduling system used by the hospital's outpatient diagnostic and treatment departments.

Hospital Inpatient and Outpatient

The schedule for the implementation was aggressive but attainable. The original plan for the hospitals was to go-live with everything—ED, clinical documentation, CPOE, and Pharmacy—on the same day. As the first hospital go-live date approached, March 15, 2003, the NorthShore project team realized that the plan for the "Big Bang" implementation needed modification. The new pharmacy system was ready to be used in the Pharmacy Department but was not yet ready for physician medication ordering.

The team made a sound decision to use a modified two-phase approach: go-live with documentation first and then CPOE. In the first phase, physicians and nurses performed all clinical documentation in the EMR. Ordering remained the same: physicians wrote orders on an order sheet, and clerical staff entered the orders. Medication orders went to Pharmacy on paper and the pharmacists entered the orders into the EMR. This gave nursing use of the eMAR at the first hospital go-live. Also, many of the hospital outpatient departments began entering their own orders between the documentation go-live and the CPOE go-live. This helped familiarize the ancillary departments with their own department's orders and helped identify any order transmittal issues prior to physician usage. The goal was for physicians to get comfortable with the system's documentation, security procedures, navigation, results and clinical information retrieval; it was also to work out any issues, and stabilize all equipment and devices before the physicians began CPOE.

At order entry go-live in May, all physicians began entering orders. Medication orders they entered were then automatically routed to Pharmacy for verification and dispensing only. Departmental orders either interfaced to or printed to an ancillary system. At this point, all paper was removed from the inpatient environment and patient charts were gone.

For each hospital go-live, NorthShore created a command center with 20 to 30 workstations, a phone at every workstation, two laser printers, a scanner, a lab label printer, a copy machine, a fax machine and 20 to 25 walkie-talkies. For two weeks, from the start of each go-live phase in each hospital, the command center was staffed 24/7 to provide support to end users and resolve any issues that surfaced.

In addition to the personnel based in the command center, support staff covered every clinical location in the hospital that was open for business. The support staffing levels were determined based upon volume and criticality. Support staff had varying degrees of knowledge and expertise, but all had more knowledge than the end users during the go-live. They included Epic personnel, consultants, and IS personnel—to resolve functionality issues and answer technical questions—and trainers and unit-based super users who had received special training.

Ambulatory

For each ambulatory off-site location, the implementation schedule included a staggered series of project plans that began four months before a site's go-live and allowed for three to five practices per month. In the first eight months, NorthShore rolled out all primary care sites, including Internal Medicine, Pediatrics, Obstetrics/Gynecology, and Family Medicine. Implementation for the remaining 30 specialties began in the ninth month and continued at the same pace.

The preparation meetings included office management and clinical staff along with project team members for registration, scheduling, billing, and the clinical system. Information Systems staff managed security, hardware, and connectivity strategy. The training team incorporated plans for training, competency testing, and allocating time to spend in the practice environment. As the go-live dates approached, appointment conversion from the older scheduling systems to the new one was completed. The team conducted dress rehearsals to test the planned workflows and hardware, from patient check-in through typical office visit scenarios to patient check-out.

Typically, the front desk operations went live at the first of the month to allow the staff time to adjust to the new routines. Two weeks later, the clinical staff began using the EMR. The ratio of support staff to clinical users was one to three for a full month. Weekly sessions with the staff worked through any workflow issues, allowed time for venting frustrations, and identified new training topics as needed.

The roll-out across the organization proceeded, as shown in Table 20-1.

The first physician office went live with scheduling (Cadence), enterprise registration (Prelude), professional billing (Resolute) and the EMR (EpicCare) Ambulatory on January 2, 2003. From this point, the ambulatory office roll-out and hospital roll-out were concurrent.

Transition to New Processes

Because this was a clinician-owned system, designed and specified by end users through the process redesign sessions, most were eager to transition to the new processes. The extensive and mandatory training prepared users for the change. Resources on hand at

Table 20-1: Timeline for EMR Roll-out Across Organization

Contract Signed	2001
Workflow Redesign, Build, Test, Training	2002
Glenbrook Hospital	2003
Evanston Hospital	2003
Highland Park Hospital	2003
50 Medical Group Offices	2003 - May, 2004
First Independent Office Go-Live	2004
25+ Medical Group Offices	2004 – 2009
Beacon Oncology Module	2005
20 Independent Office Go-Lives	2005 – 2009
Barcoding Med Administration	2007
Stork OB Module	2008
Hospital Billing Module	2009
OpTime Peri-Op Module	2009
Skokie Hospital	2009
Home Health Module	2011
Anesthesia Module	2011

go-live and beyond—super users, trainers, IS staff, supplemental IS staff consultants, and Epic staff—also supported the transition.

The culture of the organization also helped to achieve buy-in and ownership. NorthShore has a very strong leadership that made clear they were firm on this decision. The mindset among staff was to achieve the aggressive goals set by management for implementation and success. It was much easier to build enthusiasm for a project everyone was certain would come to pass than for a project that may or may not have moved forward.

For physicians, previous experience with NorthShore's successful transition to electronic x-rays and medical imaging (PACS) was helpful. This established a foundation of trust in the leadership's decision and approach to the EMR/CPOE system. It also gave them confidence that the EMR, once installed, would be reliable.

The system itself also aided the transition to the new work processes. Automation of manual processes happened seamlessly without the user needing to intervene. NorthShore and Epic Systems built navigators to pull various tools together to support specific workflows. For example, the nursing documentation navigators provided a revised electronic version of the old paper admission packet.

Training, Education, and Support

NorthShore made a massive investment in training—the largest to date for NorthShore and one of the largest in the country for healthcare. The role of the training team was not just to teach the functionality of the software, but also to introduce everyone to the new workflows and radically new ways of performing their jobs. Everyone who touched the health record across the entire organization would be formally trained and their competency verified; this exceeded Epic's specified standards for system training. Only by demonstrating competency in a given area of the system would a user be granted access to that area of the system. This included physicians, who were required to complete 16 to 20 hours of training and pass the competency test. If they did not complete this requirement, they could not admit to or treat patients in NorthShore hospitals. The professional staff passed a rule to support this.

High-level workflows served as the basis for designing the curriculum, initially developed by a group of director-level staff from operations. The curriculum was tested among users before being finalized. From the start of implementation through the end of fiscal 2004, the end result was:

- 9 general subjects, e.g., registration, office billing, pharmacy
- 53 different courses
- 143,724 training hours
- 15,854 training encounters
- 9,554 people trained an average of 16 hours each

As we have added more modules, the course selection now exceeds 80 courses.

The training team that developed and delivered the learning completed a train-the-trainer course and achieved "proficiency" status on the software over an eight-week period. The training team included during the go-live period:

- Chief Learning Officer plus
  - 9 principal trainers, pulled from operations at the director level and responsible for initial curriculum development
  - 9 core full-time trainers from the NorthShore training department
  - 40 supplemental trainers from operations
  - 1 manager of training logistics
  - 6 external consultants who served as trainers
  - 400 super users from all hospitals and medical groups to serve as local resources and training assistants
  - 200+ training coordinators prepared to register staff and track competency assessment scores
- Formal classroom training was supplemented with a variety of additional training strategies:
  - Super users, who averaged 32 hours as classroom floaters, plus time as competency assessors back in the departments
  - Review sessions
  - Validation sessions
  - Practice exercises (practice environment was available to all after class)
  - On-site support
  - Published Learning Resources
  - Five different bi-monthly newsletters
  - Physician CD-ROM for course review
  - Four quick reference guides for go-live
  - Online system announcements updated weekly for inpatient users

Training began in September 2002, five months before the first scheduled go-live date. NorthShore trained 9,554 people on the new workflows and the system. To accommodate this volume, NorthShore converted an unused, remote billing office with 17,000 square feet into a 13-“room” training center. Cubes were removed, and the staff built out the space with tables, PCs, etc. In addition, four additional training rooms were set up throughout the hospitals.

To ensure that the quality of the training and content of the curriculum met the needs of the user, each user was required to complete an evaluation form at the end of the training session they attended. More than 95 percent of the attendees, including physicians, indicated that the training met or exceeded their expectations. Of course, the success of the implementation was the greater testament to the success of the training.

A scaled-down operation remains in place today to teach new hires, students, physicians, and house staff to use the system and to prepare all users for software upgrades and enhancements. In 2007, we introduced a hospital-based trainer program that reflects the importance of training at the time of need for the clinicians. These staff members are not tied to classroom schedules. They are available on pager to come to the “elbow” of the user doing the paging. The prime purposes of this system are to respond to short-term training needs and to meet the needs especially of users who do not come to the hospital often and therefore use the system infrequently.

The training team continues to produce monthly newsletters, each targeting a different audience. These newsletters communicate updates to the system, resolve problem areas, or discuss underused features of the system. The training team has also produced a CD ROM for course review, quick reference guides and online weekly updates for all end users. An e-learning project allowed proctored training via the Internet in June 2004. Super users continue to provide support in their individual areas, and the training team, in turn, continues to support the super users and end users.

NorthShore’s chief learning officer has created an e-learning collaborative with HospitalU to share content and e-learning infrastructure with other healthcare systems.

Technology continues to be an important part of this implementation and long-term support. This project required the first install of a wireless network for NorthShore. This wireless system was necessary because we selected carts for use in the hospital to document and look up data at the point of care. The central processing function had to be performed by a high-end UNIX set of processors. NorthShore selected between the HP UX system and the IBM AIX processors. IBM was selected and the p series CPUs have continued to be our processor of choice. With the importance of the EMR in the day-to-day operation of the hospitals and offices, the CPU processors had to be backed up with a failover software. This was first put in place with a failover between two identical processor farms inside the same computer room. IBM’s HACMP software was used to failover from one group of processors to the other if the first experienced any technical issues.

Later in 2004, this failover was set up between two distant computer rooms but again from one stack of IBM AIX processors to another stack in the second remote computer room. In 2004, this failover was between our corporate data center and a small computer room in the hospital that had merged with NorthShore at the beginning of 2000. In 2006, this was further improved with a new production data center located in Skokie, Illinois. This data center is five miles from the Evanston corporate office building. This failover uses the IBM software HACMP-XD (extra distance).

In 2002, we also engaged the IT staff with an IBM study on high availability. This study documented the top 10 things our IT shop had to meet to get a "3 or 4 nines" overall uptime. This study was engaged particularly to compensate for the great changes in the clinical systems and the overall dependence that NorthShore was about to assume. Several policy and procedure changes resulted from this IBM study.

After the initial go-lives, we have:

1. Added a patient portal
2. Added new modules
   a. Oncology
   b. ICU
   c. Labor and Delivery
   d. Bar Code medication administration
3. Rolled out more than 400 additional employed physicians
4. Added more than 70 independent physicians
5. Added an enterprise data warehouse, including a clinical data mart
6. Implemented hospital revenue cycle in 2009
7. Added a fourth hospital through merger in January 2009. This 200-bed hospital went live with all NorthShore applications between January and December of 2009. Data and images were converted to NorthShore applications as appropriate.

Our patient portal (NorthShore*Connect*) is a module of our Epic EMR. It is a voluntary patient activity that has led to significant changes in how we communicate to and engage with our patients. We began the portal in 2004, once we had sufficient physician offices live and had enough data to make the portal useful.

We now have 125,000 active users with unique sign-ons for approximately one-third in any given month. The initial function was to have a secure way to release results to patients and to communicate securely by way of messaging. The portal has now expanded to:

- Request medication renewals.
- Book an appointment with a physician.
- Pay a bill.
- Update an insurance coverage.
- Download patient history (CCD format).
- See summary of all office visits.
- Plot lab results over time.
- Provide patient-specific education.
- Allow proxy access for parents of children and for adult children of elderly patients.

These activities (separate from results release) total more than 20,000 activities each month. Each of these would have taken at least one phone call if not two or even three. All of these calls have been removed from our front desks at the offices; patients can make the calls on their own schedule and not strictly between 9:00 a.m. and 5:00 p.m., and the calls are all captured in our EMR database for future use by clinicians. Our physicians are expected to answer patient messages within 48 hours.

Recently we have expanded the portal to allow patient entry of data in two areas:

1. Eight hundred diabetic patients record their home testing results for glucose for review by office staff.
2. Patients scheduled for an initial history & physical are sent a list of questions to answer before coming to the appointment.

The portal has been a very successful function for engagement of patients and families.

LESSONS LEARNED

NorthShore has realized many lessons learned from the work to install, fully implement, and support an enterprise-wide EMR over the last seven years. This system now covers the four hospitals of the health system, 650 employed medical group physicians and more than 70 of its independent physicians.

Speed/Focus

First in these lessons is the speed at which we did the initial install. We did it quickly in order to maintain the ability to maintain focus, get to the point where there was some payback from the admittedly more work that is needed up front for the initial time period of an EMR install, and to minimize the safety issues of clinicians using two different sources of patient data—paper and the online product.

Focus was necessary as we set this project up as the major activity of the corporation for the three years of the build/test and install process. We knew that this singular focus could not be continued indefinitely.

The extra work needed to start up an EMR is only returned with benefit when the data come back to users from other users so that clinicians can get information about a patient quickly from another users' input. Our decision was to install the hospitals and the offices at the same time. This resulted in more data being added to our patient database more quickly than if we had phased in the install over a longer period. By 2006, approximately 45 percent of our incoming ED patients had a full EMR—problems, allergies, and medications. In addition, the ED physicians could access other patient encounters when more data were needed. This percentage has now grown to exceed 60 percent.

In the past, with two completely different sources of data—the patient paper chart as well as the online version of at least some of the patient data, regardless of the efforts by the individual clinician—it was very difficult to keep that review in sync between two sources of information. We wanted to minimize the time we had two sources of data.

Training

The importance of training has been a major lesson of the NorthShore install. The first set of users were required to take 16 hours of in-classroom training, which led to a practical demonstration test that needed an 85 percent success rate before the clinician could get a password and ID to sign onto the EMR. As part of the initial install, we developed more than 50 different class offerings. With new products being installed over the years, we now have more than 80 classes to pick from. In addition, we continue to offer ongoing training to all users prior to the roll-out of new modules or before the annual upgrades. Also for the last three years, we have implemented a program of in-hospital trainers who have no classroom responsibility. These trainers respond to pages from clinicians and go to their floor to help at that moment with the immediate problem. Coverage is available between 7:00 a.m. and 5:00 p.m. five days a week and on Saturday morning. Night shift staff can make appointments for individual sessions.

Leadership

Corporate leadership has been essential at NorthShore to get support and focus from all users. The CEO of NorthShore, Mark Neaman, was the sponsor from the beginning and remains in that role today. He always mentions Epic in presentations as one of our corporate strengths and the "way we do business." Our senior management is challenged throughout the year to make more use of Epic to reduce the need for additional staff or to improve quality. Our professional staff leadership has been very positive in its support as well. Early on, they took steps to mandate use of the EMR to take better care of patients in the hospital. They have taken subsequent steps to mandate training for such modules as medication reconciliation. Our CMIO reports monthly to the Medical Executive Committee on EMR activities and upcoming changes.

Standard Orders/Data

An area in which we did not do well the first time around was the use of order sets. Initially, in an attempt to get acceptance, we accepted order sets from any physician, essentially. We are now working with each division or department of the professional staff to set common order sets for their members.

A second area of change for us was the failure to set a data dictionary process in place at the beginning. We are now establishing this, and it is proving more difficult than anticipated, as we have certain workflows that may need to be changed to accommodate data collection in a consistent manner across the health system.

Technical Skills

An area that should be obvious but can be difficult to maintain is the need for strong technical skills inside your department. There is also a strong need to add clinical staff to your mix of IT staff, and to utilize the technical assistance vendors in this area often offer, as part of basic support. A mix on each of your teams that allows sufficient technical programmer analysts is still necessary to provide the needed quick response to outages or to understand why a problem may be occurring. The interplay between the technical and clinical strengths of each team is an important part of developing a strong department to support the EMR.

Stay Close to Vendors' Releases

EMR vendors offer annual upgrades for their systems. It is difficult to stay current with the many changes that are offered to you. Each of them has to be tested and the users trained on how to use them. Failure to stay close to the "Model" system from your vendor or to stay current with all releases can lead to difficulty in accepting new changes from the vendor in future years and more difficulty in using support from your vendor, since they are going to think first in terms of their released product. As vendors begin releasing code to comply with Meaningful Use criteria, it will be necessary to have data values in the "right" fields to allow the proper reporting to take place and allow you to comply with the Meaningful Use criteria from the Office of the National Coordinator for Health Information Technology (see Chapter 2). We have recently set plans to get closer to Epic's "Model release" over the next three years.

Governance

During the implementation, there is normally an excess of interest from senior management, and the priorities for install are often very clear. After the initial go-lives, the conflicts between different departments or between optimization of existing functions versus adding new modules can become marked. The need for a governance model appropriate for the various decisions is essential to maximize use of staff and of the EMR by users.

NorthShore developed different structures for:

- **Request for service**—automated process for submitting smaller requests and for user management to rank requests
- **Big projects**—quarterly meeting to allow senior managers to rank these bigger projects, which are defined as more than 60 days of work
- **Annual upgrade**—annual process to get user sign-off on new functions offered in the release

All of these steps involve users significantly. In addition, we developed a process to deal with the needs of our independent offices using Epic. Often their special needs were different than those of the employed medical group physicians. While we maintain one copy of production code for all offices, we need to reflect the special needs of the independents, as well as those of our employed group.

Business Analytics

We quickly discovered that the reporting tools offered in the EMR system were specific to the needs of the day-to-day use of the EMR and did not meet needs of enterprise reporting or analysis. The analysis tools were short of the expectations of our business analytical staff. We selected a report-writing tool from one of the major vendors and placed that on top of an Oracle relational database containing cost and billing data from non-EMR systems, as well as a nightly feed from the EMR database that included whatever clinical data we chose to send over nightly. This type of function requires additional financial commitments and the need to develop a data dictionary with the EMR in mind.

Input from Other Organizations

Since we went live in 2003, we did not have a lot of peers to work with on new issues or against which to test our ideas. The EMR product is so new that it is almost always being implemented by a team that has little experience in this area. The need to talk to other users in a similar position is very useful to allow a testing of your plans, etc. This can be done by staying close to your vendor and taking part in their user group meetings. We have offered to attend site visits, and this brings us in touch with other similar organizations and gives us the opportunity to establish long-term contacts that are useful in this new area of work. We have done more than 100 site visits, providing a pool from which we can share over time. There are also HIMSS committees and Special Interest Groups to take part in to establish contacts with users that also allow the sharing of ideas. Finally, publishing or being interviewed for articles can lead to contacts from others asking for assistance that often can lead to long-term peer relationships.

Tie CDS to Your Quality Team

When we established our first set of clinical decision support tools, we dealt with the active knowledgeable physicians in that area. We have subsequently involved our quality teams, and this has led to a more systematic review of existing clinical decision support tools and a refinement or replacement of existing tools that were not making the desired impact on quality or patient safety. Involving the quality officer/teams up front can lead to better developed tools and ones that stay current with the needs of the organization.

Next Steps

1. Apply for stimulus dollars by complying with the Meaningful Use criteria for our 4 hospitals, 650 employed physicians, and our 70 independent physicians using our EMR. We expect to apply very close to the earliest date possible—April 2011.
2. Take an active role in the internal NorthShore task force to prepare for a potential Accountable Care Organization.
3. As we installed our EMR early and our vendor has recently adopted a "Model" system approach, follow a three-year plan to get closer to the current model system from the vendor.
4. Continue roll-out of independent offices.
5. Add Homecare to our list of Epic modules.
6. Expand the patient portal to engage patients and families even more by having patients submit home testing results in more areas—manually initially, but by wireless devices eventually.
7. Continue to take a leadership role with our local organizations to develop an effective Health Information Exchange.

CHAPTER 21

Case Study: Stanford Hospital and Clinics

Pravene Nath, MD, MSE, FACEP

INTRODUCTION

Stanford Hospital and Clinics (SHC) in California recently completed its four-year implementation of an integrated, enterprise-wide electronic medical record (EMR), culminating in the achievement of Stage 7 of the HIMSS Analytics EHR Adoption Model[SM] (EMRAM). This case study describes selected elements of the journey from strategic planning through implementation and post-implementation optimization, with an emphasis on the unique challenges of clinical system implementation in the highly specialized academic medical center.

Setting

SHC comprises the Stanford Hospital and its associated specialty medical clinics. The hospital is staffed by faculty physicians from the Stanford University School of Medicine, as well as affiliated community physicians. Our focus is highly complex care, and our vision is to be the best medical center in the nation. Our vital statistics follow:

- 430 active beds
- 33 operating rooms
- 30 ambulatory clinics
- 1,800 physicians
- 1,500 nurses
- 900 residents and fellows
- 24,000 hospital admissions
- 500,000 annual outpatient visits
- Multidisciplinary cancer center
- Level one trauma center

Strategy

In mid-2005, SHC recognized that its expanding network of loosely integrated, Best-of-Breed (BoB) systems, combined with a number of manual or partially-automated processes, was becoming increasingly fragmented, complex, and expensive to maintain. While these localized systems, including a partially adopted computerized practitioner order entry (CPOE) system had allowed specific departments to define and meet their needs independently, this came at the expense of cooperative optimization of clinical and business processes and resulted in information silos and other logistical barriers to the coordinated delivery of care.

The executive team responded by crafting a strategy for a single, integrated EMR built to replace essentially all existing systems and fully automate the spectrum of care delivery, including scheduling, registration, inpatient and ambulatory care, surgical services, emergency services, health information management, and billing. After a rapid but comprehensive evaluation process, the enterprise EMR vendor, Epic Systems (Verona, Wisc.) was selected and a contract was signed in March 2006.

Sequencing

Perhaps the earliest and most consequential project decision was the staging of the enterprise EMR roll-out. The core components evaluated for staging were:

- Inpatient clinicals (CPOE, MAR, pharmacy, emergency, perioperative, HIM, etc.)
- Inpatient physician documentation
- Ambulatory clinical (CPOE, physician documentation)
- Revenue cycle (ADT, scheduling, registration, billing, etc.)

Overall Staging

The overall staging analysis at SHC required consideration of a number of unique factors, perhaps the most significant of which was the pressure to begin with clinicals rather than revenue cycle. Those who had done similar projects in the past (and our vendor) strongly advised us to begin with ADT and revenue cycle components. From a strict technical and project management perspective, the advantages of establishing a solid foundation in registration, scheduling, and billing before enabling clinical functions was obvious. However, despite the importance of these core business processes, they were viewed as "back-office," out of sight and out of mind to our clinicians. Because the benefits of clinical integration were tantamount in the EMR strategy, because of significant dissatisfaction with the legacy CPOE system, and because so much clinician support had been mobilized for the vendor selection, it was essential that the immediate effects of the EMR project be visible in the daily delivery of care. Our decision to stage revenue cycle as the last component of the implementation—and in fact of our entire staging approach—was without any significant unanticipated consequence.

Inpatient Staging

As a legacy CPOE system was operable in many areas of the hospital, a staged inpatient implementation would require concurrently managing two CPOE systems, effectively doubling the number of production interfaces and requiring clinicians to navigate multiple systems as they (and their patients) moved between areas live on the existing versus the new clinical system. A big-bang implementation of inpatient clinicals was therefore required. In addition, the immediate benefits of a comprehensive online record and the desire for only a single education and transition effort for physicians led to the inclusion of inpatient physician documentation in the big-bang inpatient clinical activation.

Ambulatory Staging

The ambulatory clinical project differed from our inpatient program in two notable ways: (1) clinics were migrating from paper records, not a legacy system, and (2) few SHC clinicians practice in multiple ambulatory sites. As a result, the ambulatory clinical implementation was planned as a phased roll-out, for which each clinic was grouped into one of five successive activation dates over a one-year period. We separated the multidisciplinary cancer center, which is larger and more complex than any other single site, into a sixth activation during this same period.

Clinical Informatics

SHC's leadership team recognized early on the need for vibrant clinician involvement in planning and design. Though some organizations succeed in recruiting volunteers from the ranks of nursing and physicians, with sufficient participation incentivized only by goodwill and free meals, SHC felt that adequate participation and true accountability required the creation of paid positions. Accordingly, nurses and other clinical professionals were selected (primarily, but not exclusively from existing SHC staff) and hired into paid informatics positions under a director of Clinical Informatics. These resources were wholly dedicated to the implementation project and were assigned liaison relationships with key clinical departments based on their experience. In addition, as many as 10 physicians were engaged concurrently in paid, part-time positions as Medical Informatics Directors, also dedicated in this capacity to the EMR implementation. The physicians, along with the director of Clinical Informatics, reported to the chief medical information officer (CMIO) who, in turn, reported to the hospital chief executive officer and worked in close collaboration with the chief information officer. This structure exists today, and remains valuable for ongoing system development and optimization, though the number of physician positions has been reduced from its peak during the project, and the CMIO now reports to the CMO.

Uniqueness of the Academic Cancer Center

Our cancer center clinical implementation included clinical documentation, order entry, flow sheets, chemotherapy and infusion management, nursing, and pharmacy functions. We observed a number of characteristics unique to the academic cancer center, each of which brought specific challenges to the EMR implementation in this environment. They included:

- Multiple specialties practicing with common equipment, workspaces, and support staff, yet with widely differing workflows and expectations for roles and functions of each member of the care team.
- Decentralized governance across cancer center clinical leadership, multiple independent department chairs, hospital operational management, and nursing leadership.
- High volume.
- High acuity.

- Complex treatment regimens that combined multiple medications, chemotherapeutics, infusions, blood products, etc., spanning numerous ancillary departments and patient encounters.
- Many treatment agents with narrow therapeutic windows requiring extreme vigilance for safe administration, including complex workflows for role-based access, secondary review, co-signatures, and other safety measures.
- Frequent conversion of treatment plans from outpatient to inpatient and vice versa, each with different administration protocols for similar treatments.
- Patients referred after extensive treatment elsewhere, with complex medical record and treatment histories to integrate with our new records.
- Longitudinal and complex care, requiring unique flow sheet–style documentation of clinical events, often better represented on paper than with constrained computerized grids and limited screen real estate.
- Treatment protocols highly individualized by doctor and by patient, which change frequently.

In order to manage the challenges associated with this complexity, we leveraged and expanded close collaboration with oncology pharmacists throughout the project. Our pharmacists engaged to provide ongoing telephone support for oncologists experiencing difficulty with complex order entry. Outpatient/inpatient treatment conversions were a particularly vexing problem, as the circumstances could rarely be anticipated, and the process could not be completely automated in a reliable manner. We added coverage to allow pharmacists to complete these complex conversions upon the request of physicians. In addition, we added flexibility in our activation time line, further staging the cancer center activation into separate clinical documentation and order management phases to focus on establishing the build and safety checks required before activation. Finally, though we scanned all paper medical records to make them viewable in the EHR, we left the paper copies, and particularly the paper flow sheets, in the clinical areas to facilitate rapid review of historical information for particularly complex patients.

Training and Activation Support

Though there is limited information about their effectiveness, conventional practices have evolved for EHR activation training and support, and they are widely discussed and shared between sites implementing similar systems. We will briefly highlight our approach and provide some ideas on a few important considerations.

SHC utilized a combination of computer-based training and instructor-led training for clinicians. Training was mandatory for all nurses, physicians and other personnel that are required to use the system. We enforced the training requirements through conventional management channels and through the medical staff office with the support of the dean of the School of Medicine. A summary of the time requirements for training appears in Table 21-1.

SHC invested heavily in activation support, with uniformed personnel "at the elbow" throughout each of the large and small go-lives. Particularly valuable were the clinical resources (residents, nurses, and even attending physicians) from other institutions already live on Epic whom we paid to travel to SHC and provide this support

Table 21-1: Time Requirements for Training

	Inpatient	Ambulatory
Physicians	12 hours	8 hours
Nurses	16 hours	12 hours
Ancillary or Clerical	4–8 hours	4 hours
All Cancer Center Users		4 additional hours

during the activation period. Their problem-solving skills were invaluable, but it was the confidence and reassurance that had the most significant impact, as they told our frustrated physicians at the time, "Don't worry; it really works. I've been taking care of patients with it for years and I actually *like* it!"

The training, coupled with activation support at go-live, was adequate for a successful implementation. That notwithstanding, in general we failed to meet physician expectations for customization of the training experience to their particular specialty, and feedback was that clinicians felt the training required too much time. Most clinicians required heavy support upon initial use of the system, and many continue to struggle even after two years of use. It is unclear whether preactivation training can be drastically reduced in lieu of additional activation support, but our experience has suggested that every effort should be made to meet the educational and support needs immediately upon system activation, when users are receptive—even desperate—to learn what they might have ignored only a few days prior.

Further, successful training requires an unwavering commitment to a project plan and execution that: (1) freezes system build and changes prior to the final development of training materials, and (2) ensures adequate time and resources for the completion of these materials before the start of training. Training courses, whether computer-based or instructor-led, which end up apologizing for the fact that the training may not look like what the users will see on activation day are embarrassing time-wasters which undermine the confidence of both the users and the education and support teams.

Ambulatory Schedule Reductions

As with training and support, best practices are widely discussed about the need for ambulatory schedule reductions during EHR implementation periods. SHC followed these general guidelines, calling for 50 percent reduction in schedule during the first two weeks, with a ramp up to 100 percent over approximately four weeks. We learned quickly that these guidelines are in fact only a starting point and that the complexity of our academic and highly specialized environment called for individual negotiations with specific clinic managers, department chairs, and individual physicians. In particular, we observed the following with regard to patient volumes and staffing during our ambulatory activations:

- Most generalists appreciated the additional time afforded by schedule reductions as they began using the EHR for the first time. In general, they returned to full patient loads more quickly than all had anticipated, though some worked additional time at the end of the day to achieve this full load.

- High-volume specialists, such as orthopedics and ophthalmologists, were more resistant to schedule reductions due to revenue impact. In these cases, we negotiated individually with each physician, allowing him or her to understand and share in assuming the risk of patient delays. As such, they were able to anticipate—and staff the required personnel—for longer clinic days when they were needed.
- It was unrealistic to scale back schedules for areas of high acuity, such as cancer center patients in treatment. We increased nursing and support staff whenever possible to account for this and balanced it with more dramatic reductions in routine follow-up.
- Many academic physicians see patients for as little as one half-day per week. Extrapolating the general guidelines would suggest that these physicians may need 10 or more times as long as their full time clinical counterparts to learn the EMR navigation skills required for a return to full productivity. Though it did take somewhat longer for them, the difference was not this significant. Their return to productivity was accelerated by (1) individualized support attention provided to these limited clinical practitioners, and (2) their typical utilization of residents and fellows, whom we were able to bring up to speed much more quickly.

POST-IMPLEMENTATION SUPPORT

During the clinical system activation periods, we used an "all hands on deck" response to quickly attend to the most urgent and high-visibility issues, achieving stabilization within a few weeks. At the same time, by six months after system activation, more than a thousand other items of presumed lesser importance had accumulated in our IT ticketing system. Though our IT help desk, which had been in place for years to handle typical IT-based incidents and requests for other systems, was dutifully creating tickets, the help desk agents were not equipped to speak to end users about their EMR questions and to reliably triage the incoming calls—many of which were simply for "how-to" information. Over time, clinical users became progressively frustrated with the absence of real-time EMR help and with the fact that many of their requests seemed to be lost in a sea of tickets with no hope for completion.

Our informaticists and IT staff were similarly dissatisfied, as they were constantly working on EMR enhancements without satisfactory prioritization, and their relationships with the departments they served were deteriorating. Though a prioritization process was in place, it was lengthy, could not keep up with demand, and only separated items into groups of critical, high, medium, and low. The volume of items subjectively defined as critical and high substantially limited the value of the entire process.

Two important interventions helped us improve the situation dramatically. The first was the rapid implementation of a dedicated EMR-only help line for the sole purpose of assisting clinicians in "how-to" questions about the EMR. We established a dedicated phone number and automated call distribution system for this service, initially available only during traditional business hours and staffed by a single person highly knowledgeable in Epic, backed up by the existing informatics team for secondary coverage. This desk, unlike our outsourced general IT service desk, is physically located in the same office area as the application support, informatics, and EMR educator teams to facilitate close collaboration and problem solving. Though the primary goal is "how-to" questions, this support service also creates tickets when EMR problems or enhancement needs are discovered and provides warm-transfer handoffs to the general IT service desk as needed. This service was wildly popular with our clinicians when introduced, and we have since added a full-time agent and expanded coverage to 60 hours per week, with plans for further expansion in the coming year.

The second intervention was an overhaul of our EMR change and enhancement request prioritization process. We created a rapid-prioritization methodology (RPM) based on strict scoring criteria in the following categories:

- User productivity and satisfaction
- Patient safety
- Revenue
- Compliance
- Quality

Items are scored from zero to three in each category, based on rules required for each assigned score within a category. We also assess the scope of the request (defined by the number of events per day that would be affected). Informaticists review each new request and prepare a preliminary scoring. On a weekly basis, the requests from the previous week are presented by the assigned informaticist to the RPM group, which contains representation from informatics, quality, and various clinical and ancillary departments. Requests are presented and a final score is determined within an average time of approximately three minutes per request. The scores are combined using a weighted average formula which yields a final overall score, and the requests are then prioritized.

This process allows for timely review of requests in a way that was not previously possible and decreases the subjectivity of prioritization. *More importantly, it allows us to place all requests in rank order by overall score.* This rank ordering, which is shared openly with clinicians, other end users, and administration, allows clear understanding of enterprise priorities and of the relative importance of any request compared to others. If users feel that we have improperly scored a request, our process allows for review and modification of the score, but everyone understands that moving one item higher on the list requires displacing another. To ensure that simple, easy changes are not neglected, we also review each request for estimated effort. If the effort is thought to be small (defined by the number of minutes to build in a single environment), the request is labeled as a fast-track item. We dedicate approximately 20 percent of build resources for these types of quick-wins, which are also worked according to their rank but are pooled separately from the non–fast-track items.

Large or complex projects, particularly those which require multiple meetings to determine exactly what should be done to achieve the desired goal, are tracked separately, but the build requests from these projects are funneled into the same process and accounted for in the scoring system to yield a higher relative priority. The entire process is managed using Service-now (Solana Beach, CA), a highly-configured IT service management tool which tracks each request through intake, prioritization scoring, build, test, production, etc. The Web-based tool simplifies the entire workflow, enforces our process controls, and allows us to communicate with end users, showing with complete transparency how, why, and when work is being done.

CONCLUSION AND FUTURE DIRECTIONS

We intend to remain vigilant in our efforts to optimize the tools we have and to provide just the right kind of training for our clinicians. We intend to measure our success by the experience our clinicians have when using our tools and interacting with our service personnel, by the creativity we apply to supporting innovation in care delivery and portability of clinical information, and by the quality and usability of clinical information in our systems—and by how quickly and easily clinicians and patients can enter and retrieve it.

We now contemplate broad and ambitious changes to healthcare delivery, with innovation not just in quality and outcomes but also in appropriateness and value. As we move forward with clinical decision support in this era, it is crucial that we strike the right balance: leveraging the EHR to guide and facilitate best practice; making it easier to do the right thing when the right thing is clearly known—but without oversimplifying and overreaching in our attempts to communicate, cajole, automate, force, hard-stop, and otherwise impose a one-size-fits-all solution for circumstances in which subtle judgment and exception management may still legitimately prevail.

Although we are pleased with our accomplishment, we recognize that the achievement of Stage 7 of HIMSS Analytics EMR Adoption Model℠ (EMRAM) is not the end of our journey but rather the beginning.

CHAPTER 22

Case Study: University of Pittsburgh Medical Center

G. Daniel Martich, MD, FACP

INTRODUCTION

The University of Pittsburgh Medical Center (UPMC) is an integrated global health enterprise headquartered in Pittsburgh, Pennsylvania (see Figure 22-1). It is one of the leading non-profit health systems in the United States. As Western Pennsylvania's largest employer, with 50,000 employees and $8 billion in revenue, UPMC is transforming the economy of the region into one based on medicine, research, and technology (see Table 22-1). By integrating 20 hospitals, 400 physicians' offices and outpatient sites, long-term care facilities, and a major insurance plan, UPMC has advanced the quality and efficiency of healthcare and developed internationally renowned programs in transplantation, cancer, critical care, neurosurgery, psychiatry, orthopedics, and sports medicine, among others. UPMC is commercializing its medical and technological expertise by nurturing new companies, developing strategic business relationships with

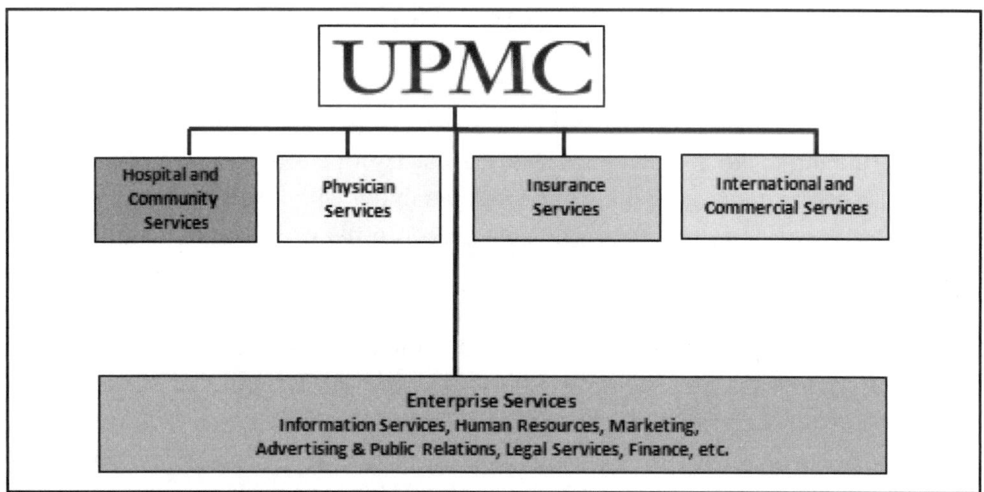

Figure 22-1: Organizational Structure

Table 22-1: Statistics UPMC—2009

Licensed Inpatient Beds (acute-hospital and subacute)	4,002
Staffed Inpatient Beds (acute and subacute)	3,430
Ambulatory and Outpatient Visits/Year (excluding ER)	4.5 Million
Emergency Department Visits/Year	500,000
Total Annual Operating Revenue (for most recent fiscal year)	$7.1 B FY08
Full-time Equivalent Employees	50,000
Full-time Employed Physicians	2,700
Graduate Medical Trainees	1,500
Affiliated Physicians (have staff privileges)	3,300

some of the world's leading multinational corporations, and expanding into international markets, including Italy, Ireland, the United Kingdom, and Cyprus.

UPMC eRECORD NAME, VISION, AND MISSION

Branding a product in a commercial sense is extraordinarily important. Kleenex (tissues) and Xerox (photocopies) exemplify the synonymous nature that can potentially be conveyed. With that in mind, we branded our electronic health record (EHR) effort, so that whatever the product or application (Cerner, Epic, Philips, dbMotion, McKesson, etc.) we continue to refer to it as the eRecord. In addition to the branding, our intent has been and continues to be providing an umbrella of services which fall under the general category of health IT. We believe that this umbrella, or mosaic, of products and applications from various vendors and homgrown solutions provide for better patient care.

In keeping with a quote by Arnold H. Glasow, "Make your life a mission, not an intermission," we posited an eRecord mission and vision statement for our new EHR effort when we embarked on this board-supported effort more than 10 years ago. Our initial vision was the following:

"To improve the quality of patient care and increase organizational efficiency through the creation of *e*Record, which will unify clinical information from the entire continuum of care across the UPMC enterprise."

This vision has grown and expanded over the last 10 years to encompass externalizing information to other sources, such as pharmacies for electronic prescribing, reference laboratories for specialized testing, interoperability with healthcare organizations outside of our own, and sharing directly with the consumer via portal strategies for ease of access, scheduling, and communications.

Our mission followed the lofty goals of our vision statement. The *e*Record mission is to be accessible to physicians and clinicians at the point of care and will ultimately allow healthcare consumers the opportunity to be informed about and participate in their own care through the appropriate use of technology. Even with a tech heavy mission and vision, we realize that there are three key factors to any successful application of new technologies, techniques, or procedures in healthcare (or perhaps any business).

The three pillars of our success rest on appropriate balance of technology, process, and people.

HISTORY OF INITIATIVE: EXECUTIVE COMMITMENT AND BOARD OVERSIGHT

Technology

As the Institute of Medicine was publishing *To Err is Human*,[1] and the Leapfrog Group announced that computerized practitioner order entry (CPOE) reduces medication errors, the UPMC executive leadership and Board of Trustees was taking its own leap. They collectively decided that the future of improved healthcare relied, at least in part, on better integration of IT into the workflow of the physicians, nurses, dieticians, and other clinicians involved in patient care. The Board of Trustee's financial commitment, to spend more than a half-billion dollars over the ensuing five years, led to the formation of the IT Committee to the Board in 1999. The IT Committee to the Board has primarily focused on the first pillar of successful IT installations, technology, while keeping in mind the other key pillars, process and people. Since its inception, the IT Committee to the Board's efforts have been many and varied but have always centered on improvement in patient care and workflow efficiency. Even when bumps in the road have been encountered, the IT committee has been fully informed, generating validated decisions made by senior leadership to stick with a vendor, jointly develop a business solution, or choose another product.

The joint ventures (JV) are intended to create new products and applications used within UPMC facilities, which could be then sold commercially outside of UPMC and Pittsburgh. UPMC's large size, broad scope of clinical services, and varied venues of care (i.e., from rural to urban, national and international, inpatient to ambulatory, and everything in between) make it a perfect test bed for these new JV products. Many of us feel that Frank Sinatra's "New York, New York" lyrics of "If you can make it here, you can make it anywhere" fit UPMC quite nicely.

This commitment to excellence and choosing another product was further validated by the board when the physician division leadership elected to switch ambulatory care eRecord applications. The IT committee voiced concerns that this change from a single vendor inpatient and outpatient might undermine enterprise-wide clinical decision support. However, the board completely understood the workflow implications and supported the move to the EpicCare EMR ambulatory application. This also led to more forward thinking related to interoperability, and the board likewise coupled this decision with support of acquisition and partnering with an interoperability vendor, dbMotion. The *technology* lesson learned is one of balance.

STANDARDIZATION EFFORTS

Process

Once the decision at a board level was made to move forward, we needed to engage as many thought leaders from across our organization as possible to build "the franchise model." Since the organization has more than 5,000 physicians and 50,000 employees representing multiple geographic areas as well as specialties, we convened 300 individuals to help build the *e*Record. In reality, even after a total of nine days spread across a six-month time period, the work had just begun. From a strategic standpoint, we came away from those meetings with many standards in place and in general agreement.

Despite standardizing laboratory systems, radiology information systems, picture archiving and communication system (PACS), emergency department, and many other IT solutions, much work was left for the clinical and IT professionals who remained involved at the local level. The hopes of accelerating implementation of the full complement of applications across all hospitals, avoiding delays associated with ongoing modifications to process and technology standards, providing IT with a predictable and repeatable delivery schedule, and providing discipline and accountability to the overall program were only partially met because of notable exceptions. Some of those exceptions to the franchise model included dealing with specific unique patient populations (i.e., pediatrics, obstetrics, oncology, and psychiatry to name a few), as well as the corresponding specialty hospitals, which required further regulatory considerations. In addition, the geographic location of an institution may have prohibited its participation in certain regional health system efforts (e.g., Reference Lab, Blood Bank). Over time, we have been successful in building to these unique requirements based on specialty, location, population etc., but as the saying goes, "The devil is in the details."

Looking back, the lesson learned from the "franchise model" experience has been one we've applied over and over again. We realize that there is a balance, or equilibrium, to every decision from total standardization across venues and specialties to full variability from individual to individual, or worse, by the same individual with the same circumstances from time A to time B. The equilibrium point for UPMC is that one size does not fit all, but one build may work per specialty or discipline despite different locales of providing similar care. Likewise, balance needs to be considered when applying rigid interruptible clinical decision support alerts to busy clinicians. Preventing egregious errors that might prevent a drug-drug fatal interaction is laudable. However, stopping the ordering process in a CPOE environment for every potential drug-drug interaction is a recipe for CPOE failure, physician frustration, and high verbal order rates. The *process* lesson learned is balance.

TOP-DOWN LEADERSHIP, BOTTOM-UP DESIGN

People

The final, and some say most important, pillar of success is people. Without hospital presidents, established attending physicians, and senior nursing leadership helping to lead the charge, no "killer app" will get a second look. Without their support of "boots on the ground" IT and clinical informatics resources, rebellions to any new technology or process become the norm and no advancement is achieved. Conversely, with executive support of initiatives and ownership of the problems and issues, the road to victory is well-paved. Likewise, engagement and buy-in of interns, residents, unit secretaries, floor nurses, and others in the trenches translates into the highest level of accomplishment for new programs. In a single hospital or office practice, this model of support helps tremendously. In a multi-hospital, multi-site organization such as UPMC, it is essential. We recognize local culture differences; hence the leadership, top and bottom, of the projects needs to be local. Politics are local; therefore each site needs to have a physician champion, nurse director of informatics, and IT manager, as well as senior administrative support of each and help under each role.

From a systemwide perspective, local hospital or ambulatory department efforts roll up to executive cabinets governing the inpatient hospital or ambulatory eRecord efforts. These executive cabinets are each chaired by the business unit (BU) president of that arm of the organization and comprises the system—CMIO, BU CIO, BU medical director of IT, and senior leadership of the respective BU. For a full view of the leadership and change control aspects of each BU, please refer to Figures 22-2 and 22-3.

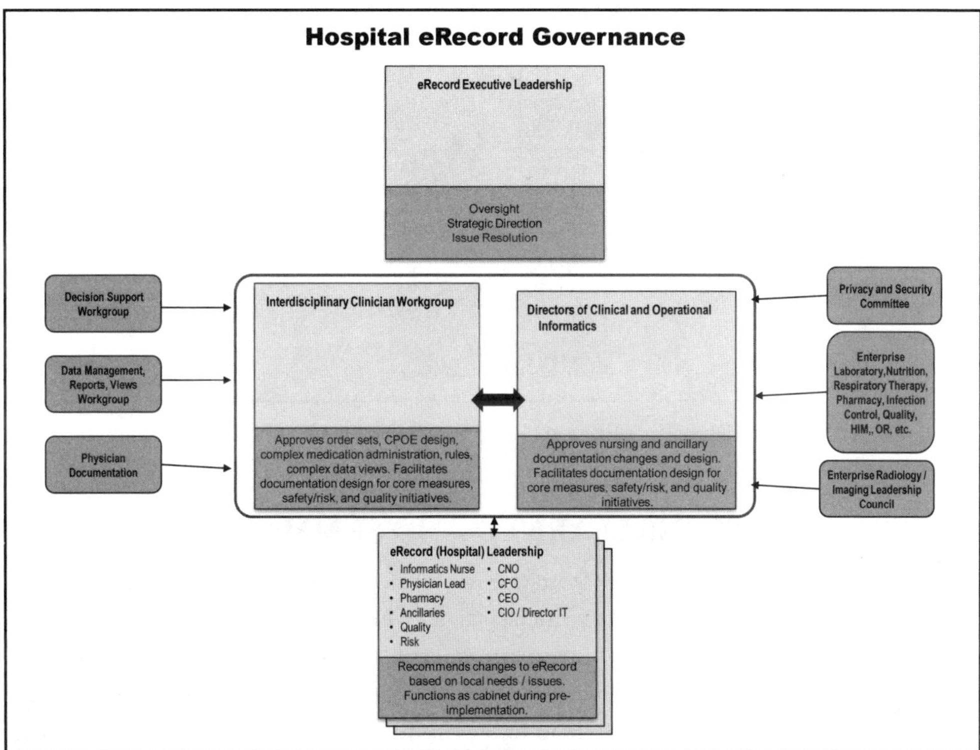

Figure 22-2: Hospital Division eRecord Governance

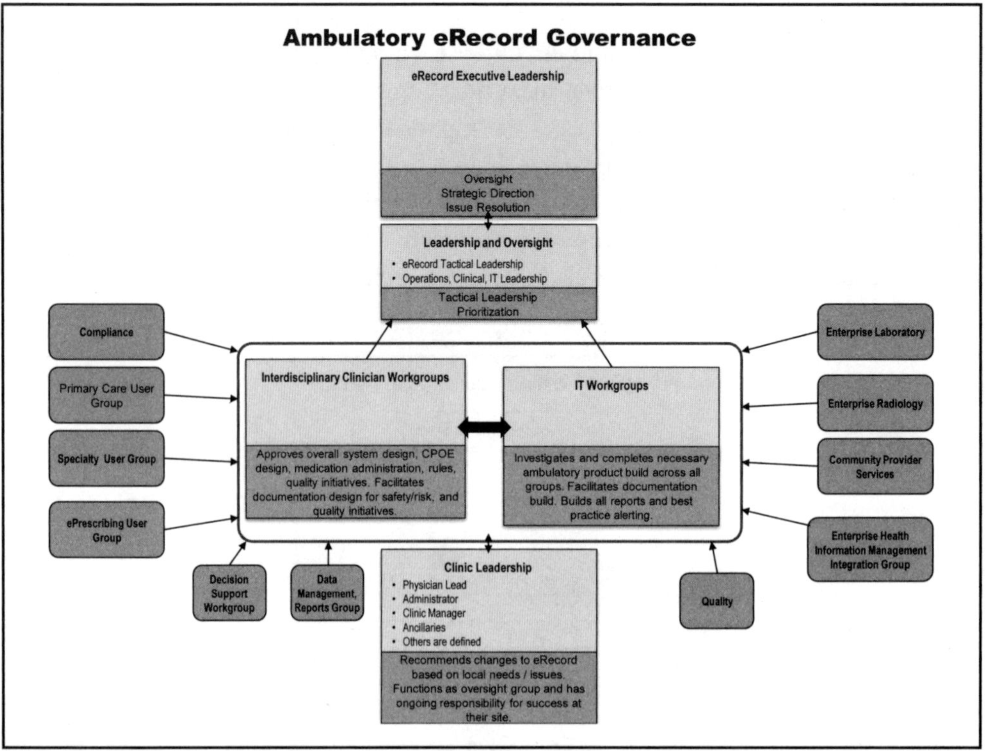

Figure 22-3: Physician Division eRecord Governance

LESSONS LEARNED AND SUMMARY

As in life, we have learned far more from our mistakes than areas in which we "nailed it" from the start. We've learned that balance is the key to every aspect, save only a few, in developing and deploying IT into clinical areas. Building, a priori, too many or too few interruptible decision support rules, too many or too few order sets, or extreme rigidity when it comes to mandating CPOE lead to inevitable problems. We've "corrected" each of these missteps over time. The most notable exception to the need for balance is that quality care, safety, and clinical decisions trump all else.

In summary, there are three vital components to any successful clinical IT deployment (see Table 21-2). Tables 22-3, 22-4 and 22-5 provide results and lessons learned from implementation of UPMC's eRecord. People, processes, and finally the IT itself are equal partners in the three-legged stool that supports clinical transformation. Put another way, installation is hard and mainly technical, implementation is really hard and mainly organizational, transition, or lasting change, is unbelievably hard and purely human. As demonstrated by Barack Obama's presidential campaign promises of 2008, it is transition, not change, which people ordinarily resist.

Table 22-2: Key Success Factors

Focus on patient safety
Unwavering support at ALL levels
Communication
Network of Champions...physician, nursing, operations, finance, IT, and administrative
All politics are local...choose physician and clinical champions who are part of the hospital/office at which you are going up with the initiative
Lack of speed kills...Ensure appropriate infrastructural support
Prevent project scope creep
Escalate issues locally and through enterprise project structure if needed

Table 22-3: Results Thus Far at UPMC's Stage 7 Children's Hospital of Pittsburgh

Serious medication errors have been reduced by 92%
Fewer than 5% of the medication orders are verbal
9.5% of all results are entered directly online, 0.5% are scanned paper
The reduction in transcription costs saves $42,800 per year for a single note typed across six service lines
From 2003 to 2009, there was a 60% decrease in medication safety events at Children's Hospital
From 2008 to 2009, the amount of time from administration of two commonly-prescribed antibiotics to documentation on the patient's chart decreased from 65–70 minutes to 10–15 minutes

Table 22-4: Monthly *e*Record Order Volumes—May 2010

Hospital	Total Orders	% Verbal	% CPOE	% Medication CPOE
All	1,344,803	8%	85%	84%
1	486,732	9%	86%	87%
2	262,233	10%	78%	76%
3	207,759	5%	91%	89%
4	152,318	3%	83%	90%
5	123,263	8%	86%	81%
6	112,498	5%	93%	90%

Table 22-5: Lessons Learned

Scalability – Establish the infrastructure, people, and processes to handle expanded functionality and user base
Performance – Ensure sub second response time is available to users, even while growing the database, functions, and user base
Reliability – Provide a high available system during disasters, technology problems, and software/hardware changes (disaster recovery site, redundancy across all components, dual power feeds, and battery backup)
Remote Access – Provide technology solutions to provide clinicians the ability to access the information anytime from anywhere with an Internet connection
Virtualization – Manage the growth and complexity of the systems by leveraging technology and virtualize process, storage, and ultimately resources
Standardization – In order to manage the growth and constant changes to the environment, when possible, to standardize in order to achieve the highest levels of economy of scale

ACKNOWLEDGEMENTS

My sincere thanks to Jody Cervenak, Chief Information Officer of the Physician Division of UPMC; Jim Venturella, Chief Information Officer of the Hospital and Community Services Division of UPMC; and Wendy Zellner, Director of Media Services, UPMC, for their thoughtful review of this chapter. Thanks also to Jennifer Brown and Lisa Welker for help in preparation of the manuscript.

REFERENCE

1. *To Err is Human: Building a Safer Health System*. Kohn LT, Corrigan JM, Donaldson MS (eds). Institute of Medicine. 2000. Available at: http://www.nap.edu/openbook.php?record_id=9728. Last accessed December 2010.

CHAPTER 23

Why Do Projects Fail?

Ken Ong, MD, MPH

"Cedars-Sinai Medical Center Suspends CPOE"
Family Medicine Notes, January 23, 2003

"Doctors Pull Plug on Paperless System"
American Medical Association News, February 17, 2003

"Cedars-Sinai Doctors Cling to Pen and Paper"
The Washington Post, March 21, 2005

"A Big Rollout Bust"
headline from CIO.com, June 1, 2003

"Hospital Shuts Down CPOE System"
Health Data Management, September 29, 2005

INTRODUCTION

The suspension of computerized practitioner order entry (CPOE) at Cedars-Sinai Hospital sent digital shock waves across the nation through the e-mail threads, list services, and blogs of health IT professionals.

The $34 million, three-year CPOE project included billing and registration. CPOE was made mandatory for all physicians. Nonparticipating physicians risked losing staff privileges. Cedars-Sinai is a highly regarded, 952-bed hospital located in Beverly Hills, California. It is one of the top 100 "Most Wired" Hospitals.[1,2]

The list of possible reasons for the CPOE project failure is long. According to reports in the media, some physicians complained before go-live that the mandatory two-hour instructor-led and online training were too long. Yet, after go-live, others reported that training was too short. Of the 2,000 physicians, 85 percent were voluntary, which may have posed a greater challenge than would have occurred with salaried residents. Medications misspelled in free text were not recognized. Common orders were excluded, such as "Clear liquids and advance diet as tolerated." There were complaints of too many questions, alerts, and reminders. Reportedly, rank-and-file physicians were not involved in design and implementation. Order entry involved too many screens with 6 to 8 seconds between each screen.[3]

The CPOE initiative did have positive aspects. More than 700,000 orders for more than 7,000 patients were placed. The system performed as designed and improved quality and safety. Uptime performance and reliability met expectations. During the hiatus, the project leadership will focus on those aspects that contributed to the failure: physician change management, workflow change management, system enhancement, and intensifying training and support resources.[4]

EASIER SAID THAN DONE

CPOE and clinical decision support (CDS) systems are technologies that serve the very intricate current healthcare environment. Medication management is one of CPOE's primary functions. A hospital's drug formulary may contain thousands of medications with tens of thousands of possible interactions between the drugs themselves (drug-drug), interactions with patient allergies (drug-allergy), and with food allergies (drug-food). Each drug has at least two names, one chemical and one brand. Each drug has its own range of therapeutic doses for children, adults, seniors, and those with liver or renal impairment. A dose that is too small will not help; a dose that is too large may do more harm than good.

Sidebar 1: The Five Rights of Drug Administration

- Right patient
- Right drug
- Right dose
- Right route
- Right time

Misspelling can lead to the administration of the wrong drug. The Institute of Safe Medication Practices compiles of list of agents that have been confused with one another.[5] For example, Cedax, which is ceftibuten, an antimicrobial given to treat infections is sometimes confused with Cidex, a disinfectant used to cleanse endoscopes. The former is taken internally by patients. The latter is used externally on equipment.

There is still more to safe medication administration than getting the right drug.[6] The dose must be correct. A medication's therapeutic dose range may be affected by a compromised liver or kidney function, body mass, or age.

The route must be correct. Medications can be given via mouth, under the tongue, intravenously, subcutaneously, per rectum, or intramuscularly (partial list only).

The final element of the "five rights" is time. The drug must be given at the right time to be effective or to prevent overdosage. Some drugs are better absorbed before meals; others are only tolerated after meals.

Replacing pen and paper with CPOE and a CDS system presents another set of challenges. A physician's illegible scrawl may be deftly delivered, but finding the right option in a drop down list may take time to learn. A required field in an electronic health record (EHR) may force a clinician to document data he or she might not otherwise choose to document in a paper-based chart.

NOT THE FIRST TIME, NOR THE LAST

The temporary setback to CPOE at Cedars-Sinai was not the first for this complex technology. Fifteen years earlier, the University of Virginia Medical Center was a pioneer when it began implementation of mandatory physician order entry in 1988.[7] In 1992, more than 550 terminals were deployed in three locations. Over 3,600 nurses, 1,200 residents, 800 medical students, and 200 attending physicians had been trained to use the new system. The program took three times longer and cost three times more than expected to install. Interestingly, the technology ("the strict, literal interpretation of rules by the computer") itself was only one of four factors that led to the system's temporary suspension. The other three factors that contributed to the "widespread organizational stress" associated with the implementation were dramatic changes in established workflow, unclear governance policies, and lack of physician understanding of the long-term strategic value of the system. Only after an executive committee with leaders from the major clinical departments was established was the initiative successfully implemented. The case study's author concludes: "[W]e may have gained a strategic and competitive advantage for the future by being forced to deal with issues of institutional change."[7]

Failed health information system projects are not unique to the United States. The lead story on the British Broadcasting Company's evening news of October 27, 1992, was the failure of a new computer system at the London Ambulance Service.[8] The deaths of 20 to 30 people were ascribed to the failure. Areas dead to radio transmission and incorrectly pressed buttons sent incorrect ambulance locations to the system. As a consequence, too many ambulances were sent to some calls and none to others. The growing error log compromised the system further. An official inquiry found that the project was underfinanced with an inadequate time line. The causes were several. It was unclear which of the contractors was primary, and the management of the project was inadequate. The software was judged to be unfinished and unstable. The emergency backup system was untested. Training was inadequate.

More recently in 2007, *The Guardian* newspaper surveyed more than 1,000 physicians and found that 59 percent of respondents were unwilling to upload any patient records to the national system without specific patient consent. Another 30 percent were unsure about doing so, and only 11 percent indicated they likely would comply. Seventy percent of respondent physicians did not believe the electronic records program were a good use of National Health Service (NHS) resources, and only 1 percent rated its progress as good or excellent.[9]

The departing head of the NHS IT program, Richard Granger, has said he is "ashamed" of the quality of some of the systems put into the NHS by Connecting for Health suppliers. Likewise, Milton Keynes, the Connecting for Health lead has said "Sometimes we put in stuff that I'm just ashamed of." He said a key reason for the failings of systems was that contractors had not listened to end users.[10]

On the other side of the world, in 1996, a major health IT failure occurred in the New South Wales public health system in Australia.[11] An information systems steering committee commissioned a consulting firm to devise their IT strategy. The consultants recommended a Best-of-Breed (BoB) approach to purchase three core systems: financial, pathology, and patient administration/clinicals. Scenarios with predetermined scripts were given to each vendor. Ultimately, a vendor was selected who had installed software in 100 sites in the United States. Five pilot sites were selected, none of which had taken part in developing the strategy or selecting the system. The sites pressed for more software customization than the vendor was willing to deliver. Nurses had difficulty arranging time for training, and not all adopted the new system, while physicians had limited time for training. Managers found the report generator inadequate. Clinicians found logging into the system cumbersome with four levels of login. Navigation was complicated, with up to 11 screens and 43 keystrokes to order one test. Orders were not linked with results reporting. The character-based system appeared archaic to end users accustomed to Windows-driven systems. The IS staff was highly dependent on vendor support. After just six weeks in one institution and 15 months in another, with problems continuing without resolution, the $110 million project was terminated.

Aarts and Berg describe two CPOE projects in the Netherlands; one was terminated and the other limited only to nurses and clerks.[12] A terminal emulator in a Windows environment was chosen to expand the incumbent IBM technology infrastructure. Though a mouse was adapted in the new system to replicate the light pen in the old, its movements were cumbersome. The screen was limited to a maximum of 24 x 40 characters, a fraction of the size of today's Windows or Web browser-based graphic user interfaces. One clinic nurse reported that "the characters look like Braille."

As a navigation aid in the old registration system, the patient ID number was persistently visible. The absence of such data in the new system led to delays in the ambulatory clinics. More staff was required to mitigate the computer-generated delays. The delays in the clerical workflows of the system dissuaded physicians from implementing the system's CPOE application. Inaccurate reports that underestimated patient throughput frustrated departments whose budgets were dependent on the numbers of patients treated.[13]

While the health IT initiatives that failed in the 1990s could be ascribed to the recognized risk in building rather than buying software applications, three studies reported negative outcomes after implementing commercially developed CPOE applications. The Veterans Administration Hospital in Salt Lake City, Utah, reported increased rates of adverse drug events associated with CPOE without a related CDS system for drug selection, dosing, and monitoring.[14] After implementing CPOE, a pediatric hospital reported increased mortality that the authors attributed to issues centered on "systems integration" and "human-machine interface."[15]

The third such study, written by Koppel et al. from the University of Pennsylvania, surveyed and interviewed house staff and concluded that a leading CPOE system facilitated 22 types of medication error risks, with many reported to occur frequently.[16] The Koppel study "generated a tremendous amount of attention and discussion within the informatics community."[17] Bates[17] cautioned that Koppel's study did not count errors or adverse events, but the perception of errors. The study failed to count errors that CPOE prevented. Thus, the study failed to demonstrate whether the medication error rate was lower or higher with CPOE. In addition, the CPOE system in use was very old (1997) and required multiple screens for many activities, causing many of the problems reported. A new system has since replaced the old one.

The ambulatory EHR has faced challenges too. According to a study by the Medical Records Institute, nearly 19 percent of respondents to the survey indicated they either have in the past experienced the de-installation of an EMR system (12%) or are now going through a de-installation (7%). Slightly more than 8 percent of those surveyed indicated they'd ripped out their EMRs and gone back to paper.[18]

Garg et al. reviewed 100 published studies on computerized CDSS.[19] CDSS is that portion of software in health IT that provides the intelligence or the rules for an application. In most pharmacy and CPOE systems, the CDSS governs alerts for drug-drug interactions, drug-allergy interactions, and dose-range checking. In an EMR in acute or ambulatory care, emergency department or other setting of care, the CDSS consists of order sets, reminders, alerts, and clinical documentation. If CPOE is the hand that writes, CDSS is the brain that tells it what to write.

Garg's literature review included a broad assortment of trials. The trials were published between 1973 and 2004. While 32 percent of the studies provided training prior to implementation, another 42 percent offered training *during* implementation. Only a small percentage of the trials had a graphic user interface. The CDS system communicated its recommendations directly to the clinician via the computer in 41 percent of the trials and indirectly via reports placed in charts in 45 percent. The desired patient outcomes included cancer screening, vaccinations, and mammography. The review's authors concluded, "Many CDS systems improve practitioner performance. To date, the effects on patient outcomes remain understudied and, when studied, inconsistent."

In an accompanying editorial,[19] entitled "Waiting for Godot," the editor comments that while

> "The literature in these fields has been characterized by frequent reports of success, often accompanied by predictions of a bright new (and near) future; however, the future seems never to arrive. Behind the cheers and high hopes that dominate conference proceedings, vendor information, and large parts of the scientific literature, the reality is that systems that are in use in multiple locations, that have satisfied users, and that effectively and efficiently contribute to the quality and safety of care are few and far between."

WAITING FOR GODOT VS. THE INEVITABLE REALITY CHECK

Adherents of the Gartner theory of the Hype Cycle of Emerging Technology might argue that the surprise that accompanied the Cedars-Sinai CPOE suspension was inevitable.[20] The theory holds that there are five phases to a technology's popularity or visibility (see Figure 23-1). The first phase of a Hype Cycle is the "technology trigger" or breakthrough. The media predicts that a technology may be the next big thing.

The next phase is the "Peak of Inflated Expectations" when the buzz is overpowering and expectations go far beyond reality. The third phase is the "Trough of Disillusionment" when expectations are dashed and media attention wanes. Despite the relative silence in the press, some businesses press on to better understand the actual benefits and limitations of the technology. They persist on the "Slope of Enlightenment," as shown in see Figure 23-1.

The last and final phase is the "Plateau of Productivity." The technology has a growing history of successes. The technology has matured beyond its first generation. Its appropriate application and usefulness is better understood.

In an editorial, Wears and Berg tried to put the studies reporting contrary CPOE results in perspective: "There is a long-standing, rich, and abundant literature on the

Visibility

Five Key Phases of a Technology's Life Cycle:

1. **Technology Trigger:** when a technology breakthrough peaks stakeholders' interest in the technology
2. **Peak of Inflated Expectations:** when publicity produces a number of success stories and often scores of failures
3. **Trough of Disillusionment:** when interests wane, as implementations fail to deliver
4. **Slope of Enlightenment:** when the benefits of the technology become more widely understood
5. **Plateau of Productivity:** when mainstream adoption begins to take off

Maturity

Adapted from: Hype Cycle. www.gartner.com/technology/research/methodologies/hype-cycle.jsp.

Figure 23-1: Hype Cycle of Emerging Technology.[21]

problems associated with the introduction of computer technology into complex work in other domains, as well as occasional notes in healthcare. Clearly, there is no reason to expect healthcare, that from an organizational standpoint probably the most complex enterprise in modern society, to be immune to them."[22]

Indeed, we should not be too surprised to hear of speed bumps on the path to CPOE. Research from the Standish Group in 1994 revealed that IT project failure was not unusual. Their study, the CHAOS report, revealed that 31.1 percent of projects were canceled before completion. Further results indicated 52.7 percent of projects cost 189 percent of their original estimates.[23]

The CHAOS report found that three factors were associated with success: (1) small projects were more likely to succeed than large projects; (2) shorter timeframes with early and frequent delivery of software components had a greater chance for success; and, (3) smaller project teams performed better than larger teams. The level of success was attributed to the degree of user involvement, executive management support, and the participation of an experienced project manager.[24]

CPOE system installations are large, multifaceted projects. A CPOE system may cost from $8 million to $12 million.[25] Projects of similar size in Fortune 500 companies have been reported to have only an 8 percent success rate (see Figure 23-2).[26]

Another factor in the success or failure of a software installation is the quality of the software itself. KLAS, a provider of customer satisfaction reports for health IT, conducted a recent study of vendor and provider perspectives on software quality. Sixty-one acute care providers and seven vendor executives representing 12 firms were interviewed. The providers represented 211 acute care hospitals, each with more than

Over $10 million	0%
$6 million to $10 million	8%
$3 million to $6 million	15%
$1.5 million to $3 million	25%
$750K to $1.5 million	33%
Less than $750K	55%

Figure 23-2: Success By Project Budget[27]

200 beds. Given the aggregate number of beds, the hospitals comprised 0.5 percent of the industry segment.

The participating vendors were among the top 20 in customer satisfaction in 2004. They included many of the more established in health IT, e.g., Cerner, Epic, GE, McKesson, Mediware, Misys, PeopleSoft, Per-Se, Picis, SCI Scheduling.com, Siemens, and Unibased Systems Architecture.[28]

Vendors and providers ranked the characteristics of quality similarly. Stability and uptime were ranked first. Response time, ease of use, release management, maintenance cost, and certification and benchmarking followed. Though the scoring was most different for maintenance cost, providers scored each of the characteristics higher in importance than the vendors (see Figure 23-3).

When queried how poor software quality may impact an organization, 18–56 percent of the providers acknowledged severe to intolerable negative effects on outcomes such as end user disruptions, downtime of software systems, time spent recovering and fixing, testing releases and IT effort on other quality issues (see Figure 23-4).

Not all software is created equal, and different vendors will have different on-time delivery rates. The more difficult the technology and the greater the clinical transformation required, the longer an application may take to install. The 2005 On-Time Delivery Report from KLAS gathered delivery times for clinical data repositories (CDR), CPOE, nurse charting, pharmacy, and physician notes.[29] Physician notes projects were the most likely to be reported on-time (67%). The other project types were reported to be 45–54 percent on schedule.

Providers reported that late projects could be ascribed to vendors half the time, to providers 13 percent of the time, and both to vendors and providers 37 percent of the time. CPOE projects were the most challenging, while pharmacy projects were the

Ranking Characteristics of Software Quality (on a scoring scale of 1.00 to 9.00)		
Characteristic of Software Quality	Vendor Scoring	Provider Scoring
Stability, Uptime	8.65	8.80
Response Time, Efficiency	8.18	8.21
Ease of Use, Human Factors	7.47	7.72
Release Management	6.63	6.82
Maintenance Cost	5.82	6.92
Certification and Benchmarking	4.82	5.15

Adapted from KLAS Enterprises. *Software Quality Study: vendor and provider perspectives.* January 2005.

Figure 23-3: Characteristics of Software Quality[28]

End User Disruptions	
Vendor	**Provider**
13% no issue 38% nuisance 31% tolerable 19% severe	8% no issue 25% nuisance 43% tolerable 21% severe 3% intolerable
Downtime of SW Systems	
19% no issue 19% nuisance 44% tolerable 13% severe 6% intolerable	20% no issue 20% nuisance 43% tolerable 11% severe 7% intolerable
Time Spent Recovering & Fixing	
6% no issue 25% nuisance 50% tolerable 19% severe	11% no issue 23% nuisance 36% tolerable 23% severe 7% intolerable
Testing Releases	
6% no issue 25% nuisance 38% tolerable 31% severe	2% no issue 8% nuisance 34% tolerable 46% severe 10% intolerable
IT Effort on Other Quality Issues	
7% no issue 20% nuisance 53% tolerable 13% severe 7% intolerable	3% no issue 16% nuisance 44% tolerable 31% severe 5% intolerable

Adapted from KLAS Enterprises. *Software Quality Study: vendor and provider perspectives.* January 2005.

Figure 23-4: Effects of Software Quality on Provider Organizations

least. CPOE implementations were an average of 12 months late. Physician notes implementations were 10 months late; nurse charting 9 months late; CDR 7 months late; and pharmacy 5 months late (see Table 23-1).

Implementing on-time and on-budget is hard. Yet, even when implemented, inpatient EHR adoption does not in and of itself necessarily improve care. As shown in Figure 23-5, DesRoches et al. compared the degree of EHR adoption with certain quality metrics, e.g., acute myocardial infarction, pneumonia, surgical care improvement practices, length of stay, 30-day readmission rates, and observed-to-expected cost ratio. However, CPOE, clinical reminders, and clinical practice guidelines were generally associated with marginally better performance on each of the Hospital Quality Alliance quality metrics.[30]

Metzger et al. applied a simulation tool to assess how well a national sample of 62 hospitals use of safety decision support worked when applied to medication orders in computerized order entry. Their simulation picked up only 53 percent of the medication orders that would have resulted in fatalities and 10–82 percent of the test orders that would have caused serious adverse drug events. The findings suggest that meaningful use should account for how well CPOE and clinical decision support are being used and not just whether these technologies have been deployed.[31]

Another study reported similar findings with adoption of the ambulatory EHR. A study from Harvard and Stanford examined records of 50,574 patient visits collected as

Table 23-1: On-Time Delivery of Software Projects.[29]

Overall Averages:	Percent On-Time	Percent Live On-Time	Percent On-Schedule	Average Months Late
CDR	45%	29%	16%	7 Months
CPOE	54%	8%	46%	12 Months
Nurse Charting	54%	20%	34%	9 Months
Pharmacy	50%	29%	21%	5 Months
Physician Notes	67%	9%	58%	10 Months

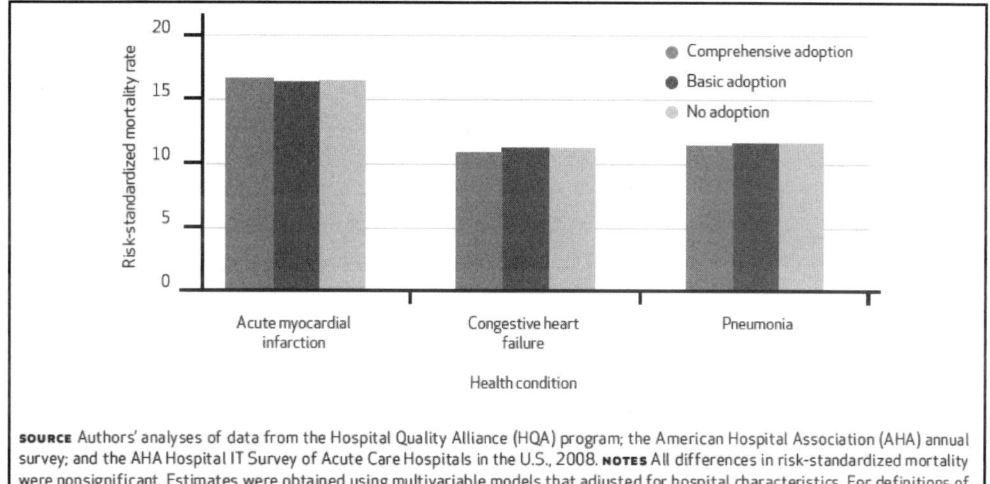

Figure 23-5: Thirty-Day Risk-Standardized Mortality Rates For Three Health Conditions, By Hospitals' Level Of Electronic Health Record (EHR) Adoption, 2008

Copyrighted and published by Project HOPE/*Health Affairs* as Catherine M. DesRoches, et al. Electronic Health Records' Limited Successes Suggest More Targeted Uses, *Health Affairs,* Volume 29, No. 4, pp. 639-646, April 2010. The published article is archived and available online at www.healthaffairs.org. Used by permission.

part of the National Ambulatory Medical Care Survey in 2003 and 2004 and compared how physicians with and without EHRs did on 17 quality measures. The researchers concluded that EHR-using physicians had significantly better scores on only 2 quality indicators, had no significant difference on 14, and did significantly worse performance on 1. The study's authors bluntly surmised: "As implemented, EHRs were not associated with better quality ambulatory care."[32]

Linder commented, "They're not magic. You just can't plug it in, turn it on and watch quality magically improve." He said, "There's that old axiom that a fool with a tool is still a fool. And, if you don't change your processes, (implementing technology) will just help you make the same mistakes faster and more efficiently."[33]

A national study on electronic prescribing is illustrative. Center for Studying Health System Change found that little more than two in five physicians reported that electronic prescribing was available in their practice in 2008. Of those with E-prescribing capabilities, only about a quarter of the physicians used it. Fewer than 60 percent of physicians with E-prescribing had access to three advanced functions, e.g., drug-drug interaction checking, formulary information, and electronic transmission to pharmacies. Fewer than a quarter used all three features regularly.[34]

Our cursory review of the literature shows that the Cedars-Sinai CPOE project suspension was neither an isolated nor an unexpected event, given the prevalence of IT project failure both inside and outside healthcare. The KLAS, CHIME, and Standish Group reports established project failure as common, and the surveys propose why projects fail.

KEYS TO SUCCESS

The industry press is replete with advice to those implementing health IT. One observer warns of six deadly mistakes to avoid: (1) raising expectations too high; (2) providing skimpy training; (3) doing the "Big Bang" implementation; (4) leaving physicians to their own devices; (5) disregarding dissidents; and (6) giving physicians a choice.[35]

Another commentator speaks of "The Yoda Factor," admonishing those who seek CPOE to "do" rather than simply "try." The do-ers follow four basic principles: set high expectations for clinician participation and do not relent; plan for hospital-wide, phased-in implementation and stick to a unit-by-unit roll out schedule; spend massive amounts of time on workflow design, testing and training; and have 24/7 support.[36]

John Glaser, vice president and CIO of Partners HealthCare, Boston, prescribes six success factors for clinical information system implementation: (1) strong organizational vision and strategy; (2) talented and committed leadership; (3) a partnership between the clinical, administrative, and IT staffs; (4) thoughtful redesign of clinical processes; (5) excellent implementation skills, especially in project management and support; and, (6) good-to-excellent IT.[39]

Other principles provide guidance that applies to all IT projects. A roundtable on IT failures at the University of Houston struck a common chord with advice given elsewhere:[40]

- Shrink the development cycle time by breaking projects into smaller bites and making sure that value is delivered at each bite.
- Don't get caught in the "throwing good money after bad" trap. If value isn't being delivered, ignore the sunk costs and look only at future dollars versus benefits.
- Focus attention on the opinion leaders and the change agents.
- Vendors and business partners can help in diffusing technologies.
- Customers may sometimes serve as a change agent.
- Be sure you understand the current state completely before attempting to introduce change.
- Demonstrate the value of the systems by using the worst critics as the earliest adopters.
- Know to whom you are selling.
- Have proper incentives for adoption.
- Take advantage of beta testing opportunities.

Sidebar 2: Ten Steps for Success Recommended by Physicians Who Implemented CPOE Successfully at University of Pennsylvania Health System, NorthShore University HealthSystem, and Cincinnati Children's Hospital[37]

1. All hands on deck: Make CPOE a top organizational priority with full support from the executive leadership to unit staff.
2. Pay physician champions: Value and protect time for a physician to design, plan, and lead CPOE implementation.
3. Analyze your workflow: New, more efficient workflows should be designed to replace inefficient extant workflows.
4. Build adequate order sets: Order sets can help standardize care and speed adoption. The number of needed order sets can number in the hundreds.
5. Recognize politics: The chief medical information officer or director of medical informatics must get buy-in from the clinical department chairs.
6. Set a deadline and mean it: Delays and postponed deadlines dampen physician and organizational enthusiasm.
7. Train, train, train: Train before, during, and after implementation. Train in formal sessions, online and on the patient care units.
8. Exploit physician resistance: Go one-on-one and find out why physicians resist and use the knowledge to improve training, create more order sets, or improve usability.
9. Sell the benefits: It is about quality care and patient safety. This is not just an IT project.
10. Crack the whip: If CPOE is mandatory, enforce it.

Sidebar 3: Lessons Premier Hospitals Learned About Implementing EHRs[38]

1. Challenge of Culture Changes
2 Value of Clinical Champions
3. Need for Medical Staff Training
4 Integration of Alerts and Reporting of Measures
5. Rigorous Security
6. Clear Policies To Document Communication
7. Flexible Budgets

Copyrighted and published by Project HOPE/*Health Affairs* as Susan D. DeVore, et al. Lessons Premier Hospitals Learned About Implementing Electronic Health Records, *Health Affairs*, Volume 29, No. 4, pp. 664-667, April 2010. The published article is archived and available online at www.healthaffairs.org.

- Make sure you understand company culture and the degree that you will be affecting it.
- Make your systems as reliable as is possible within the given restraints.
- Develop measurement/reporting processes to monitor the success of diffusion.

A number of quality improvement organizations sponsored by the Centers for Medicare & Medicaid Services (CMS) offer CPOE Readiness Assessment for participating hospitals ("Identified Participant Groups"). The readiness assessment tool identifies executive and physician commitment to CPOE and analyzes the IT infrastructure readiness as well.[41]

During any software selection process, the site visits and reference calls can serve as an introduction to clients of the selected vendor who installed the product successfully.

The users group can serve as a community with a depth of experience and knowledge of the product unavailable otherwise.

WHEN THINGS GO WRONG

Though good planning and rigorous implementation can mitigate potential problems, problems will arise. Information technology is complicated and expensive. The nature of healthcare in the 21st century is in and of itself complex. Any successful IT project is the result of paying meticulous attention to workflows and people.

The tools of performance improvement can be well applied to the challenges of health IT projects. Root cause analysis, workflow diagrams, the Shewhart Cycle, Failure Modes and Effects Analysis, and cause-and-effect diagrams can reveal the nuances of the human–computer interface and clinical transformation.

Horsky et al. applied a novel workflow analysis to study a dosing error related to computer-based ordering of potassium chloride (KCl). They reconstructed events chronologically from practitioner order entry usage logs, semi-structured interviews with involved clinicians, and examined interface usability of the ordering system.[42] They found errors in the drug ordering process, confusing on-screen laboratory results review, system usability difficulties, user training problems, and suboptimal display of intravenous (IV) bolus injection and medicated fluid drip orders.

In response to their findings, they determined that the screens for ordering continuous IV fluid drips and drips of limited volume needed to be clearly distinct, so that the ordering of each is unambiguous; screens that list active medication orders needed to list IV drip orders; the laboratory results review screen needed to clearly visually indicate when the most recent results are not from the current day; an alert should be added that would inform users of existing potassium administration; another alert should be added informing users ordering potassium when there has not been a serum potassium value recorded in the past 12 hours or the most recent potassium value is greater than 4.0; and other minor changes should be made to increase the consistency of ordering screen behavior.

Cause-and-effect diagrams can identify the policies, procedures, people, or technology issues that need intervention.[43] Caudill-Slosberg and Weeks report a case study of inadequate Coumadin therapy related to clinical documentation in an electronic medical record.[44] They employed a fishbone diagram to pinpoint opportunities for improvement (see Figure 23-6).

Their analysis discovered that the ambiguity of the warfarin (Coumadin) dosing on the medication order list resulted in inaccurate interpretation of warfarin dose and administration, the use of templates created visual barriers to identifying important information because of extraneous details, and the availability of both readable documentation and a copy-and-paste function gave false assurances that the available information was correct and facilitated its promulgation.

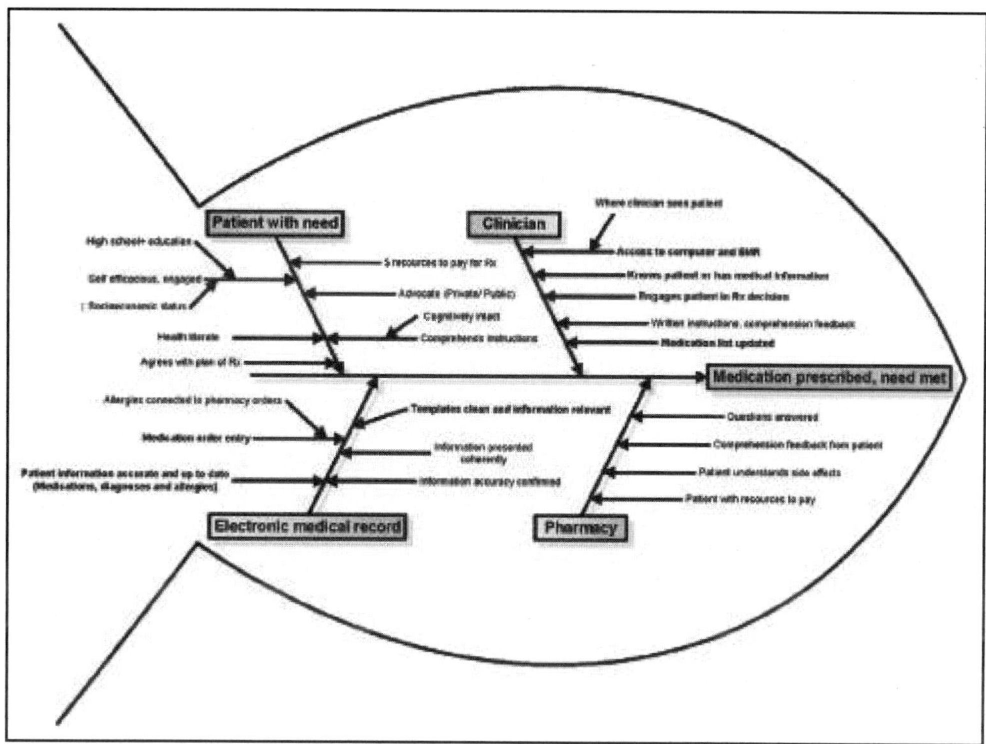

Figure 23-6: Cause-and-Effect Diagram of Coumadin Error

Margaret Caudill-Slosberg and William B. Weeks, *American Journal of Medical Quality*, Volume 20, No. 6 pp. 353-357, copyright © 2005 by American College of Medical Quality. Reprinted by Permission of SAGE Publications.

CONCLUSION

Knowing why projects fail can help projects succeed. No matter what the technology, getting the people, policies, and workflow right are always critical. No matter how grand the plan, without scrupulous attention to execution, no innovation can succeed.

From a policy perspective, the American Medical Informatics Association (AMIA) sponsored a workshop on IT project failure and made the following recommendations:

- Research and Publication: Support and publish qualitative and longitudinal studies of all project phases in addition to outcomes for a variety of applications, including for failed projects
- Best Practices: Create databases and an AMIA White Paper translating general principles into practice
- Advocacy: Advocate for regulatory changes to facilitate using best practices of health IT
- Education: Develop curriculum on project management and organizational issues to maximize success
- Certification: Partner with certifying bodies to include guidelines for better health IT development and use
- Databases and Knowledge Integration: Develop repositories (database, blog) for project histories and outcomes and for best practices

HITECH allocates funds that adopt many of these recommendations to improve the likelihood of successful health IT implementations:[45]

- CMS will certify EHR products for defined functionality. Providers who purchase a CMS-certified EHR can be assured that product meets basic standards and can achieve meaningful uses of the EHR.
- The Health Information Technology Regional Extension Centers (RECs) situated across the nation will assist priority physician practices in selecting, implementing, and maintaining their EHRs.
- The Health Information Technology Research Center (HITRC) will collect and disseminate knowledge about best practices for EHR adoption and use.
- Grants supporting work force development will help train the some 50,000 health IT professionals the nation needs to deploy and maintain this technology.
- Beacon Communities will demonstrate meaningful users of health IT among patients, hospitals, and eligible professionals.

The CMS EHR incentives are not really about paying for technology as much as using technology to get to better patient outcomes:

> "The focus on meaningful use is a recognition that better health care does not come solely from the adoption of technology itself, but through the exchange and use of health information to best inform clinical decisions at the point of care." – *Health and Human Services*[46]

Health IT is still maturing. Technologies such as CPOE with CDSS are evolving and growing in sophistication. Ongoing research into optimizing workflow and human factors will enable smarter implementations of this essential technology in the future.[47-49]

REFERENCES

1. Chin T. Doctor involvement key to success of computerized order entry. *American Medical News.* March 17, 2003. Available at: http://www.ama-assn.org/amednews/2003/03/17/bisc0317.htm. Last accessed August 2010.
2. Versel N. Cedars-Sinai learns from its CPOE mistakes to improve workflow. *Health IT World.* September 9, 2004. Available at: http://www.bio-itworld.com/newsletters/healthit/2004/09/09/20040909_10115. Last accessed August 2010.
3. Connolly C. Cedars-Sinai doctors cling to pen and paper. *Washington Post.* March 21, 2005; Section A, page 1. Available at: http://www.washingtonpost.com/wp-dyn/articles/A52384-2005Mar20.html. Last accessed August 2010.
4. Langberg ML. Challenges to implementing CPOE. *Modern Physician.* February 1, 2003. Available at: http://www.modernphysician.com/article/20030201/MODERNPHYSICIAN/302010715#. Last accessed August 2010.
5. Institute for Safe Medication Practices. Confused drug name list. Available at: http://www.ismp.org/Tools/confuseddrugnames.pdf. Last accessed April 2006.
6. Mutter M. One hospital's journey toward reducing medication errors. *Jt Comm J Qual Saf.* 2003; 29(6):279–88.
7. Massaro TA. Introducing physician order entry at a major academic medical center: Impact on organizational culture and behavior. *Acad Med.* 1993;68(1):20-5.

8. Beynon-Davies P, Lloyd-Williams M. When health information systems fail. *Top Health Inf Manage.* 1999;20(1):66–79.

9. English IT. Effort losing support. *HDM Breaking News.* November 26, 2007.

10. Granger says he is 'ashamed' of some systems provided. *eHealthInsider.* July 10, 2007.

11. Souton G, Sauer C, Dampney K. Information technology in complex health services: organizational impediments to successful technology transfer and diffusion. *JAMIA.* 1997;4:112–24.

12. Aarts J, Berg M. Same systems, different outcomes—comparing the implementation of computerized physician order entry in two Dutch hospitals. *Methods Inf Med.* 2006;45(1):53–61.

13. Aarts J, Doorewaard H, Berg M. Understanding implementation: the case of a computerized physician order entry system in a large Dutch university medical center. *JAMIA.* 2004;11(3):207–16.

14. Nebeker JR, Hoffman JM, Weir CR et al. High rates of adverse drug events in a highly computerized hospital. *Arch Intern Med.* 2005;165:1111–6.

15. Watson S, Nguyen TC, Bayir H et al. Computerized physician order entry system unexpected increased mortality after implementation of a commercially sold. *Pediatrics.* 2005;116;1506–12.

16. Koppel R, Metlay JP, Cohen A et al. Role of computerized physician order entry systems in facilitating medication errors. *JAMA.* 2005;9;293(10):1197–203.

17. Bates DW. Computerized physician order entry and medication errors: finding a balance. *J Biomed Inform.* 2005;38(4):259–61.

18. Conn J. Failure, de-installation of EHRs abound. *Modern Healthcare.* October 30, 2007. Available at: http://www.modernhealthcare.com/article/20071030/FREE/310300002. Last accessed August 2010.

19. Garg AX, Adhikari NK, McDonald H et al. Effects of computerized clinical decision support systems on practitioner performance and patient outcomes: a systematic review. *JAMA.* 2005;293(10):1223–38.

20. The hype cycle. Available at: http://www.gartner.com/technology/research/methodologies/hype-cycle.jsp. Last accessed August 2010.

21. Available at: http://24.222.53.223/printed.asp?active_page_id=94. Last accessed October 2010.

22. Wears RL, Berg M. Computer technology and clinical work still waiting for Godot. *JAMA.* 2005;293; 10:1261–3.

23. The Standish Group International, Inc. The CHAOS report (1994). Available at: http://www.standishgroup.com/sample_research/chaos_1994_1.php. Last accessed August 2010.

24. Schwartz E. Six myths of IT: Myth 5—Most IT projects fail. *Infoworld.* August 2004. http://www.infoworld.com/t/application-development/six-great-myths-it-384. Last accessed August 2010.

25. First Consulting Group. *Computerized Physician Order Entry: costs, benefits and challenges.* January 2003.

26. The Standish Group International, Inc. CHAOS: a recipe for success. ©1999.

27. Available at: http://www4.informatik.tu-muenchen.de/lehre/vorlesungen/vse/WS2004/1999_Standish_Chaos.pdf. Last accessed October 2010.

28. KLAS Enterprises. *Software Quality Study: vendor and provider perspectives.* January 2005.

29. KLAS Enterprises. *On-time Delivery Report 2005.* August 2005.

30. DesRoches CM, Campbell EG, Vogeli C et al. Electronic health records' Limited successes suggest more targeted uses. *Health Aff.* 2010;29.4: 639–46.

31. Metzger J, Welebob E, Bates D et al. Mixed results In the safety performance of computerized physician order entry. *Health Aff.* 29, 2010;4: 655–63.

32. Linder et al. Electronic Health Record Use and the Quality of Ambulatory Care in the United States. *Arch Intern Med.* 2007;167(13):1400-1405

33. Robeznieks A.Vendors dispute EHR, ambulatory-care report. *Modern Healthcare.* July 18, 2007. Available at: http://www.modernhealthcare.com/apps/pbcs.dll/article?AID=/20070718/FREE/70718003/0/FRONTPAGE. Last accessed August 2010.

34. Grossman JM. Even When Physicians Adopt e-Prescribing, Use of Advanced Features Lags. Center for Studying Health System Change. No. 133, July 2010:1-5.

35. Baldwin G. Avoid six deadly mistakes. *Healthleaders.* January 2005;51–54. Available at: http://www.billthecomputerguy.com/itsupport/help%20desk/Avoid%20six%20Deadly%20Implementation%20Mistakes.PDF. Last accessed August 2010.

36. Gaillour FR. Why do health systems flop with CPOE? Ask Yoda: the "Yoda factor" is the difference between "trying to do CPOE" and "doing CPOE." *Physician Exec.* 2004;30(2):28–9.

37. Baldwin G. Bring Order to CPOE With 10 Make or Break Steps (and 5 myths). *HealthLeaders Magazine.* November 14, 2005. Available at: http://www.methodisthealth.org/static/files/1184770136997/baldwin_cpoe_steps.pdf. Last accessed August 2010.

38. DeVore SD, Figlioli K. Lessons premier hospitals learned about implementing electronic health records. *Health Aff.* 29,4(2010):664-7.

39. Glaser J. Success factors for clinical information system implementation. *Hospital and Health Network's Most Wired Magazine.* June 2005. Available at: http://www.usafp.org/CHCSIIFiles/ImplementationFiles/Success%20Factors%20for%20Clinical%20Information%20System%20Implementation.pdf. Last accessed August 2010.

40. Information Systems Research Center, College of Business Administration, University of Houston. Project implementation, technology diffusion, adoption and acceptance: an ISRC roundtable discussion lead by Peter A. Todd and Wynne W. Chin. *ISRC Notes.* January 2001. Available at: http://www.uhisrc.com/pdf/jan01.pdf. Last accessed August 2010.

41. Computerized Physician Order Entry (CPOE) Readiness Assessment Version 1.0. By Health Care Excel, QIO for Indiana and Kentucky. http://www.hce.org/Education/ToolKits/CPOE_Toolkit/03_TOOLS/05-CPOE-ReadinessAssessment-DRAFT-Tool.pdf. Last accessed August 2010.

42. Horsky J, Kuperman GJ, Patel VL. Comprehensive analysis of a medication dosing error related to CPOE. *JAMIA.* 2005;12:377–82.

43. Fishbone, Ishikawa. The cause and effect diagram. Available at: http://www.isixsigma.com/index.php?option=com_k2&view=item&id=1416:the-cause-and-effect-aka-fishbone-diagram&Itemid=200. Last accessed August 2010.

44. Caudill-Slosberg M, Weeks WB. Case study: Identifying potential problems at the human/technical interface in complex clinical systems. *Am J of Med Qual.* 2005;200(6):353ff.

45. Available at: http://healthit.hhs.gov/portal/server.pt/community/healthit_hhs_gov__hitech_programs/1487. Accessed August 2010.

46. Available at: http://www.thehealthcareblog.com/the_health_care_blog/2009/08/meaningful-use-criteria-as-a-unifying-force.html. Last accessed August 2010.

47. Feldstein A, Simon SR, Schneider J et al. How to design computerized alerts to ensure safe prescribing practices. *Jt Com J on Qual and Saf.* 2004;30(11):602–6.

48. Shah NR, Seger AC, Seger DL et al. Improving acceptance of computerized prescribing alerts in ambulatory care. *JAMIA.* 2006;(1):5–11. Epub 2005; October 12.

49. Karsh BT. Beyond usability: designing effective technology implementation systems to promote patient safety. *Qual Saf Health Care.* 2004;(5):388–94.

Appendix

Acronyms Used in This Book

AACN	American Association of Colleges of Nursing
AAFP	American Academy of Family Physicians
AAP	American Academy of Pediatrics
AARP	Association for the Advancement of Retired Persons
ABMS	American Board of Medical Specialties
ABMS MOC®	ABMS Maintenance of Certification®
ABN	advance beneficiary notice
ACEI	angiotensin-converting enzyme inhibitor
ACP	American College of Physicians
ADT	admit discharge transfer
AEHR	ambulatory electronic health record
AHA	American Hospital Association
AHIMA	American Health Information Management Association
AHRQ	Agency for Healthcare Research and Quality
AMA	American Medical Association
ANA	American Nurses Association
ANCC	American Nurses Credentialing Center
ANI	Alliance for Nursing Informatics
ANSI	American National Standards Institute
AOA	American Osteopathic Association
ARB	angiotensin receptor blocker
ARRA	American Recovery and Reinvestment Act of 2009
ASC	accredited standards committee
ASP	application service provider
ASTM	American Society for Testing and Materials
BCMA	barcode medication administration
BMCC	Borough of Manhattan Community College
BMDI	bedside monitor device integration

BoB	best-of-breed
BoS	best-of-suite
BU	business unit
CAD	coronary artery disease
CAH	critical access hospital
CCD	continuity of care document
CCHIT	Certification Commission for Health Information Technology
CCN	CMS certification number
CCOW	clinical context object workgroup
CCR	continuity of care record
CDA	clinical document architecture
CDC	Centers for Disease Control and Prevention
CDR	clinical data repository
CDS	clinical decision support
CEO	chief executive officer
CFO	chief financial officer
CHF	congestive heart failure
CHITA	Community Health Information Technology Adoption Collaboration
CHPL	Certified HIT Products List
CHIPRA	Children's Health Insurance Program Reauthorization Act Of 2007
CIC	clinical informatics committee
CIO	chief information officer
CMH	Citizens Memorial Healthcare
CMIO	chief medical information officer
CMO	chief medical officer
CMS	Centers for Medicare & Medicaid Services
CMV	controlled medical vocabulary
CNM	certified nurse-midwife
CNO	chief nursing officer
COO	chief operating officer
COP	Conditions of Participation
COPP	Council of Pediatric Practice
CPHIMS	Certified Professional in Healthcare Information and Management Systems
CPMRC®	CPM Resource Center

CPOE	computerized practitioner order entry
CPT	current procedures and treatments
CQM	clinical quality measure
CSHCN	children with special healthcare needs
CUI	common user interface
CY	calendar year
DASNY	Dormitory Authority of the State of New York
DBV	design, build, and validation
DOH	Department of Health
DVT	deep vein thrombosis
ECG	electrocardiography
eCW	eClinicalWorks
ED	emergency department
EDC	executive design committee
EH	eligible hospital
EHR	electronic health record
EHRA	HIMSS Electronic Health Record Association
EHR Demo	electronic health record demonstration
eMAR	electronic medication administration record
EMPI	electronic master patient index
EMR	electronic medical record
EMRAM	HIMSS Analytics EMR Adoption Model℠
EOC	executive optimization committee
EP	eligible professional
ERP	enterprise resource planning
FDA	U.S. Food and Drug Administration
FFS	fee for service
FQHC	federally qualified health center
F-SHRP	Federal State Health Reform Partnership
FTE	full-time employee
GPS	global positioning system
HAC	hospital-acquired condition
HEAL NY Program	Health Care Efficiency and Affordability Law for New Yorkers Capital Grant Program
HEDIS	Healthcare Effectiveness Data and Information Set
HF	heart failure
HHC	Health and Hospitals Corporation

HHS	Department of Health & Human Services
HIE	health information exchange
HIM	health information management
HIMSS	Healthcare Information and Management Systems Society
HIPAA	Health Insurance Portability and Accountability Act of 1996
HITECH	Health Information Technology for Economic and Clinical Health Act of 2009
HITRC	Health Information Technology Research Center
HITSP	Healthcare Information Technology Standards Panel
HIV	human immunodeficiency virus
HL7	Health Level 7
HP	Hewlett Packard
HPSA	health professional shortage area
HQID	hospital quality improvement demonstration project
HRSA	Health Resources and Services Administration
ICD-9	International Classification of Diseases – Ninth Revision
ICDL	International Computer Driving License
ICU	intensive care unit
IHI	Institute for Healthcare Improvement
IHTSDO	International Health Terminology Standards Development Organization
INPC	Indiana Network for Patient Care
IOM	Institute of Medicine
IPA	Independent Practice Association
ISMP	Institute for Safe Medication Practices
IT	information technology
IVD	ischemic vascular disease
IWA	integrated Windows authentication
LAN	local area network
LDL	low density lipoprotein
LMRP	local medical review policy
LOINC®	Logical Observation Identifiers Names and Codes
LOS	length of stay
LVSD	left ventricular systolic dysfunction
MA	Medicare Advantage
MA	medical assistant

MIPPA	Medicare Improvements for Patients and Providers Act of 2008
MOU	memorandum of understanding
MPI	master patient index
NANDA	North American Nursing Diagnosis Association
NCD/LCD	national and local coverage determination
NCQA	National Committee for Quality Assurance
NHS	National Health Service
NHTSA	National Highway Traffic Safety Administration
NIC	Nursing Interventions Classifications
NIFA	National Institute of Food and Agriculture
NIST	National Institute of Standards and Technology
NPI	national provider identifier
NIST-ATL	NIST-accredited testing labs
NLM	National Library of Medicine
NMDS	nursing minimum data set
NOC	nursing outcomes classifications
NorthShore	NorthShore University HealthSystem
NP	nurse practitioner
NPPES	National Plan and Provider Enumeration System
NQF	National Quality Forum
NYC DOHMH	New York City Department of Health and Mental Hygiene
NYCLIX	New York Clinical Information Exchange
NYHQ	New York Hospital Queens
OASIS	Organization for the Advancement of Structured Information Standards
OCR	Office for Civil Rights
OM	office manager
ONC	Office of the National Coordinator for Health Information Technology
ONC-AA	ONC-approved accreditor
ONC-ATCB	ONC-authorized testing and certification body
OPD	out-patient department
PA	physician assistant
PACS	picture archiving and communication system
PAG	physician advisory group
PAL	Public Authorities Law

PC	personal computer
PCIP	Primary Care Information Project
PCMH	patient-centered medical home
PDA	personal digital assistant
PDCA Model	"Plan, Do, Check, Act" Model
PDE	patient data entry
PECOS	provider enrollment, chain and ownership system
PHI	protected health information
PHR	personal health record
PIN	personal identification number
PMBOK	project management book of knowledge
PMO	project management office
PMS	Practice Management System
POAG	Primary Open Angle Glaucoma
POS	prevention outreach specialist
PPACA	Patient Protection and Affordable Care Act
PQRI	physician quality reporting initiative
QHN	Queens Health Network
QI	quality improvement
QIO	quality improvement organization
REACH	Regional Electronic Adoption Center for Health
REC	regional extension center
RFID	radio-frequency identification
RFI	request for information
RFP	request for proposal
RHQDAPU	Reporting Hospital Quality Data for Annual Payment Update
ROI	return on investment
RPM	rapid-prioritization methodology
SaaS	software as a service
SAML	security assertion markup language
SBS	small business services
SCD	sequential compression devices
SDLC	system development life cycle
SDO	standards developing organization
SHARP	strategic health IT advanced research project
SHC	Stanford Hospital and Clinics

SINI	Summer Institute in Nursing Informatics
SME	subject matter expert
SNOMED	Systematized Nomenclature of Medicine—Clinical Terms
SPML	service provisioning markup language
SSN	Social Security number
TCO	total cost of ownership
TIGER Initiative	Technology Informatics Guiding Education Reform initiative
TIN	taxpayer identification number
UDS	uniform data system
UMG	Uptown Medical Group
UPMC	University of Pittsburgh Medical Center
VA	Veterans Administration
VNSNY	Visiting Nurse Service of New York
VOI	value of the investment
VP	vice president
VPN	virtual private networking
VR	voice recognition
VTE	venous thromboembolism
WBS	work breakdown structure
WHO	World Health Organization
wRVU	work relative value units

Index

f=figure entry
t=table entry

F

H

I

J

K

M

Q

R

S

T

U

V

W